OXFORD MEDICAL PUBLICATIONS

Primary child care: Book Two

A guide for the community leader, manager, and teacher

Primary child care
Book Two
A guide for the community leader, manager, and teacher

MAURICE KING

M.D. (Cantab.), F.R.C.P. (Lond.)

Staff member, Deutsche Gesellschaft für Technische Zusammen-
arbeit (GTZ),
Lately WHO Staff Member, the Puslitbang Pelayanan
Kesehatan, Surabaya, Indonesia; Professor of Social Medicine in
the University of Zambia, and Visiting Professor in Johns
Hopkins University.

FELICITY KING

B.M. (Oxon.), M.R.C.P. (Lond.)

Senior Lecturer, Tropical Child Health Unit, Institute of Child Health,
London University.

SOEBAGYO MARTODIPOERO
M.D. (Airlangga)
Director of Basic Health Care Research, Puslitbang Pelayanan
Kesehatan, Surabaya, Indonesia.

Illustrated by Soenarto Timoer

OXFORD UNIVERSITY PRESS
OXFORD   DELHI   KUALA LUMPUR
1979

Oxford University Press, Walton Street, Oxford OX2 6DP

OXFORD LONDON GLASGOW NEW YORK
TORONTO MELBOURNE WELLINGTON CAPE TOWN
NAIROBI DAR ES SALAAM KUALA LUMPUR
SINGAPORE JAKARTA HONG KONG TOKYO
DELHI BOMBAY CALCUTTA MADRAS KARACHI

Published on behalf of the World Health Organization

Published without author's royalty

British Library Cataloguing in Publication Data

King, Maurice
    Primary child care, a guide for the community
    leader, manager and teacher. – (Oxford medical
    publications).
    1. Underdeveloped areas – Child health services
    I. Title II. King, Felicity
    III. Martodipoero, Soebagyo IV. World Health
    Organization V. Series
    362.7'8'1091724 RJ101 79–40146

    ISBN 0–19–264230–8

The opinions in this book are those of the authors, and do not necessarily reflect the opinions and policies of the World Health Organization.

Phototypeset by Burgess & Son (Abingdon) Ltd.
Printed in Great Britain
by Spottiswoode, Ballantyne Ltd., Colchester

Preface

This is the second of two books on Primary Child Care. The first is a Manual for Health Workers. This Guide for the Community Leader, Manager, and Teacher has one major theme—quality of primary care: its definition and measurement, and above all its improvement. The guide is also concerned with the need to integrate and improve a worker's initial education, his continuing education, and his supervision; to link his education and re-education with service requirements, and to abandon such old-fashioned methods as copying off the blackboard and learning by heart.

The guide provides managers, such as district medical officers, senior nurses, and midwives, with a wide variety of instruments for measuring some variables that determine the quality of primary child care. With these you can make a service diagnosis to find out where your present services fell short of what they might reasonably be. You can also choose what targets you would like to achieve to improve the care your services give. You can then read how you can run a programme to improve the primary care in your district, and so achieve your chosen targets.

The largest, but not necessarily the most important, parts of this guide are the three matched sets of multiple-choice questions in Booklets A, B, and C. *These booklets can be cut from copies of the guide for distribution round a class.* For each of the 26 chapters in the workers' manual there is a pretest (in Booklet A), a set of questions for the students to practise on and teach themselves (in Booklet B), and a post-test (in Booklet C). Nobody need write in these booklets, so they can be used again many times. The multiple-choice questions in them are all coded to one of eight answer codes, they can all be corrected with the same plastic overlay, and they can all be done on self-correcting answer-sheets which go red when the right answer is marked. You will probably find these multiple-choice questions even more useful for teaching workers than for evaluating them. We have prepared large numbers of questions because we have found that schools have great difficulty in preparing a sufficient number of good ones. We look forward to developing these questions further, and will welcome any new ones, either completed or as problems or ideas that we can use to construct further questions ourselves.

Ten sets, each of 24 35 mm transparencies, have been prepared and are available from TALC (Teaching Aids at Low Cost). These illustrate the contents of the manual and are cross-referenced to it. With them is a leaflet giving suggested questions to ask a class and the answers a teacher should expect.

All these components (descriptions of technologies, evaluation instruments, teaching aids, etc.) are integrated with one another so that they form a system of a particular kind. We have called this system a 'microplan'. Its main purpose is to enable you as a manager to achieve objective, and therefore measurable, improvements in the average quality of primary child care in your district. Until now it has only been applied in an incomplete form. How effective it will be, now that it is complete, will depend on the practicality of its components, and particularly on how carefully they are adapted, on the energy with which you implement it, and on the opportunities and constraints of your particular services.

Microplans are not static systems, but need to be continually improved. The instruments we provide here are what they are as our project ends in Indonesia and we go to press. Some instruments have been intensively developed, some less so. Those for which trials have so far been limited have been labelled as experimental. For the improvement of the whole microplan we need your help, so we look forward to your comments and suggestions. We shall also be interested to know what scores your workers get with the instruments we have provided, what their basic education is, and how long they take to achieve given levels of competence.

Few tasks are more laborious than improving other people's multiple-choice questions, so we would like to thank the many kind people who have helped in this task, particularly Jim Smith, John Biddulph, David Curnock, and Jon Rohde. We would also like to thank Christopher King, father of one of us and a retired colonial civil servant, who, when he heard that the Rockefeller Foundation were unable to do so, kindly contributed half the cost of the word processor, on which this microplan can be adapted.

Finally, we should like to thank both the World Health Organization, and the Government of Indonesia for providing us with the opportunity to spend five years in the exacting task of attempting to provide you with some of the tools you need in an integrated and systematic form. You and the children you care for have our good wishes in their use.

Any queries about this book should be addressed to the authors c/o Oxford University Press, Walton Street, Oxford OX2 6DP.

Soebagyo Martodipoero   Maurice and Felicity King

Contents

Chapter 7 Implementing the microplan 39

7.1. Levels of implementation. **7.2.** A six-months 'in service' implementation programme. **7.3.** What are the faults of our services?—the service diagnosis. **7.4.** Choosing priority targets. **7.5.** Changed attitudes through group discussion. **7.6.** Implementation in a district—the district medical officer. **7.7.** The first district meeting for health-centre managers. **7.8.** Implementation in a health-centre—the health centre doctor. **7.9.** The final district meeting—evaluation. **7.10.** Some problems.

Chapter 8 A look at the workers' manual 45

8.1. Introduction. **8.2a.** Disease in the child and the community. **8.2b.** Beliefs and customs. **8.2c.** The community diagnosis. **8.2d.** Health education. **8.2e.** Health with the people. **8.3a.** Drugs. **8.3b.** Equipment. **8.4.** Immunization. **8.5a.** The ten steps. **8.5b.** Arranging the clinic. **8.6.** Recording, reporting, and sterilizing. **8.7a.** When should a child first be given porridge? **8.7b.** Weight charts. **8.7c.** Nutrition education. **8.8.** Cough. **8.9.** Diarrhoea. **8.12.** Leprosy. **8.15.** Fits. **8.17.** Ears. **8.18.** Mouth and throat. **8.22.** Anaemia and jaundice. **8.23.** Urinary and genital symptoms. **8.24.** Not walking and talking. **8.26.** The newborn baby.

Chapter 9 Some other aspects of microplanning 52

9.1. Can primary child care be cheap enough? **9.2.** On educational theory. **9.3.** Using the health information systems to promote quality of care. **9.4.** Job descriptions. **9.5.** Language. **9.6.** What is the best kind of algorithm? **9.7.** Medical students and the microplan. **9.8.** Adapting the microplan.

Equipment and supplies—TALC 57

References 58

Booklet A Pretests 61

A.1. READING PRETEST. **A.2.** MATHS PRETEST. **A.3.** Instrument MCQS—EASY. **A.4.** Instrument MCQS—VARIED. **A.5.** OVERALL PRETEST. **A.6.** Instrument BREAST- AND BOTTLE-FEEDING. Pretest multiple-choice instruments of the CHAPTER SERIES.

Booklet B For the student to test and teach himself 97

B.1. For workers implementing the microplan. **B.2.** For students learning the microplan. **B.3.** Joint targets for workers and managers. **B.4.** Measuring your skills. Self-evaluation multiple-choice instruments of the CHAPTER SERIES AND SICK CHILDREN SERIES.

Booklet C Postests 161

C.1. MANUAL POSTEST. **C.2.** OVERALL POSTEST. **C.3.** DOSES POSTEST. **C.4.** WEIGHT-CHART POSTEST. Postest multiple-choice instruments of the CHAPTER SERIES. DEDICATION.

A message to our community's leaders

From a District Medical Officer

Our children are our most precious possession. Here are two books which will help them. The workers' manual describes the primary health care these children need. This guide describes how we can measure how good the care is that they are getting now, and how we can find out which children are getting it and which children are not. We health workers care for children, but we cannot do this adequately without the support of their fathers and mothers, and of you, the people's leaders. This is why we send you this message and why we give you these two books. We hope that you will help us to train, encourage, and support the health workers of our community so that *all* our children get health care of at least the quality you see here. The children in our district now get some health care, but they do not get enough, and the care they do get is not as good as it might be. Can we help you, and you help us, to improve both the quality and the quantity of this care? Can we plan together what kind of workers should give it, and how we should recruit, train, supply, discipline, reward, and retrain them?

Training. Can we train new health workers? We do not have enough and we need more. These workers might work full time or part time, they might work closely with other workers, or they might work mostly on their own. Training should not be difficult, because the workers' manual is easy to read and contains everything a worker needs to know. If we can find recruits who can read it, we can probably teach them to use it.

Retraining. Can we help the workers we already have to give better care? The care that many of them give now is far below that which most children could reasonably have, which is the care described in the workers' manual. Chapter 7 of the Guide describes a programme for improving the quality of child care in a district. Can you and the people help us to find the money for the training, retraining, equipment, and drugs that this programme needs?

The guide lists a number of measuring instruments and targets (Section 2.5) which measure the quality of primary child care and which children get it. We have used some of these to find out how good and how bad primary child care is in our district. In doing so we have made a service diagnosis (Section 7.3) and will be delighted to show it to you. We would like to run a programme for improving primary child care (Section 7.2), and we would be happy to discuss it with you. If you could join us at its opening meeting (Section 7.7), we should be delighted. Between us we have great responsibility and a most difficult task—to give all the children in our community the health care they need. I am sure that if we work hard we can succeed, but I am also sure that we can only succeed if we work together.

District Medical Officer.

1 Introduction

'Daddy, what are people for?'
          Dominic, aged 4, born in Java during the project.

'To praise their creator; to conserve, enjoy, and study his creation; and most especially to love and care for one another.'
    His parents, after much consideration, and on good authority.

1.1. Primary health care

Primary health care is part of that love. It has several meanings. It was first used to mean the care given to the patient by the first health worker who saw him. If the patient was referred to hospital that was called 'secondary care'. More recently, WHO and UNICEF have given primary health care a wider meaning. This is how they summarize it in their report to the 1978 International Conference on Primary Health Care at Alma-Ata, in the USSR [1].

Primary Health Care is essential health care made universally accessible to individuals and families in the community by means acceptable to them, through their full participation, and at a cost they can afford. It forms an integral part of both the country's health system, of which it is the nucleus, and of the overall social and economic development of the community.

This definition implies that primary health care is part of a co-ordinated multisectoral fight against poverty, and that it promotes health through helping the community to help itself. Since health depends on enough food and water, an adequate house, a clean environment, and a just society, the first task of primary care is to provide these things. It exists to satisfy our fundamental human need to be helped to lead a socially and economically productive life, and to be relieved from sickness, suffering, isolation, unemployment, and an untimely death. It provides promotive, preventive, and curative care. It defines and measures the quality of care. Above all it is compassionate and is accessible to those in greatest need.

By this definition primary health care is equally valid for all countries from the most to the least developed, although it takes varying forms in each of them. It means much more than the mere extension of basic health services, since it has social and developmental dimensions, which if properly applied, influence the way the rest of the health system works, and indeed the rest of society.

†In the guide we give references in the same way as in the manual: 1.2 or one *dot* two is the second section in Chapter One; 3–6 or three *dash* six is sixth figure in Chapter Three. 5:1 or five *colon* one is the first table in Chapter Five.

This microplan deliberately covers only part of primary care—the clinical part of primary child care —and says little about water, sanitation, housing, employment, or a just wage for his father, important though these are. It is likely to be most effective in promoting development and improving the quality of life, if it is applied in conjunction with improvements in these other sectors.

1.2. The whole is more than the sum of its parts

Primary health care services are made of many components (parts). These components include administrative arrangements, buildings, workers, technologies (methods), knowledge, equipment, drugs, teaching aids, and evaluation instruments. If primary care is going to be good, these components must exist, and they must all work well together. For example, if workers are taught a technology, they must be given the equipment to do it with. A microplan takes *some* of these components, or makes them (evaluation instruments, for example), and integrates (joins) them together. The most suitable components for making a microplan are the technologies and the components which immediately support them, such as the necessary theoretical knowledge, equipment lists, and evaluation instruments.

The workers' manual contains many technologies which are linked to and support one another. They are also linked to the essential anatomy, physiology, microbiology, and pharmacology. These links are well shown by the many cross-references in the workers' manual. There are more links between the technologies, the teaching aids, the multiple-choice questions and the other instruments in this guide. Many components of a health service are however outside a microplan. For example, we say nothing here about buildings, or about how health care is paid for.

'A microplan is an integrated set of components, prepared nationally, to support a particular part of the health-care system' [2]. Primary child care is the part of the whole health care system supported by this microplan. Because the components of a microplan support one another, they are more useful together than they would be alone.

1

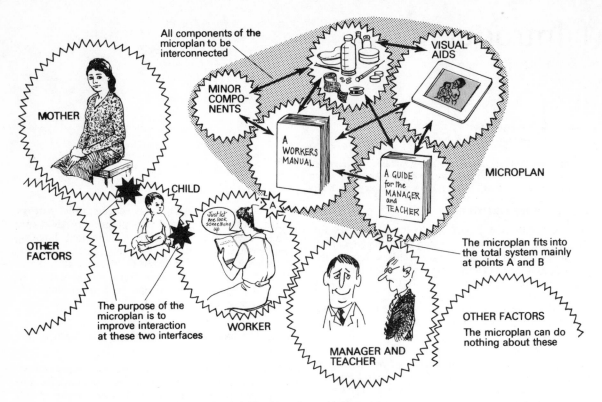

Fig. 1-1 The microplan as a subsystem

Another way of saying this is that the whole (microplan) is more than the sum of its parts (components). For example, the multiple-choice questions would be useful by themselves. But they are even more useful when they are used to increase a worker's understanding of the manual, and his willingness to read it. Thus the multiple-choice questions and the manual interact with one another and are *more useful together than they would be alone*. The same is probably true for the other components also.

So a microplan is more than a manual, or even two manuals. It is called a *micro*plan because it is concerned with many small details. It is a micro*plan* because it is a way for governments to plan national systems of appropriate technology.

Microplans try to answer questions like these —What technologies should health workers use? What technologies are appropriate to them? What should they do? What equipment should they do it with? How should we teach and evaluate them? Many of the answers to these questions are the same, or nearly the same, all over the world. Acute dehydrating diarrhoea, for example, can be diagnosed and treated in the same way everywhere. This

therefore is an international or 'master microplan'. We hope that it will be adapted and translated by any developing country that wants to plan its own system of appropriate technology for primary child care.

A master microplan is mostly appropriate technology, because this is the only way to make it a widely useful health-service tool. It contains no routine administration, because this is different in each country, each district, and sometimes in each clinic. It says nothing about how health workers should be recruited or disciplined, or what they should do each day of the week, because these things vary so much. A national microplan can say something about them, but the details must be left for local standing orders.

ALTHOUGH MOST OF THE TECHNOLOGY IN A MICROPLAN IS UNIVERSAL, ITS APPLICATION IN A COUNTRY IS LIKELY TO BE UNIQUE

The model in Guide 1-1 may make a microplan easier

2

to understand. It was originally made in plastic for use with an overhead projector. If a health-delivery system is seen as a series of cogs (components) which mesh together (interface or interact with one another), then this figure shows some of those interactions. The cog for the child is the focus of the system and interacts with the cog for his mother. The main purpose of the microplan is to improve the way the worker interacts with the child—to improve what he does. It does this by providing a special manual for the worker to interact with, and, by providing this guide to improve the way his manager and teacher interact with him. These two books interact with one another, with the teaching aids, with the equipment, and with other minor components, such as the relevant part of the health information system (Guide 9.3). In this model the microplan is a sub-system of five intermeshing cogs which fit into the whole health care delivery system in a particular way. Making a microplan [2] involves selecting or making the components, and ensuring that they interact. Inevitably the model has limitations. It does not, for example, show the many subcomponents inside both manuals, and it only hints at the many 'other factors' in the total system.

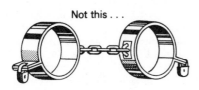

Not this . . .

. . . but this!

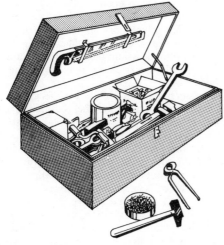

Fig. 1-2 A microplan is a box of tools not a pair of handcuffs

A microplan fits into the total health-care system in several ways. Among them are the following.

A microplan is a means whereby a Ministry of Health can plan a system of appropriate technology for a particular field of health care.

This microplan can show a community's leaders the kind of care its children could get and indicates some of the ways in which the community can provide this care.

This microplan is a tool which a manager can use to *change* his services so as to improve the *average* quality of the primary child care that is given in his district. Chapter 7 describes how a district medical officer or senior nurse can improve the quality of the care their services give by running an intensive implementation programme lasting a few months. This programme can be part of a national programme, or you can do it on your own.

Look on a microplan as a tool for improving health services and not a pair of handcuffs. Adapt or improve it in any way you wish. Microplans define minimum standards—do better if you can.

Teachers can use most of the components of this microplan in training schools. For convenience, we discuss the uses of the microplan by managers and teachers together. Sometimes what we say in this guide applies only to managers in their districts, sometimes only to teachers in schools, oftern it applies to both. Where we say 'workers', we mean districts, where we say 'students', we mean schools.

Finally, and most importantly, a microplan enables a worker to improve the quality of the care he gives.

A microplan is a new way of nationally planning the technologies for primary health care. It is thorough and systematic. Its components are integrated. Its edges are carefully defined—it covers a particular field thoroughly. It defines and measures quality and coverage. It contains only the administration necessary for its own implementation. It is dynamic not static, so that it should be improved upon every few years. Most importantly, it is, we hope, practical. We hope also that this one will help to give MCH programmes something of the rigour and quantification which they have hitherto lacked, compared with programmes for, say, malaria or TB.

1.3. Microplans for primary care

The workers' manual describes a child's primary care from the time he is born until he goes to school. It says little about his mother, because there is not enough room in one manual to describe care for both of them. Mother care is the subject of another microplan which is presently being prepared for WHO. The separation of child care from mother care is necessary, but it is unfortunate, because a child is part of his mother. We have, however, done all we can to describe the child with his mother. For example, every treatment in the manual includes the explanation she needs. We have also made family planning one of the ten steps in caring for a child.

If health workers are going to give good primary child care, they must have a good knowledge of nutrition. For microplanning, nutrition has two parts. First, clinical nutrition, or the care of the malnourished child, and secondly, general nutrition, which includes growth, and food composition, etc. Chapter 7 of the workers' manual describes the care of the malnourished child, but it contains very little general nutrition. So health workers need a manual on general nutrition. We have had to choose a nutrition manual to refer to, so we have given cross-references to *Nutrition for developing countries* [3]. This was written for Central and East Africa, but most of it is useful in other places also. Because each country has its own foods and customs, each country needs its own nutrition manual. If your country does not have such a manual, one should be written, or *Nutrition for developing countries* adapted and translated. A general nutrition manual like this is useful for many other kinds of workers, besides health workers.

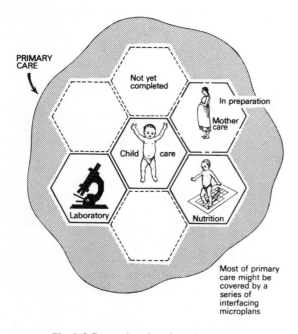

PRIMARY CARE

Not yet completed

In preparation

Mother care

Child care

Laboratory

Nutrition

Most of primary care might be covered by a series of interfacing microplans

Fig. 1-3 Some microplans for primary care

Some simple laboratory methods are essential for good primary care. So the workers' manual is cross-referenced to *A medical laboratory for developing countries* [4]. This describes the methods for a health-centre laboratory. Because laboratory methods are nearly the same everywhere, this manual needs little adaptation. It only needs translating. Unfortunately at least one of the instruments it describes is no longer manufactured (the MRC grey wedge photometer), and it also describes some procedures (blood transfusion) suited only to hospitals. Even so, it probably gives the most complete

descriptions of the simple procedures necessary for primary health care.

You can think of these two manuals on nutrition and laboratory methods as simple microplans. They were made for national adaptation and translation, and are made of more than one component (manual and equipment list). Fig. 1-3 shows that these microplans cover only part of primary care. 'Mother care', for example, is still in preparation, and there is nothing on 'Adult care'. There are manuals on some of these, but we have not found any which fit in well with the three we already have. We hope that there will eventually be master microplans for most of the clinical aspects of primary care, and we are ourselves about to embark on one for district hospital surgery—'primary surgery'.

1.4. Choosing the technologies

We started with the question 'What could a primary care worker reasonably do for the children who come to him?' Our answer is the workers' manual. What he could reasonably do depends on the diseases children have. It also depends on the technologies that exist for preventing or curing them, and the money available for health care. Answering the question was usually easy, and we have found widespread agreement on what workers could 'reasonably do'—if they were suitably trained. The manual describes a high level of primary care that many groups of workers could give. Other kinds of worker might only give part of it. Some methods, such as lumbar puncture, might seem difficult and even dangerous. They are, however, regularly and safely done by many auxiliaries.

It is commonly said that the wishes of the community should be considered in choosing the technologies. We have not found this to be practicable. Instead, we have included all the technologies that we have found to be suitable for primary child care. The community may however set priorities within these, and will certainly be concerned with how services are delivered (Manual 1.1, and Guide 7.6).

For a master microplan, such as this one, diseases are of three kinds. First, there are the diseases that are common everywhere, such as skin sepsis, scabies, measles, and whooping cough. These are all included.

Secondly, there are the less common diseases found all over the world, such as the backward child, the prolapsed rectum, the nephrotic syndrome, and talipes. Many of these are included because there is always some help or explanation a health worker can give. Also, although they may individually be uncommon, they do in aggregate make up a significant fraction of primary child care. We have not however found space for such comparatively rare diseases as rheumatic fever, heart failure, cirrhosis, or any tumours.

The technologies for these two first kinds of disease form the 'core technologies' of a master microplan.

Thirdly, there are diseases that are found in some places only, and which require 'local technologies'. In this master microplan we have described some of the local technologies for sub-Saharan Africa—for sickle-cell anaemia, the 'tumbu fly', pyomyositis, and *Schistosoma haematobium,* for example.

Inevitably, this version of the microplan is not perfectly suited to any region, so we look forward to hearing that countries are making their own exact adaptations. Since most of the technologies for primary child care are applicable all over the developing world, the changes required will be few. For example, a teacher of medical auxiliaries in New Guinea reviewed all the multiple-choice instruments. He found that, of the hundreds of technologies referred to by these instruments, only the following six alterations were required for New Guinea —intramuscular for subcutaneous chloroquine, the deletion of vitamin A deficiency, a simpler classification of burns, the removal of hypernatraemic dehydration, a different treatment regime for tuberculosis, and less emphasis on the dangers of bottle feeding.

When adaptations are made, we hope that they will bear the names of the adaptors and translators, acknowledge the part played by WHO, and make no reference to ourselves.

1.5. Who is this microplan for?

It is conventional wisdom that a manual should be written for one level of worker only. We have deliberately broken that rule, and tried to write for a broad spectrum of readers. Fortunately, there is good evidence that wide readership is possible. Not only are many other books successful in reaching many levels of reader, but we found that our own nutrition manual was required reading for postgraduate students at Michigan University, and for dressers in Zambia. Similarly, we are interested to hear that the workers' manual for this microplan is to be required reading at Yale University. It remains to be seen how far its readership will extend in the other direction.

As the workers' manual shows, the microplan describes a high standard of primary care. Potentially, this standard of care can be given by anyone who can read and use the workers' manual, and teach himself with the multiple-choice questions. This is why we have written it in the simplest English, and have made it as far as possible completely freestanding on primary education. To promote wide readership further, we have referred where possible to roles (worker, manager, teacher) rather than to staff categories (community health worker, doctor, or midwife).

The ability of a group of workers to read the workers' manual can easily be measured by testing them with the READING PRETEST (Guide A.1). Several of the instruments test their ability to use it. These instruments promise to be very useful when measuring how well individual workers or groups of workers can use the microplan.

Although primarily intended for application by nurses, medical assistants, and midwives, the microplan promises to span a wider range of workers than this. Many doctors have found it useful, and indeed it describes a better standard of care than some doctors practise. At the other extreme it may possibly be useful to some traditional practitioners and to some community health workers —provided they are sufficiently literate. The manual has also been read with interest by some mothers and fathers with no medical training. Unfortunately the illiterate mothers who need it most cannot use it—health workers must use it for them.

The most critical groups of workers, some of whom may be able to use the microplan, are such literate community health workers as are permitted to give injections, and traditional practitioners. We emphasize these workers because, at the present time, so many children get no medical care of any kind. Training community health workers and improving the skills of existing traditional practitioners promise to be practical ways of caring for them.

IT DOES NOT MATTER WHO DOES A TASK AS LONG AS IT IS DONE CORRECTLY

1.6. How 'microplan competent' should doctors, or senior nurses, or teachers be?

As we have said, the workers' manual is mainly written for medical assistants, nurses, and midwives. Consequently, most of us doctors and senior nurses think that, unless we score high marks with the multiple-choice questions, we are disgraced. That is, we think we should be fully 'microplan competent' (Guide 2.7). In practice, however, the only people who have been found to score high marks regularly with the multiple-choice questions, are those who are either practising or teaching a high standard of tropical paediatrics. Most doctors, who may be practising with high competence in some other field, usually score about 15 marks out of a possible 25. This is not surprising, since much of the knowledge in the workers' manual is specific to tropical paediatrics and some of it is comparatively new. This is well shown by the quotation at the top of Chapter 3 which concerns the drug for treating tapeworms. The optimum drug for treating these worms has recently changed from dichlorophen to niclosamide. Any doctor who does not treat children with tapeworms regularly can well be excused from knowing this. It is however simple and highly relevant knowledge for community health workers who treat these worms. As for ourselves, *we could not have answered all the multiple-choice questions, or indeed written them, until we came to collect the knowledge for the workers' manual from many highly specialized and expert sources.* As doctors or senior nurses we should not therefore be frightened to do these questions, or be ashamed of our own low scores. Much less creditable would be a low score and unwillingness to learn—if primary care or teaching it was our job.

WE SHOULD NOT BE ASHAMED TO LEARN WITH OUR WORKERS OR STUDENTS

1.7. An explanatory dialogue

The following conversation, which took place between a colleague and one of the authors, illustrates certain features of the microplan.

'You over-emphasize technology. Surely the social processes that determine the recruitment, motivation, and support of the health worker are much more important.' 'Indeed they are, but once there are health workers and managers they require the tools that we have tried to provide here. Your concern with the grand strategy of development policy, and mine with the nuts and bolts, are highly complementary.'

'I taught auxiliaries, but I did not use the instruments and targets I see here and we hardly had any manuals.' 'You taught them admirably, I remember. Here we try to help indirectly the learning of much larger numbers of people, whom we can never meet. Also, we are writing for people who may not have had the good luck to enjoy the learning experiences that both you and I have had. Unfortunately, there are many workers and managers who have no means of knowing what targets they might reach. Also, I am sure you had many targets, although you did not recognize them as such.'

'There is so much detail, why not confine yourself to guidelines?' 'Good clinical medicine, even in primary care, depends on the successful application of much minute detail and this has to be described somewhere. Where it is missing it will be invented and primary health workers have insufficient basic education to do this reliably. There is nothing like the privilege of being very ill to show one how necessary the details are. We have done our best to convey the importance and indeed the beauty of simple things well done. Guidelines too often disguise an inability to fill in the detail.'

'To provide such a detailed system denies managers the valuable learning experience of thinking through the process themselves.' 'The targets we provide are only suggestions, we encourage managers to make their own targets and instruments. Also, when managers and workers sit round a table to define their targets, they have inevitably to think them through in the same way that we have done.'

'You describe things as if your way was the only way of doing them.' 'We can only describe one way, which was the best way we could find. If anyone can find ways that really are better, I hope they will use them and tell us.'

'Surely there is a danger that once all this is printed it will become too much fixed and immutable. I have seen manuals from the 1930s still in use.' 'We emphasize the plastic nature of the microplan by stressing its adaptation to the needs of a particular country, its use as a box of tools and not a pair of handcuffs, and its frequent revision.'

'Surely, it makes countries much too dependent?' 'Dependent on one another perhaps, but we all inevitably depend on one another. The microplan was produced in a developing country, and there could hardly be a better example of WHO's policy of TCDC—technical cooperation among developing countries.'

'Many of the technologies here, such as the weight chart, are not of proven value.' 'Certainly, but this is so for much of medicine. To have awaited for rigorous proof would have denied technologies of widely accepted value to the people who need them.'

'What, do you think, are the most useful features of this microplan?' It appears to make several innovations. It trains auxiliary workers to use a manual to solve clinical problems. It links retraining to objective changes in the way children are cared for. And it links evaluation procedures to groups of technologies, rather than to grades of worker.

'What are going to be the main criticisms of this approach?' I am sure that it will be said that there is too much emphasis on multiple-choice questions, merely because they inevitably occupy so much space. The range of targets and instruments needs to be extended to include more dimensions of primary child care. Valid practical ones are however very difficult to construct.'

'Is not this systematic linking of tangible components, which is the principle behind the microplan, rather obvious? Why has it not been done before?' 'It certainly seems obvious. One of the reasons why it has not been done before, is the great labour involved—there is a year's work in the multiple-choice questions alone. Also, many things only seem obvious once they are done.'

'Might not this microplan be ahead of its time?' 'Possibly, this may perhaps explain why its production has been so difficult and so painful, and why it is so little understood. It will certainly be far behind whatever comes afterwards. It is to be hoped that eventually all the clinical aspects of primary care will be systematized in this way.'

'If this way of improving the quality of primary care is as useful as it seems, this microplan urgently needs to be monitored, developed, and promoted. What steps are being taken to do this?' 'None, we are urgently looking for any person, organization, or source of money interested in continuing where we have been obliged to stop.'

2 Quality of care

'Health services are likely to have a beneficial effect only to the extent that they reach a minimum level of quality.'
A report on health services in Ghana.

2.1. Quality

Our final purpose is to reduce sickness (morbidity) and death (mortality). Unfortunately, measuring morbidity requires special surveys. Measuring mortality requires the registration of births and deaths. Often this is not done. Even more unfortunately, there is no generally recognized way of measuring health. Also, health, sickness, and death depend on much else besides primary child care. So, instead of trying to measure them, we shall try instead to measure the 'quality' of the care we give and its coverage. We will assume that, if we give high-quality care, we are doing all we reasonably can to promote health and reduce sickness and death. Mostly, we shall be concerned with quality and we will only describe two methods for measuring coverage.

One great advantage of a microplan is that its workers' manual describes good quality primary care in great detail. It defines what workers should do for a child (process). It assumes that, if the process has been correct, what happens afterwards (outcome) will be as satisfactory as it could be with the technologies available. Thus, if a child is dehydrated and we treat him in the way the manual describes, we assume that the chances of his getting well are as good as they could be with the technologies we have. We do not in this microplan use any record of whether he lived or died to evaluate our care, because this is not easy to do. He might live even if we treat him badly, and die even if we treat him well. But, if we treat him well, his chance of living is as good as it could reasonably be.

If we consider only process and if we define it exactly, we can simplify quality enough to be able to measure it. We can say that a child gets high-quality primary care—care of 100 per cent microplan quality—if he gets everything described in the workers' manual. For example, his history should be taken in the way the manual describes. He should be examined by the methods the manual gives. The right diagnosis should be chosen from among the diagnoses it lists. A sick child must be able to get any of the drugs in the manual. The workers who care for him must be competent (Guide 2.7). They must know, or be able to use, the knowledge in the manual, and have the skills it describes. They must be kind and interested in him and his family. He must have both continuity of care and integrated care (Manual 5.2). If he is seriously ill, he should be able to get any of the treatments in the manual at any hour of the day or night, seven days a week. All these things are *variables*. They are called variables (factors or things which vary or differ) because they are ways in which the care in one clinic can vary from the care in another clinic. They are ways in which good-quality care differs from poor-quality care. We can easily measure some of these variables. For example, we can easily find out if a clinic has the right drugs. Other variables, such as kindness, are more difficult to measure. We can easily measure knowledge with multiple-choice questions. Although doing the right thing is more important than knowing about it, a worker cannot care for a child in the right way unless he first knows what to do. So knowledge, or knowing where to look it up, is an important variable deciding quality of care.

2.2. Instruments and targets

When we measure any variable, such as temperature, weight, or knowledge, we need a measuring **instrument,** and a scale to make the measurements on. A thermometer, for example, has a scale and measures heat. The multiple-choice instruments measure knowledge and have a scale of 25 points. The check-lists for measuring skills (Booklet B) usually have scale of about 10 points. There are many things we want to achieve which have a scale of only two points. For example, '0' the clinic has no soap, and '1' it has soap. We do not need special instruments to measure things like this. We can easily look to see if there is soap or not.

**AN INSTRUMENT IS SOMETHING WE
MEASURE WITH
A TARGET IS SOMETHING WE TRY TO REACH**

Targets are objectives that managers try to reach. They are sometimes called 'management objectives'. We want our workers to know about diarrhoea. So one of our targets is to make sure that they get good scores with multiple-choice instruments for diarrhoea. Good scores

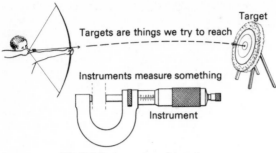

Targets are things we try to reach

Instruments measure something

Instrument

Target

Fig. 2–1 Instruments and targets

with any of the instruments are among our management targets. We do not need any instruments to measure some of our other targets, such as whether our clinics have torches which work. So, some of our targets need instruments to measure them, and some do not.

Every instrument has some kind of scale or score. There is a good score for it and a bad score. Somewhere along that scale we must fix our target score. So for every instrument there is a target.

SOME TARGETS NEED SPECIAL INSTRUMENTS TO MEASURE THEM AND SOME DO NOT
EVERY INSTRUMENT HAS ITS TARGET SCORE

Our instruments to measure quality of care and coverage must be quick to use, practical, and objective. By objective we mean that different people should easily agree about the score with an instrument. So we do not ask 'Is the attitude of the health worker sympathetic?' Instead we might ask 'Was the child's mother praised for something?' People would more easily agree about this, and it would show sympathy objectively. Because the instruments of the microplan must be quick and easy to use, they are not necessarily 'research' instruments.

The instruments have some or all of the following five uses. The last two concern teaching and learning, not measuring.

(1) The instruments tell us about our services. They are useful for making the service diagnosis (Guide 7.3).
(2) Getting good scores with an instrument can be one of the targets of a manager.
(3) Getting good scores with an instrument can be one of the objectives of a teacher.
(4) The instruments are useful teaching aids for students or workers.
(5) We ourselves learn from the instruments.

We must use measuring instruments in a way which gives reliable results. This means that they must give the same or nearly the same results when they are used on more than one occasion to measure the same thing. The 15 POINTS instrument (Guide 4.14), for example, should give the same, or nearly the same score, when it is used more than once on the same worker—provided he has not been learning more meanwhile. It should also give the same score when it is used by different observers on the same workers. This will only happen if it is always used in the same way, so follow the instructions for each instrument carefully.

INSTRUMENTS MUST BE USED IN THE SAME WAY EACH TIME

Each instrument should measure one kind of variable only. It should measure knowledge, or drugs, or waiting time, or something else, but not mixtures of these things. A score which mixes many different variables has little meaning. So we seldom use mixed scores and we usually measure each variable by itself. The only exceptions are the 15 POINTS instrument (Guide 4.14) and the quality score (Manual 6.8). Some of the points in the 15 POINTS instrument are questions or instructions, and others are methods of examination. We have put these 15 different variables together in one instrument, because most children coming to a clinic need most of them.

If we keep variables separate, we do not need to weight them. To weight a variable means giving it more weight or importance than another variable. For example, is penicillin more useful than glucose saline? Arguing does not help, and we cannot find out by experiment. Both are necessary, so we must measure each of them separately. Even so, some parts of child care are so much more important than others that we must weight them when we set management priorities (Guide 7.4). So some of the targets we suggest as being especially important have stars beside them—the **star targets—★.**

THE TARGETS ARE THE MOST IMPORTANT PARTS OF THE MICROPLAN

2.3. Pretests and postests

We give pretests to students or workers to find out how much they know before we train them. After we have trained them we give them a postest. The difference between a pretest and a postest tells us how much they have learnt. Unless we test workers or students like this, some of them will not try to learn, and we shall not know how successful we have been in teaching them.

Some instruments, such as the MATHS PRETEST (A.2) and the READING PRETEST (A.1) are pretests only. We use them to *find out* if workers can read the manual, and if they know enough maths to work out doses before we start to train them. Other tests are postests only. We use the MANUAL POSTEST to find if workers can use the manual after they have been trained. This test has no meaning before workers have learnt to use the manual. Many tests can be used as pretests or postests. The CHAPTER TESTS A, B, and C can be used like this. The pretests do not have targets.

GIVE THE PRETESTS BEFORE TEACHING STARTS

2.4. Positive and negative targets

A positive target is something which we want to happen. A negative target is something which we do not want to happen. It is a 'no' or 'not' target. Examples of positive targets are—workers use an auriscope, or get good scores with multiple-choice instruments, or rehydrate children before sending them home.

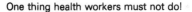

One thing health workers must not do!

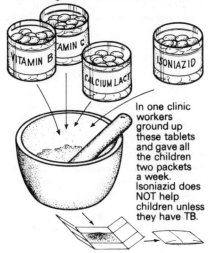

In one clinic workers ground up these tablets and gave all the children two packets a week. Isoniazid does NOT help children unless they have TB.

Fig. 2-2 A negative target

Negative targets include *not* giving injections to children who don't need them, *not* making more records than you need, *not* using the same syringe for more than one child, and *not* using amidopyrine.

Positive targets are usually easier to reach. You can easily teach workers to make glucose–salt solution, or to use weight charts. Making them change their bad habits is more difficult. We have listed many positive targets but very few negative targets because they vary from country to country.

2.5. Workers' targets, managers' targets, and joint targets

A worker is more likely to work to reach a target if he helped to make or choose it himself, so we should let workers help to choose targets wherever possible. To make this easier we have divided targets into workers' targets, joint targets, and managers' targets. Needless to say, these divisions are not exact. Although managers and teachers should help workers and students to reach their knowledge and skills targets, these targets have for convenience been considered as 'workers' targets'. All the workers' targets and the joint targets, start with 'We . . .'.

Workers' knowledge targets. These are the targets we test for with the multiple-choice instruments. For example, 'We must show that we understand "coughs", by passing instrument COUGHS A, B, or C,' is a workers' target, because workers can choose and reach it. Each student has a score sheet for these instruments at the back of his manual. These instruments go from the DIFFICULT WORDS tests A, B, and C for the first chapter of the manual through to NEWBORN BABY A, B, and C for the last chapter.

Workers' skills targets. There are check-lists for the skills workers should have the at front of Booklet B. They are check-lists for things that workers should be able to do. They all start 'We must be able to . . . count the respirations . . ., or treat a child for scabies, etc.'

Joint targets. These are also at the front of Booklet B. They are targets which workers and managers can try to reach together.

Managers' targets. These are targets which the worker cannot reach alone. Many of them concern supplies which the manager must provide. The numbers after the major headings refer to the chapters in the workers' manual. Here are some suggestions with spaces to fill in your findings.

MANAGERS' TARGETS

INTRODUCTION (1)

Examine the workers' manuals six months after they have been issued. Are they dirty, and 'dog-eared', and finger-marked? Are there notes in the margins? (This is valuable objective evidence that manuals are being read and used. It could easily be falsified if it was listed as a workers' target.)..
....

DISEASE IN THE CHILD AND THE COMMUNITY (2)
★*Primary care services are (a) planned in collaboration with community leaders; and (b) responsible to them. (c) Regular meetings are held with community leaders*..........
....

Health activities are linked to and integrated with other development programmes for raising living standards.......
....

★*Primary child care is being taught to new workers, and to existing ones.* ....
....

Community volunteers are helping in clinics.................
....

DRUGS (3)

★All the 'important 50' drugs are available (Manual 3.7) .. ..

★All the 'important 20' items of equipment are available (Manual 3.50)... ....

All drugs are purchased by and prescribed by generic title... ....

Not more than ...per cent (say 20 per cent) of the children who come to a clinic are given an injection. ....

HEALTHY CHILD (4)

Every time the clinic opens the following vaccines are available: BCG, measles, polio, DPT. ....

80 per cent or more of children are immunized with BCG, measles, polio, and DPT. ....

Where the relevant diseases are sufficiently prevalent, malaria is suppressed, children are routinely treated for Ascaris or hookworms, prophylactic vitamin A is given six-monthly, and goitre is prevented with an injection of iodized oil every three years. ....

SICK CHILD (5)

★Every task has been delegated to the most humbly trained (and least expensive) worker capable of doing it adequately. Highly trained expensive professional staff do not spend their time doing simple routine jobs, such as weighing or keeping the clinic register. This is done by clerks or helpers. ....

RECORDING AND REPORTING (6)

Record-keeping requires the equivalent of less than one full-time person per 100 out-patients per day. ....

Less than 2 per cent of weight charts are lost. ....

Standard shorthand is used (Manual 6:1). ....

No old or unnecessary record systems in use. ....

Syringes and needles sterilized in a pressure cooker. ....

NUTRITION (7)

★All children take home weight charts in plastic bags. ....

Weight charts are in stock. ....

Plastic bags are in stock. ....

People in the community, such as members of mothers clubs, are being taught to weigh children and use the weight charts.. ....

Breast pumps and nipple shields available in the clinic for sale or hire. ....

A child's length is NOT measured routinely. ....

DIARRHOEA (9)

Clinics able to test the stools for lactose. ....

FITS (15)

(a) Some sterile disposable needles and (b) Pandy's, solution available. ....

Lumbar puncture undertaken in the clinics when neces-sary. ....

EARS (17)

The clinics have auriscopes which work. ....

MOUTH AND THROAT (18)

The clinic has spatulae and a torch which works. ....

WORMS (21)

Clinics are able to examine a child's stools for worms. . ...

ANAEMIA (22)

★The clinics are able to measure the haemoglobin. ....

URINARY AND GENITAL (23)

The clinic is able to (a) count pus cells in the urine and (b) examine pus for Gram negative intracellular diplococci. .. ..

MORE MANAGERS' TARGETS

Workers do not spend more than a quarter of the time idle. ....

★Staff meetings, for all staff, the main purpose of which is teaching, are held at least once each month. ....

MCH clinics are held on all market days. ....

At least 50 per cent of vehicle mileage spent taking health care (outreach clinics) to the people. ....

Average waiting time less than one hour (Guide 4.17). ....

WHAT OTHER TARGETS HAVE YOU?

....
....
....
....

2.6. Many variables determine quality

Quality of care depends on many variables. Some of these variables are large—Has the clinic any penicillin? Other variables seem to be small—Do mothers have a chair to sit on? Does the health worker touch the shaft of a needle when he gives an injection? Even though these detailed variables seem to be small, they all add to the quality of care a child gets.

QUALITY DEPENDS ON MANY DETAILS

One or two variables by themselves are not enough to measure quality. Enough drugs in a clinic and enough knowledge in its workers do not make sure that the children who go to that clinic get high quality care. But if a clinic and its workers score well with many varied instruments, it is probably giving high quality care. It is certainly giving better care than another clinic which gives low scores with these same instruments. So we measure quality with many *different* instruments, each of which measures some part of it. A mixture of different instruments is better than several instruments of the same kind. Thus some 'skills check-lists', MCQs VARIED, and the WEIGHT CHART SCORE (Guide 4.10) would be better than several instruments which tested knowledge only.

MANY VARIABLES DEFINE QUALITY

An example of another kind may help. If something has a simple shape, such as a square, one variable (the length of a side) tells us everything about it. If it is a rectangle we need two variables (length and width). We can picture quality as a very complex shape, like the child in Guide 2–3. We can only draw this shape if we know where all the dots are. Even then we have to guess where the line goes between the dots.

This microplan contains 107 multiple-choice instruments for measuring knowledge or the ability to find it in the manual. There are more than 150 instruments and targets of other kinds. But even this number of instruments and targets only measure some of the variables which determine quality of care. It is as if we could find out where some of the dots are in Guide 2–3, but not all of them. For example, we have no practical instrument to measure whether a health worker will treat seriously-ill children at night, or on Sunday. This would be difficult to measure, although we might get some help by asking people in his village.

The variables determining quality of care are probably linked in part to one another. Thus a good score with one instrument probably means a good score with another, even though we cannot measure it. For example, if a

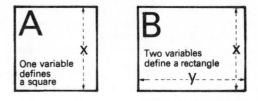

MANY VARIABLES DETERMINE QUALITY OF CARE

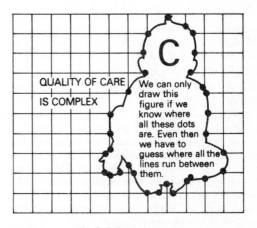

Fig. 2–3 Quality of care

worker gets a high score with instrument DIARRHOEA A (knowledge about diarrhoea), and instrument USING A 'CARING FOR' SECTION, he will probably make the right diagnosis also. He will probably do this, even though our instruments don't measure it. It is as if, by knowing where two dots are in Guide 2–3, we can guess where the line goes between them. So by measuring as many of the variables as we can measure, we are probably getting some knowledge of the variables we cannot measure.

Quality of care also depends on the speed with which children are seen. A worker who has an average of only 3 minutes to see a child cannot do as much for him as a worker who has 7 minutes for each child. Even so, we have not tried to relate the scores with particular instruments to the time a child spends with a worker. Also *we are not trying to judge workers.* Instead, we have looked at quality from the point of view of the child—What is he getting when he comes to a clinic? If workers are too busy to give reasonable care, more workers must be trained. Because better care makes people want more care, more people will come for care. Because more people come for care, we shall need to train more workers.

2.7. 'Microplan competence' or 'microplan mastery'—the student or worker

A student or worker can be 'microplan competent'. This means that he knows what he should know in the workers' manual, and can do the tasks it describes. If he knows and can do everything perfectly, or nearly perfectly, he is 100 per cent microplan competent. The microplan can be implemented by many levels of worker, so that scores that would be good for dressers would be bad for medical students. So you may need to choose different levels of competence depending on your workers. In Guide 3.7 we describe standard ways of setting these levels for multiple-choice questions. Unfortunately, there are no standard ways of setting them for skills check-lists.

A worker is only competent at a particular level for the instruments against which he has been tested. If you want to know how competent a worker is for the microplan as a whole, test him against as many instruments as possible, especially instruments of different kinds.

2.8. A quality-of-care profile—'microplan quality'

Each of the many targets in this guide tells us about one of the variables which help to decide the quality of care. Some of these variables describe the competence of the worker. Other variables describe what happens in the clinic. They do not tell us everything about the quality of our services, but they tell us as much as we can measure.

When we have measured quality as completely as we can, we must list our successes and failures with each target, so as to make an outline or profile of quality of care. The managers' targets are in Guide 2.5. Make your own summary of the multiple-choice questions. Booklet B summarizes the skills check-lists and the joint targets. With each target there is a dotted line on which you can write in how far you have succeeded in reaching it. Fill in all the dotted lines as far as you can for your services and your workers. Where there is no numerical score, 60 per cent for example, estimate it from 0 to 100 per cent (the target completely reached). Probably there will be many instruments you have not used. Put a line through these as 'not known'. Fill in as many dotted lines as you can.

When you know where your workers and your services are in relation to as many targets as possible, work out the percentage scores for each group of targets and write them on the dotted lines below. These percentages are 'percentages of microplan quality'. Do this as part of your service diagnosis before implementation of the microplan, and again afterwards. Work out the percentage of total targets reached. Because weighting targets is so difficult, this is less meaningful than the groups of targets, and these in turn are less meaningful than each target by itself.

AVERAGE SCORES	IMPLEMENTATION BEFORE	AFTER
Workers' knowledge targets	.........%	.........%
Workers' skills targets	.........%	.........%
Joint targets	.........%	.........%
Managers' targets	.........%	.........%
Star targets reached	.........%	.........%
Percentages of total targets reached	.........%	.........%
Total numbers of targets assessed	.........%	.........%

2.9. We none of us like being evaluated!

Although the evaluation instruments are intended to evaluate the workers, they threaten ourselves as managers and teachers. We think that, because we are managers or teachers, we should score 100 per cent always and are worried if we score less. We are also worried if our clinics score badly with the instruments measuring quality of care. We should not be worried. Where we or our clinics start from is not important. But the targets we reach are important.

Some knowledge in the manual is new. Some comes from experts in special subjects, or from recent WHO Expert Committee Reports, such as the recommendation to start dapsone at full dosage, and not to start at a low dose and increase it gradually. We hope therefore, that as teachers and managers you will do the multiple-choice questions—under a pen-name if necessary! One teacher averaged 24 per cent on a large number of multiple-choice instruments, and his third-year paramedical students 17 per cent. Can you, and your students do better?

WE MUST NOT BE AFRAID TO EVALUATE OURSELVES
WHAT ARE *YOUR* SCORES WITH THE MCQs?

After diagnosis comes treatment. When we have diagnosed what is wrong with the quality and coverage of our services, we need to 'treat' or improve them. We describe this in Chapter 7 'Implementing the microplan'.

2.10. Three targets for which there are no instruments

The instruments and targets in this microplan measure much of child care, but they do not measure all of it. They do not ask three important questions. There is no universally right answer to these questions, and there are no instruments for measuring them. The answers and the 'pass marks' to these questions are special for ourselves. They depend on who we are, what we are, and where we are.

Are our staff, money, and buildings being used to care for the children who most need it? Perhaps some of our staff have very little work and could easily be moved to another clinic? Perhaps our clinic belongs to the army, the port authority, the airways, a factory, or an oil company, and only cares for children whose fathers have good jobs? Can we also care for the children of the daily labourers and for those whose fathers have no jobs?

Are all our staff doing the most skilled jobs they can? Perhaps a highly trained public-health nurse is only giving routine injections, which could easily be done by someone with much less training? Perhaps weighing and record keeping is being done by someone who could easily be trained to do something more difficult? Perhaps sweepers could be taught to make records or weigh children?

Are we always trying to increase the skills of our staff, so that there are more skills for child care in our district? When a sick child is referred to us, is the person who sent him present when we examine the child, so that he can learn how the child should be examined and cared for? How much teaching do we give our staff? What books do we give them? Do we try to make our own staff as broadly competent as possible, so that that one worker can substitute for another if necessary?

2.11. Some dangers

There are dangers that the evaluation instruments in this microplan will be used in the wrong way. Most of these dangers can be prevented. For example, if there were only a few multiple-choice questions, students or workers could easily learn the answers to them. We have overcome this danger by providing very many questions. Students will find it easier to learn the manual than the answers to all the questions.

Some instruments can easily be used in a way which gives false results. For example, there are very many variables which determine how a child should be examined and how a history should be taken from his mother. But the 15 POINTS instrument only scores a few of them. Its usefulness depends on the variables that are being observed (Is an explanation given? Is a child's mother told when to return?) being linked to those which are not being observed (kindness, making the right diagnosis, etc.). The worker must not know what he is being observed for. If he does, he can easily get a good score with the 15 POINTS instrument without improving the rest of the way in which he cares for a child.

It would be possible to train workers and arrange a clinic so as to deliberately get good scores with all the instruments. There are so many of these, that if you do, your clinic will certainly be giving high quality care. This is exactly what is wanted. The instruments are designed for making a service diagnosis and as management objectives. However, because some important variables cannot be measured, even high scores do not guarantee perfect services. Nevertheless, if you do get high scores, your services must be very good.

Make your own instruments and try to improve on ours. We suggest, however, that, if you make more than one or two small changes, you give the instrument a new name. It is important that MANUAL POSTEST, or MCQs EASY should always mean the same or nearly the same instrument.

***

WHAT INSTRUMENTS AND TARGETS CAN YOU MAKE?

3 Multiple-choice instruments (MCQs) for learning and evaluation

'I would have to look this up! Even though I did write a chapter on parasites for ...'s textbook.'

A distinguished paediatrician commenting on a multiple-choice question asking for the appropriate drug to treat tapeworms.

3.1. Measuring knowledge

Each child who comes to a health worker presents him with the problem 'What can I do for this child?' If the worker is to solve the problem, he must have the necessary knowledge, and be able to apply it. If he does not know something, he must be able to look it up. The best way to teach and evaluate the worker is to use real children. In practice students seldom get enough experience with real children. So we need other methods of teaching and evaluation. Lifelike multiple-choice questions are useful for both of these purposes. They are simple and objective. You can use them 'manual shut' to find out what a worker remembers, or 'manual open' to find out what he can look up.

The manual contains all the knowledge necessary for primary child care. If workers are going to practise with complete competence they must know it all, or be able to look it up. Workers who are microplan competent (Guide 2.7) should get most of the multiple-choice questions right. The use of test instruments in this way is called **criterion reference testing.** We define the necessary knowledge or skill (the reference criterion), and the students either know something or can do something, or they cannot. If all the students are good, they all pass. If they are all bad, they all fail. This is different from the older way of testing which compares students with one another (**norm reference testing**). In the old way the same percentage of students passes or fails, even if the class as a whole is very good or very bad.

Knowledge is necessary and is comparatively easy to measure. This is why the microplan makes the most of multiple-choice questions. *But doing is what matters. Don't over-emphasize these questions, merely because there are so many of them!* They do not tell us if workers are able to *use* their knowledge.

We have not given any open-ended questions, for example, 'How would you promote breast feeding?' or 'Describe the dangers of bottle feeding'. We have not given any, because there is no standard way of marking them. Also, schools can more easily make their own.

What should a student learn, and what should he look up? Doses are the only things he should *not* learn. If possible he should know everything else, starting with the more common diseases. He should *not* try to learn the manual by heart. He should learn it as he reads it, as he gains experience, and as he does the multiple-choice questions.

3.2. The questions

Unfortunately, because multiple-choice questions have to be written in a special way, the language in them is sometimes more difficult than the language in the manual. Some students who can understand the manual may have difficulty with the questions. Guide 6.3 describes an instrument to measure reading ability. A line at 50 per cent separates somewhat arbitrarily those who read easily from those who need help. It would be possible to draw a line further to the right at, say, 60 per cent separating those who can read well enough to understand the multiple-choice questions from those who cannot. How far to the right this line lies we do not yet know.

To save paper the questions and the answer-sheets are laid out in lines rather than in columns. *All questions are entirely confined to the knowledge in the manual—all the right answers can be found there.* Most of the wrong answers come from the manual also. This particular version of the microplan is primarily adapted to sub-Saharan Africa (Guide 1.4). So the multiple-choice questions assume that sick children come from a district where malaria is holoendemic. They do not always say each time that there is malaria in the district. The same applies to *Schistosoma*, etc.

If you do not like some questions, use the others. Ask the class to cross out or alter the questions you do not want. Before you decide that a question is wrong, be sure you are not wrong!

CROSS OUT THE QUESTIONS YOU DON'T WANT

3.3. A standard format

We have tried to make the questions easy to use, and easy to mark. To help this they are all done on the same answer-sheet. You can use the same plastic overlay to correct them all. Each multiple-choice instrument has 25 questions. Each question has up to five answers A, B, C, D, E. Only one answer is right. Usually, all five options are used, sometimes only two. Some questions are of the 'matching' kind, for example, 'MATCH these worms ... with the drugs used to treat them.' Some are of the style 'All the following are true EXCEPT one ...' We have tried to minimize the number of questions with 'NOT' in the stem, but some are inevitable.

Guide 3–1 shows a piece of A4 paper stencilled with two answer-sheets. Each answer-sheet has 32 questions. In practice we only use 25 of these questions.

The transparent plastic overlay shown in Guide 3–2 has holes over the right answers. You can use it in four different ways to give eight different answer codes. Codes 1 and 2 are with the overlay in the position shown in Guide 3–2. Codes 3 and 4 are with the overlay turned back to front. Codes 5 and 6 are with the overlay turned upside down. Codes 7 and 8 are with it upside down and back to front. You can find the right code to use by looking at the top-right-hand corner of each multiple-choice instrument. The codes on the overlay are

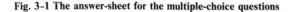

Fig. 3-1 The answer-sheet for the multiple-choice questions

15

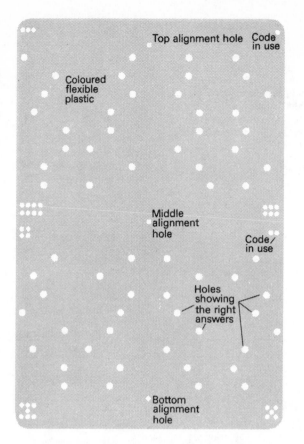

Fig. 3–2 The plastic overlay for the answer-sheet

numbered with holes, because overlays are easier to make like this.

Where there are less than five answers in a question, they do not always start with A. Sometimes they start with B, C, or D. This is necessary because of the coding. Students soon understand it.

3.4. Answers which correct themselves

If possible, a worker should know immediately if his answer to a multiple-choice question is right or wrong. There is an easy way of telling him this.

Phenolphthalein (a commonly used drug) is colourless in a neutral solution. But in an alkaline solution, such as a solution of sodium carbonate (not bicarbonate), it goes red. If we put some phenolphthalein over the right answers on an answer-sheet it remains completely invisible—we cannot see it. If the worker marks his answer-sheet with a swab dipped in alkaline brown ink, the wrong ones stay brown, but the right answers go red.

You can put phenolphthalein on the right answers by dissolving it in spirit. Make a cloth damp with the solution of phenolphthalein in spirit and dab it through the holes of the plastic overlay onto the answer-sheets.

The spirit soon dries and you cannot see the phenolphthalein.

SELF-CORRECTING QUESTIONS

ALKALINE INK. This can be any colour except red. Add sodium carbonate (or some other alkali) to ink, or poster paint, or distemper, water paint, or strong coffee, or even soy sauce! Use plenty of sodium carbonate. Experiment, you may need to add 20 per cent of sodium carbonate to ink, and to use equal quantities of sodium carbonate and poster paint. With sticky fluids, such as soy sauce, add water (3 parts or more). Soy sauce is sticky, and sinks slowly into the paper. Adding water makes it sink in faster and brings up the red colour quicker. If it evaporates, so that it becomes sticky again, add more water.

Two teaspoonfuls of instant coffee and two teaspoonfuls of sodium carbonate in a quarter of a cupful of water make a good 'ink'. If the red colour is too pale, the sodium carbonate solution may be too strong or too weak. So more sodium carbonate or more water may help.

Put about 5 ml of alkaline ink in many small plastic pots. Keep these pots on a tray. Add water when they become dry. Small volumes of ink make less mess when they spill.

16

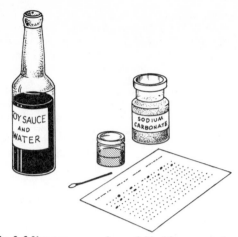

Fig. 3–3 You can even make an 'ink' with soy sauce!

SWABS. Make 'ear swabs' by wrapping a little cotton wool round the end of a small stick or tooth pick. Dip a swab in the alkaline ink, and smear it over the questions on the answer-sheet.

ALCOHOLIC 2 per cent PHENOLPHTHALEIN. Dissolve 2 g of phenolphthalein in white surgical spirit (96 per cent alcohol) or methylated spirit. The concentration is not important. If it becomes too strong, you can see where it is on the paper.

MAKING A STENCIL FOR ANSWER SHEETS. Type out Guide 3–1 on to a stencil as carefully as possible. Space out the letters and the lines as shown. The top and bottom '0' must be the same distance above and below the lines. The middle '0' must be exactly in the middle. If possible, use a 10-pitch typewriter. Stencils are also available from TALC.

MAKING PLASTIC OVERLAYS. Take a stencilled double answer-sheet. Put large dots over the right answers for Code One on the top answer-sheet. Put dots over the right answers for Code Two on the bottom answer-sheet.

Get one or more sheets of thick coloured plastic. Plastic file-covers are the right size. Clip the marked answer-sheet to the plastic sheet with paper clips. Go to a shoemaker. Choose a 5 mm leather punch. Ask him to punch holes through the plastic over the right answers. You can also use a laboratory cork borer. If necessary make 5 mm-square holes with a scalpel. The plastic sheet must not slip over the paper. The holes must be *exactly* over the right answers. If necessary the shoemaker can punch through several sheets of plastic at the same time.

Mark the plastic with numbers 1,2,3,4,5,6,7, and 8 in the places shown in Guide 3–2. Use a felt pen. To prevent the numbers rubbing off, cover them with a piece of transparent sticky tape.

If you have not got plastic, make a paper overlay by cutting holes in an answer-sheet. Overlays are available from TALC.

MAKING SELF-CORRECTING ANSWER-SHEETS. Turn the overlay so that the code you want is in the top-right-hand corner. Put the central hole in the overlay over the '0' in the middle of a stencilled answer-sheet. Make sure that the top and bottom holes are over the top and bottom '0's on the answer-sheet.

Dip a piece of clean cotton wool into a small bowl of alcoholic phenolphthalein. Squeeze it well so that it is just damp. It must not be too wet. Dab the cotton wool onto the paper through every hole in the overlay, so that the paper is just damped. If the swab is too wet, phenolphthalein solution runs onto the wrong answers also. Write the code number on the answer-sheet immediately. If you do not do this, you will not know which code it is when the alcohol has evaporated.

Try out an occasional answer-sheet by smearing alkaline ink over every question. The right answers should be easily seen, with no red colour on the wrong ones.

If the same piece of cotton wool is used many times, the spirit evaporates and leaves the phenolphthalein in the wool. This makes the solution stronger each time you use it. If the solution becomes too strong or gets dirty, it makes a mark on the answer-sheet which you can easily see. Prevent this by using clean cotton wool.

THE CODES. Codes One and Two are in Guide 3–1.

Code One is—1A, 2E, 3C, 4A, 5D, 6D, 7C, 8B, 9C, 10E, 11B, 12D, 13B, 14C, 15D, 16A, 17E, 18C, 19D, 20B, 21E, 22A, 23B, 24A, 25C.

Code Two is—1D, 2E, 3A, 4C, 5B, 6B, 7D, 8A, 9C, 10E, 11A, 12D, 13A, 14D, 15B, 16C, 17E, 18C, 19D, 20E, 21B, 22A, 23A, 24B, 25E.

Code Three is—1E, 2C, 3A, 4E, 5D, 6C, 7B, 8B, 9B, 10D, 11A, 12C, 13E, 14B, 15C, 16D, 17D, 18B, 19C, 20A, 21E, 22D, 23E, 24A, 25B.

Code Four is 1C, 2E, 3A, 4B, 5E, 6B, 7D, 8D, 9B, 10E, 11A, 12C, 13C, 14D, 15B, 16E, 17A, 18B, 19C, 20A, 21D, 22E, 23E, 24D, 25E.

Code Five is 1E, 2C, 3D, 4B, 5E, 6D, 7C, 8A, 9B, 10A, 11A, 12B, 13E, 14C, 15D, 16E, 17A, 18D, 19B, 20C, 21C, 22E, 23A, 24D, 25B.

Code Six is 1C, 2A, 3E, 4B, 5C, 6E, 7D, 8D, 9E, 10A, 11B, 12A, 13E, 14C, 15D, 16B, 17B, 18C, 19D, 20A, 21C, 22E, 23B, 24D, 25D.

Code Seven is 1D, 2B, 3C, 4A, 5E, 6C, 7B, 8A, 9D, 10E, 11E, 12D, 13A, 14B, 15C, 16A, 17C, 18D, 19B, 20E, 21B, 22E, 23A, 24C, 25E.

Code Eight is 1D, 2A, 3E, 4C, 5B, 6B, 7A, 8C, 9E, 10D, 11E, 12A, 13D, 14B, 15C, 16A, 17E, 18B, 19C, 20D, 21B, 22D, 23A, 24C, 25D.

CODING YOUR OWN MULTIPLE-CHOICE QUESTIONS. Get eight answer-sheets, the plastic overlay and a felt pen. On each sheet mark the correct answers for one code. You will then have all the right answers for each code. Clip these answer-sheets together to make a booklet, as shown in Guide 3–4.

Questions of the 'matching' kind can only be done on some parts of the code. There has to be an A, a B, a C, a D, and, if necessary, an E in a sequence of four or five numbers. Start 'matching' questions in question 13, 18, 23, and 28 of Code One; questions 13, 18, 23, and 28 of Code Two; questions 9 and 17 of Code Three; questions 13 and 18 of Code Four; questions 5, 11, 16 and 21 of Code Five; questions 11 and 20 of Code Six; questions 1, 6, 11, 23, and 28 of Code Seven; and questions 1, 6, 11, and 16 of Code Eight. Although a five-letter sequence (A B C D E, but not necessarily in this order) starts in each of these places, most of the 'matching' questions use only four letters.

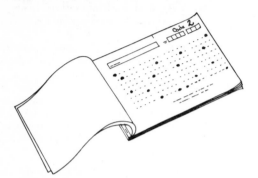

Fig. 3–4 Make yourself a booklet of answer-codes

Put questions where the right answer is 'None of these' against a question in the code where the right answer is 'E'.

When you have made your own multiple-choice questions, you can soon teach a clerk to code them. Write out the questions and number them. Make sure that the 'matching' questions are in the right places. Put a mark against the right questions. Let him code them. The right answers must have the right letter. The wrong answers can have any of the other letters.

These self-correcting answer-sheets cause few problems. Workers can, however, easily cheat by seeing each other's right answers. They can also put a very small spot of ink in a letter, wait to see if this changes colour, and then make a larger spot if it does change. Repeated scores of 25 should make you suspicious! Often, cheating is not important. But, if it prevents you evaluating the workers, separate them, ask them to do the questions with an ordinary pen, and correct their answer-sheets with an overlay. Afterwards, they can see which questions they got right with the self correcting ink.

Workers like these self-correcting multiple-choice questions, and ask for more. This is one reason why we have provided so many.

3.5. Three sets of multiple-choice questions

There are three kinds of multiple-choice instrument distributed between the three Booklets A, B, and C.

One. The SICK CHILDREN INSTRUMENTS. All 18 of these instruments are in Booklet B. They are based on short case-histories and come in random order from all over the manual. Workers or students can do them with manuals open or shut. They are, however, intended for use with an open manual. When used like this they help students to learn to use their manuals. Students can also use them to play 'the clinic game' described in Guide 3.8.

Two. The CHAPTER INSTRUMENTS. There are 81 of these instruments. There are three for each of the 26 chapters of the workers' manual, with three extra ones for Chapter 26 (The newborn child) which is very long. One instrument for each chapter has gone into each booklet, with two for Chapter 26. Instruments for the shorter chapters contain revision questions from the preceding part of the manual. Questions for a particular chapter have been randomly allocated between booklets so that the three instruments for, say, diarrhoea (Chapter 9) are matched.

Three. The SPECIAL SET. These are all either pretests in Booklet A or postests in Booklet C.

MCQs VARIED (Booklet A). This contains questions from all over the manual. Some are very easy. Most of them are as difficult as we have been able to make them within the limitations of the microplan. MCQs VARIED is intended as a short general test of microplan competence, particularly for senior workers. It is useful for introducing a discussion or workshop on the microplan. If workers are anxious about their scores, do it anonymously, or ask them to choose borrowed names.

MCQs EASY (Booklet A). This contains 25 of the easiest questions we could make, taken from all over the manual. Low scores with this instrument mean that workers know nothing—provided they can read and understand multiple-choice questions. The pass mark (Guide 3.7) for MCQ's EASY should be 25 (100 per cent).

OVERALL PRETEST (Booklet A) and OVERALL POSTEST (Booklet C). These are a matched pair of instruments made from questions taken at random from all those in the 81 CHAPTER INSTRUMENTS. They are for use as pre- and post-tests of knowledge of the whole manual. OVERALL PRETEST for example, might be given before the implementation of a microplan in a district, and OVERALL POSTEST after it. They can also be used before a course in child care and after it. The limitations of these instruments is their small sample size—only 25 questions each out of a total of 2025, or a little more than 1 per cent. If there is time for workers to do more questions than this, choose more questions at random, and make two more instruments.

MATHS PRETEST (Booklet A). This is a pretest of the elementary maths needed to use the microplan (Guide 6.3).

MANUAL POSTEST (Booklet C). This measures how well a student can use the manual (Guide 6.3).

DOSES POSTEST (Booklet C). This postest must be done with an open manual. It tests a worker's ability to use the dose tables only. Make sure that workers have studied Fig. 3–11b carefully first (Guide 6.3).

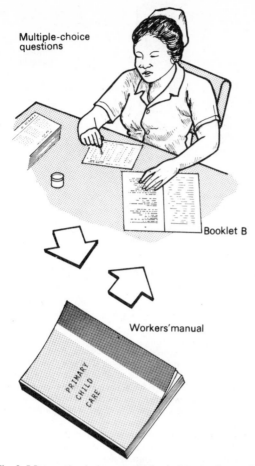

Multiple-choice questions

Booklet B

Workers' manual

Fig. 3–5 Interaction between multiple-choice questions and the manual

WEIGHT-CHART POSTEST (Booklet C). This postest measures how much workers know about the weight charts. It is also a very useful teaching aid.

KEEP THE SPECIAL SET FOR EVALUATION DON'T USE THEM FOR ORDINARY TRAINING

USING THE BOOKLETS DURING A COURSE IN CHILD CARE

CHAPTER INSTRUMENTS. Give one Booklet B to each student. Let the students keep the booklets during the course. Ask them to sign for them. Ask them to keep the booklets clean and not to write in them. They will be used again by next year's class of students.

Keep Booklets A and C yourself and issue them only during a class as required.

Use the instruments in Booklet A as a pretest. Find out how much the students know about a particular chapter

before they start to learn about it. Tell the students to read the chosen chapter in the manual during a few days or a week. Let them test themselves using Booklet B. Keep a stock of answer-sheets, ink, and swabs where students can find them.

Then give them a postest in class with Booklet C to find out how much they have learnt. If possible use the statistical method in Chapter 5 to find out if there has been a real improvement, or if it is probably only due to chance. The graphical method in Guide 5.3 is particularly easy.

THE SICK CHILDREN INSTRUMENTS. There are 18 of these instruments in Booklet B for students to do in their own time from an open manual. They can do the questions in any way which is convenient. You can test students in class to see how good they are at doing them from an open manual. They come from all over the manual, so they are not suitable for pre- and postests, before and after reading particular chapters.

If you see marks opposite the right answers in these booklets, add more marks against the wrong answers!

At the beginning workers take about an hour for each instrument. If they are learning to use an index and doing one of the sick children instruments from an open manual, they may take 15 minutes for one question. Later, they can do a whole instrument in 20 minutes. They are soon able to do five instruments in a morning. Probably, about 50 hours are needed for all the instruments. If there is not time for all of them, do the most important ones.

There is little relationship between the number of questions on a subject and its importance. For example, there are about the same number of questions on diarrhoea and on the backward child.

3.6. Analysing multiple-choice questions

Sometimes, we do not only want to know how many questions a student gets right. We may also want to know which questions he gets right, and which of the answers A,B,C,D, or E he marks. Analysing answer sheets to find this out takes time, but you can easily teach a clerk to do it.

ANALYSING MULTIPLE-CHOICE QUESTIONS BY HAND Stencil some papers with questions 1 to 25 on them. For every question write A,B,C,D, and E with a row of dots about 3 cm long after each letter.

Ask a clerk, or a cleaner, to take each of the students' answer-sheets and to make a tally for each answer that a student marks, like that in Guide 3–6

You can soon see which questions everyone gets right, which questions students only get right by guessing, and which answers nobody thinks are right. You can also see which of the distractors (wrong answers) are chosen by the students.

The multiple-choice questions in this edition of the guide have not been analysed in detail. We do not know

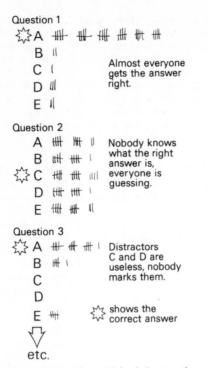

Question 1

Almost everyone gets the answer right.

Question 2

Nobody knows what the right answer is, everyone is guessing.

Question 3

Distractors C and D are useless, nobody marks them.

shows the correct answer

etc.

Fig. 3–6 Analyse the multiple-choice questions

which questions are easy and which are difficult, and for which kind of students. We do not know which are the best questions for distinguishing the good students from bad ones. Also, there may be some wrong answers which all students know are wrong, and which are therefore not useful. We can only find out these things for large numbers of questions by using a computer. Arrangements are being made for the computer analysis of question papers from representative groups of students. If you would like your students or workers to participate in this scheme please write to us. It is probably going to be possible to design special answer-sheets which are visually self-correcting, and can be read automatically.

3.8. The clinic game

Each of the questions in the SICK CHILDREN

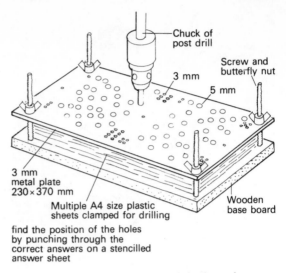

find the position of the holes by punching through the correct answers on a stencilled answer sheet

Fig. 3–7 The mass production of plastic overlays

instruments is made from a child's case-history. You can use these histories to play a game.

THE CLINIC GAME
Choose some multiple-choice questions from the SICK CHILDREN instruments in Booklet C. Type them out and stencil them. Type onto one side of the paper only. Use the codes (Guide 3.4) to find the right answers to these questions. Dip a swab into alcoholic phenolphthalein and smear it over the letter A, or B, or C, etc. of the right answer. Cut up the sheets and, where necessary, clip the pieces together, so that all the questions about each child are together. Each piece of paper is a 'child'. Allow about ten 'children' for each pair of students.

Arrange the class in pairs. On a table put a pile of 'children' (questions with the right answers invisibly marked with phenolphthalein). These are the children waiting to be seen in a clinic. Ask one member of each pair to go to the clinic and collect a 'child', from the *top* of the pile. Let the pair discuss him, and use the alkaline ink to answer the questions about him. The game can be played manual open or manual shut. Students usually take about five minutes for each question.

Give one mark for each right answer. Subtract one or two marks for each wrong answer. The pair getting the most marks wins.

4 Some more instruments for evaluation

'Evaluation is not just research or study, but a necessary component of good service, so those who are too busy to evaluate, must be too busy to do good service. An unevaluated service is a poor service.'

G.W. Steuart.

4.1. Births and deaths

If births and deaths are recorded for your district, use this information. If they have to be reported to the chief or headman, ask his clerk to report them to a clinic. You may be able to work out the birth rate (births per year per 1000 people) or infant mortality rate (deaths in the first year of life per 1000 live births), or other rates. Try to find the age of each dead child, and his symptoms. Even if deaths are not reported, try to find out about them. Most child deaths are preventable, especially those from severe dehydration, or diseases we can immunize against. So, if a child dies, try to prevent other deaths from the same disease.

4.2. Surveys

Surveys are the only way we can obtain some kinds of data on health and disease in children. They need more time and transport than most readers will have, so we will not say more about them, except about the weight-chart survey in the next section. *Some* of the things you *may* be able to survey are—weight for age, arm circumference, haemoglobin, the length of breast feeding, the percentage of children breast- or bottle-fed, the birth interval, and the percentage of children immunized.

Surveys to answer such questions as 'What do mothers know about diarrhoea?' are difficult to do well. Questions must be carefully chosen, asked in exactly the same way each time, and tried out before they are used.

If you do a simple survey, here are a *few* of the points to remember—

INSTRUMENT—SIMPLE SURVEYS
Ask the permission of the village leader first.
Give each house an equal chance to be visited. Go from one house to the house closest to it.
Collect a little data well.
Don't collect more data than you can analyse.
Survey enough children. Usually 100 children is the smallest useful sample.
If the survey has been well done, publish it somewhere.
Good survey data are valuable.

4.3. Coverage of care by weight-chart survey

We try to provide health care for *all* the children in our community. So we must look at our community and see who is getting it. The manual uses a rough measure of coverage—the average yearly visits per child under five. But this does not tell us if many children are coming only once, or a few children are coming many times. Also, it does not tell us how coverage decreases with the distance of a child's home from the clinic.

Fortunately, we can get another estimate of coverage by doing a simple survey. We can go from house to house to find out what percentage of children have a weight chart. These are the children who are covered by the clinic servics. Attendance at a health unit decreases logarithmically with the distance of a patient's home from a clinic [6]. The children who live near a clinic come to it much more often than those who live further away. When we plot this with a linear scale we get a curve like that in Graph A, Guide 4–1. When we plot it on a logarithmic scale in Graph B the curve becomes a straight line. If necessary, we can draw this line from two points only, although more are better. Try to get at least three. We can take one village close to the clinic and others up to five kilometres away. When we know the position and slope of the line, we can find out the percentage of children with weight charts at any distance from the clinic.

Unfortunately, our graph does not tell us the percentage of the children in the whole community who have weight charts. To find this out we need to know how many people live at each distance from the clinic. This information may be very difficult to get.

You will find that the percentage of children with weight charts decreases very rapidly the further they live from the clinic. In Guide 4–1 about 50 per cent of children close to the clinic had weight charts. Three kilometres away, only 5 per cent of them had charts.

When you do a weight chart survey you can record any other information on the weight charts you find, especially a child's immunizations. This is necessary for the immunization targets.

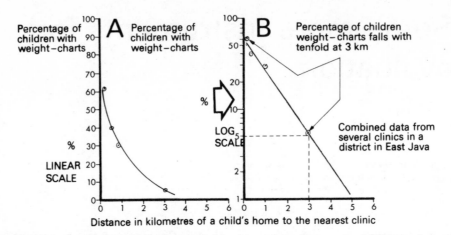

Fig. 4–1 The relationship between the possession of a weight-chart and the distance of a child's home from the clinic

INSTRUMENT—COVERAGE BY WEIGHT CHARTS

Start with the houses closest to the clinic and move outwards. Go from one house to the house closest to it. By doing this you will go to houses at random with the minimum of bias (unfair choice). At each house ask to see the children's weight charts. Make a tally of all the children under five who have weight charts. Make another tally of the children without weight charts. Tally any other data you want to collect, such as children's immunizations.

Do the same thing at a village one to five kilmetres away. Choose a place less than half way to the next clinic. Try to count at least 100 children in each place. If possible, survey a third village.

Work out the percentage of children with weight charts near the clinic and at your chosen village.

Plot your points on logarithmic paper, or plot them on Guide 4–1. In your district, how does the distance of a child's home from a clinic influence coverage, as shown by the possession of a weight chart?

DIFFICULTIES. There are many of these. This instrument assumes that all children at a particular distance from a clinic have an equal chance of going to it. Charts may have been given for a short time to some children only. Charts may have been out of stock sometimes in the past. Some weights may be written on cards of another kind and not charted. Mothers' clubs may be weighing children in the villages.

HOUSE TO HOUSE VISITING HELPS YOU TO KNOW YOUR COMMUNITY

4.4. Observation in the clinic

We do not need a special instrument to measure every target. We can measure many of them by simple observation. For example, one of the targets is 'Workers treat pyogenic infection with an adequate dose of antibiotics lasting not less than three days.' We can only see if workers reach this target by observing what they do in a clinic. Most of these targets are carefully defined. For example, the manual tells us what an 'adequate' dose of an antibiotic is. These targets which we measure by simple observation in a clinic are both easy and valuable. Some targets are much less carefully defined. For example, one of the targets only says that 'The community diagnosis of malnutrition is made and recorded'. We do not try to measure if this is done well or badly.

4.5. Skills check-lists

We can use a check-list to measure a worker's skill in doing things such as counting a child's respirations or measuring his temperature, etc. There are 48 check-lists in Booklet B. They are mostly for use in training schools.

INSTRUMENT—EXAMPLE OF A SKILLS CHECK-LIST, Booklet B

Workers able to—

—resuscitate a new born baby, **Manual 26.3** *(Hands washed*, clock looked at, baby held head downwards, sucked out, 'Your baby does not breathe', cord clamped, and cut quickly, baby's head bent backwards, worker blows gently from his cheeks, 40 times a minute, worker's mouth over baby's nose and mouth, worker does NOT blow from his lungs, oxygen tube in worker's mouth, oxygen tube left in baby's nose—13 points)

'Hands washed' has been put into many of the check-lists to emphasize its importance. If you are not sure what is meant by one of the phrases between commas, for example, ... baby's head bent backwards ..., look in the manual.

SCORING FOR SKILLS

Tick off the check-list in pencil, either as it is, or typed out on another sheet of paper.

Except for phrases with NOT in them, and phrases in quotes, count one point for each phrase between commas. In the example above there are 13 of these phrases, so there are 13 points for this skill.

Some instruments start with 'procedure explained'. Score this positive if a worker says anything to a child or his mother about what he is going to do, or says any kind words to the child.

A worker scores no points (1) if he disobeys a NOT phrase, or (2) if he leaves out an italic item (Hands washed, ...).

Phrases in quotes, such as, ' ... your baby does not breathe, ...' are instructions from you to the worker. They tell him what has happened or what to do. Don't count these phrases in quotes for points.

Test workers for several skills and add up the points they get. We suggest 80 per cent, as a pass mark (Experimental).

We can use these skills instruments in several ways.

One. We can evaluate workers who undertake these tasks during their work.

Two. We can ask a worker in a clinic to show us how some task should be done while we score for it using one of these check-lists.

Three. We can simulate the real-life situation in a classroom and use these check-lists to evaluate students. For this we need a co-operative child, or a doll, or sometimes another student.

Four. Students can use the check-lists to teach and evaluate one another in a 'skills lab', as described in Guide 6.6. This is why the check-lists are in Booklet B.

We can use the first and second ways to make a service diagnosis and as management targets.

These skills check-lists have their limits. Unfortunately, we can only check for what we can observe. For example, we cannot check that a worker is observing if a child is 'well' or 'ill'. If a task is very simple, such as making a child vomit by putting a spatula down his throat, or very complex, such as lumbar puncture, a check-list becomes meaningless. Some skills can be simulated in class much more easily than others. For example, students in a skills lab can simulate examining for meningeal signs more easily than they can simulate sewing up a cut. For these, and other reasons, we cannot make a check-list for every skill. Booklet B contains the check-lists which we hope will be practical either in the clinic or in the classroom, or both.

MAKING YOUR OWN SKILLS CHECK-LISTS

Describe the skill in detail. Make sure it contains everything you want the worker to do. Follow the bold type style of the manual, and use the imperative. (Hold ...', not, 'The worker should hold ...', etc.). Underline all the things you can see the worker doing, and thus check for objectively. Make a skills check-list from these (Experimental).

4.6. Using a 'Caring for ...' section

There is a 'Caring for ...' section or algorithm at the end of most chapters in the manual from Chapter 7 onwards. If a worker or student can use one of these sections correctly, he can probably use the others correctly also, so we only need test for one of them. Unfortunately, there is no objective way of finding out if a worker makes the right diagnosis. However, if he can use one of these sections and gets good marks with the multiple-choice instruments, he will probably make the right diagnosis.

INSTRUMENT—USING A 'CARING FOR . . .' SECTION

Choose a child with a symptom which has one of the longer 'Caring for . . .' sections. Let the worker ask the mother what the child's symptoms are, then look them up in the manual. He must find the right 'Caring for ...' section in the manual and then go through all its steps, as far as the diagnosis. When the diagnosis is reached he should turn to the correct section on treatment and follow the steps there also. He can be observed to follow some steps, but not others. For example, we can observe him feeling a child's cervical glands, but not when he looks to see if a child's eyes are sunken. Give one point for each step that can be observed to be done correctly. A worker who gets more than 80 per cent does well (Experimental).

4.7. Attitudes to breast- and bottle-feeding

The instrument BREAST- AND BOTTLE-FEEDING is the only one which is first a measure of attitudes, and second, a measure of knowledge. It provides a way of measuring the attitudes of the workers, and a way of improving them through discussion afterwards. There is no target score with this instrument, because to make a target would defeat its purpose.

INSTRUMENT—BREAST- AND BOTTLE-FEEDING. Booklet A.

Apply this instrument early before workers have had time to read the manual and find out the attitude taken by the microplan to breast-feeding.

Give out Booklet A at a meeting and ask workers to turn to this instrument. Ask workers to take a pencil and paper and write '1' to '20' down the left hand side. Ask them to read the 20 statements in the instrument and to write 'Agree', 'No opinion', or 'Disagree' beside each. Don't let them know what opinion is expected of them. Discuss the questions with the class afterwards.

There are 20 questions. 'Disagree' in the first ten questions and 'agree' in the second ten questions shows an attitude favourable to breast-feeding. So the 'right' answer with this instrument is 'disagree' with the first ten, and 'agree' with the second ten questions.

4.8. Dots on the growth curve

Mothers are good judges of the quality of care in a clinic. They come often if it is good and seldom if it is bad. We can measure how often mothers bring their children to a clinic by making a tally of the numbers of dots on children's weight-charts.

INSTRUMENT—DOTS ON THE GROWTH CURVE

Ask workers to make a tally of the number of dots on the weight-charts of the children who come to their clinic.

The tally should look like Guide 4–2B not Guide 4–2A. Two years or more after the introduction of the weight chart there should be an average of at least six dots per child.

done to encourage mothers to feed their children more often and give them better meals. Unless mothers do this, they cannot break the vicious circle of malnutrition and infection. Often, the most practicable advice to them is, 'Feed him more often'. The answer, 'Oh, he won't eat' will not do. He *must* be made to eat. Workers must do all they possibly can to encourage mothers to get more food into anorexic children with flat growth curves. This is the only way to make them grow.

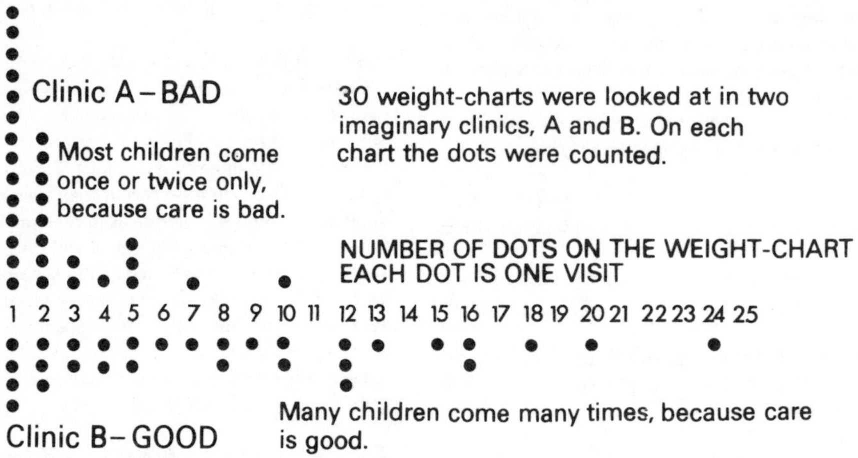

Clinic A – BAD

Most children come once or twice only, because care is bad.

30 weight-charts were looked at in two imaginary clinics, A and B. On each chart the dots were counted.

NUMBER OF DOTS ON THE WEIGHT-CHART
EACH DOT IS ONE VISIT

1 2 3 4 5 6 7 8 9 10 11 12 13 14 15 16 17 18 19 20 21 22 23 24 25

Many children come many times, because care is good.

Clinic B – GOOD

Fig. 4–2 Dots on the growth curve

4.9. On and off the road to health

The children's tally (Manual 6–4) records the percentage of children who have gained weight since they last came to the clinic. A high percentage gaining weight is a very important target. Another target is to try to keep as many children as possible on the 'road to health' (Manual 7.2). They must not lose weight and 'fall off' it. If they fall off, they should gain weight and 'climb back' on to it again. 'Falling off' shows that we have failed. Keeping him on it, or helping him climb back after he has fallen off, shows that we have succeeded. We can define and measure both 'falling off' and 'climbing back'.

INSTRUMENT—ON AND OFF THE ROAD TO HEALTH

'Falling off' is two dots above the 'lower line' (Manual 7.1) followed by two dots below it.

'Climbing back' is two dots below the lower line followed by two dots above it.

Dots on the line don't count. Two dots are chosen rather than one because there is so much random error in weighing.

If most children stay on the 'road', and most children who have fallen off it climb back, the clinic is doing well (Experimental).

In some communities many children fall off the road to health and stay off it. They may come to the clinic and have their weight charted, and there may be enough food in the community. But no *effective* health education is

4.10. How well is the weight-chart used?

Workers can use weight-charts well or not so well. This instrument is a simple tally for the items that should be seen on a weight-chart if it is being used well.

INSTRUMENT—WEIGHT-CHART SCORE

Type out the items in the list below as a column down the left-hand side of a page. Visit a clinic, take 25 or 50 weight charts and make a tally for each item. The maximum is eleven points.

Inside the chart. Any record of—an illness; a family event, such as the birth of brother or sister; family planning; drugs given; malaria suppression; vitamin A given; or a food supplement. Is the birth month in every thick-lined box? Is the calendar filled in completely?

Outside the chart. Any record of—a child's name; his address; his brothers or sisters; or his father's work.

Immunization is not scored because this is another target (2.5).

An average score above 7 items per weight chart shows that weight charts are being used well (Experimental).

4.11. What do mothers know about the weight-chart?

Weight charts should help mothers to understand the growth of their children. They should also know several other things about weight charts. We can measure what they know. Here are some suggestions.

INSTRUMENT—WHAT DO MOTHERS KNOW ABOUT WEIGHT-CHARTS?

(1) Take two weight charts. On Chart A, draw the growth curve of a child going along the road to health. On Chart B copy out Manual 7:7b. Ask mothers which chart they would like their children to have. At least 90 per cent of them should choose A.

(2) Do mothers understand that they should go on breast-feeding their child until his growth curve has reached the level of the breast-feeding picture on his weight chart?

(3) What does the porridge picture show? (Experimental).

4.12. How much have mothers learnt?

One of the most important parts of a mother's visit to a clinic is what she learns from it. We can measure this by asking her.

INSTRUMENT—HOW MUCH HAVE MOTHERS LEARNT?

1. Question ten mothers leaving a clinic and ask them what they have learnt. If most of them have learnt something, care is good.

2. Ask a mother after she has been to a clinic—What do you know about the drugs you have been given? What are you going to do with them? At the same time ask the same questions to the health worker who saw the child. If the health worker and the mother give good answers, care is very good.

4.13. Questions about the presenting symptoms

If a worker is going to diagnose and manage a child correctly he must ask the right questions about the presenting symptoms. Often no questions are asked. This instrument is simpler than the next one.

INSTRUMENT—QUESTIONS ABOUT PRESENTING SYMPTOMS

Listen to a worker caring for children. Make a tally of the number of questions asked about presenting symptoms. For example 'How long has his cough lasted?' 'What do his stools look like?'

More than three questions per child shows good quality care (Experimental).

4.14. Fifteen points on a child's visit

History-taking and examination are difficult to evaluate, because each child has a different history and needs a different examination. It is not practical to make separate score-sheets for every common symptom or combination of symptoms. This instrument overcomes this difficulty by scoring for 15 important things most of which should happen to most children on their first visit to a health worker.

INSTRUMENT—15 POINTS ON A CHILD'S FIRST VISIT

(1) Any questions asked about previous illnesses?
(2) Any questions asked about previous treatment?
(3) Any questions asked about other members of the family?
(4) Duration of symptoms asked about?
(5) Child examined naked?
(6) Lips or conjunctivae examined for anaemia?
(7) Throat examined with spatula and torch?
(8) Ears examined?
(9) Anything said about food or feeding?
(10) Any mention of immunization?
(11) Any explanation given about anything?
(12) Anything said about family planning?
(13) Was the child's mother praised for something?
(14) Was she told when to return?
(15) Mother asked if she had any questions to ask?

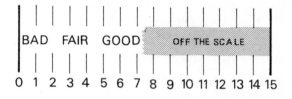

Fig. 4–3 Fifteen points on a child's first visit

Points 10 to 15 are required by almost all children, well or sick. Points 7 and 8, are required by all 'ill' children with fever. Points 5 and 6 are part of any good examination. Points 1, 2, and 3 apply to most children, well or sick. Family planning (point 12) is not commonly thought of as being part of child care. But we should make full use of every possible opportunity to promote it.

Most items apply to all children on their first visit, whether they are well or sick. The only items which do not apply to well children are items 4, 7, and 8. So we can use this instrument for both well and sick children at their first visit. It does not apply to children coming for follow-up visits, since they usually need only a few of the items it contains.

We do not expect average scores of 15 points for a child to be having 'good care'. Good care is shown by a score of five or six. Some workers have an average score of less than one, which certainly shows very bad care.

This is a simple, rough, quick instrument that is useful for measuring quality of care at its lowest levels on a child's first visit. Other points could be used. You might like to use instead 'Anything said about a child's milestones?' or, where this is culturally appropriate, 'Mother or child spoken to by name?' One of the disadvantages of this instrument is that workers can change their practice if they know what they are being observed for.

You can use this instrument yourself and make a tally for each point you are observing, or you can train observers to do a quick survey. If you train observers you will have to define exactly what is meant by point 11, for example, 'Was there any mention of immunization?' Is it to include looking at a child's immunizations on his weight chart? You can decide these things in any way you like, and we will not discuss them further. You must however decide on them before you train workers and do a survey. If you train observers you will find role play very useful. If 15 points is too many for an observer to look for, shorten the instrument to 10 points.

4.15. New diagnoses

Manual 6.1 advises that few records be kept, and that diagnoses should not be recorded. However, if diagnoses are recorded, you can use them to see if workers make new diagnoses after you have implemented the microplan. If the microplan has improved the knowledge and skills of the workers, they should make new diagnoses that they did not make before. Their diagnoses may not be right, but new diagnoses show that they are thinking about new diseases.

INSTRUMENT—NEW DIAGNOSES

If workers do not record diagnoses routinely, ask them to record them for a short period. This will tell you what diagnoses they make.

BEFORE. Examine the record books from before the introduction of the microplan. Make a tally of several hundred diagnoses. Don't bother to make a separate category of each of the more common 'diagnoses', such as 'cough', 'hotness of the body', or 'sores'. Group all these together. Make separate categories for the less common diagnoses only.

AFTER. Do the same thing after the introduction of the microplan. There should be new diagnoses derived from the manual.

There will be many diagnoses that are common to BEFORE and AFTER. There will be some that are in BEFORE and not in AFTER and the other way round. If the microplan has been successful in helping the workers to make new diagnoses there should be more kinds of diagnoses in AFTER than in BEFORE. Since the new kinds of diagnoses may be rare you will need to tally many diagnoses—several hundreds at least.

If it is not possible to make a tally in this way, even looking at the record books may show that new kinds of diagnosis are being made.

4.16. Changes in the way children are referred

The successful introduction of a microplan into a district should change the kind of cases that are referred to hospital and the way in which they are referred. This could be measured, but it is enough to ask the doctor in charge of the local hospital what changes he has noticed. One doctor observed that since the inplementation of the

microplan he no longer saw severely dehydrated children with abdominal swelling. This was because they were now being given glucose–salt solution instead of papaveretum (an opiate) and tea. The implementation of the microplan should cause cases of meningitis to be referred before they reach the stage of coma. It should also cause much better letters to be sent with the patients (Manual 5.22). Improvement will probably not be noticeable in less than a year.

4.17. A mother's average waiting time

A mother's time is valuable to her, so she should waste as little of it as possible waiting in a clinic. This instrument measures her approximate average waiting time. It is easier and more accurate if mothers know how long they have waited. If they don't know how long they have waited, use Method B.

INSTRUMENT—WAITING TIME

METHOD A, WHERE MOTHERS KNOW HOW LONG THEY HAVE WAITED

Each hour ask each worker to ask the first mother they see how long she has waited. For example, if the clinic opens at 7 a.m., the worker should ask the first mother seen at 7 a.m., 8 a.m., and 9 a.m. through to the end of the clinic.

Work out the average of these waiting times.

METHOD B, WHERE MOTHERS DON'T KNOW HOW LONG THEY HAVE WAITED

Ask a clerk to count the number of mothers waiting when the clinic opens at, say, 7 a.m. Ask which mother came first. Estimate how long she has been waiting. Halve this time. Multiply it by the number of mothers who were waiting when the clinic opened. This will tell you, approximately, the number of 'mother hours' waited *before* the clinic opened.

One hour later, say at 8 a.m., count the number of mothers again. This is the number of mother hours waited *since* the clinic opened at 7 a.m. Add this to the mother hours waited before the clinic opened.

Do the same thing each hour.

At the end of the clinic, say, there were 5 mothers waiting at 5 p.m., and the last mother went at 5.45 p.m. Multiply 5 mothers by 3/4 of an hour and divide by two. This equals 1.9 mother hours waited since 5 p.m. Add this to the sum of the mother hours waited so far.

Divide the total number of mother hours waited by the number of mothers who came to the clinic during the day. This is the average time each mother waited.

Do this each day for a week and average it.

If possible, a mother should not wait for more than one hour.

Usually the distribution of waiting time is 'peaked'. Mothers coming early wait a shorter time, and mothers coming late wait a shorter time. Mothers coming in the middle of the clinic wait the longest time. If your waiting curve is peaked, try to flatten it by asking some mothers to come earlier, and some later. The average waiting time is shorter when the curve is flat, and there is less difference between the longest and the shortest waiting times. Try to make the curve for your clinic as flat as possible. Make the average waiting time as short as possible. Are there workers who are specially busy and who could give tasks to workers who are less busy? Could work start earlier in the morning?

5 What do the instruments tell us?

5.1. These methods are easy

When we give some students a pretest we get a column of figures showing the marks for each student. When we give them a postest we get some more marks. The postest marks may look better, but we want to know if the students are really (significantly) better, or if they are only better by chance. How much better are they? We can easily find out. The methods we are going to show you are mostly for the multiple-choice instruments, but you can use them for some of the other instruments also. You need only know how to add, subtract, and divide, and understand decimals. You need some squared paper and a pencil and rubber. A simple calculator is useful, but not essential.

A LIST OF NAMES AND MARKS IS NOT ENOUGH

5.2. The chance-mark for multiple-choice instruments

Most multiple-choice questions have five answers (A, B, C, D, and E). Some questions have four answers. A few have three answers and some have only two answers. On average there are about 4·8 answers for each question. If someone who knows nothing about child care answers a multiple instrument, he has about one chance in 4·8 of getting a question right. If he does 25 questions, he gets an average of 25 divided by 4·8 = 5·2 questions right. So even a monkey would get about five questions right by chance! With these multiple-choice questions the 'no knowledge', or chance-mark for 25 questions is not 0, but about 5 marks. If a class of monkeys did the instrument, some unfortunate monkeys would get less than five questions right, and a few fortunate monkeys would get more than five questions right. The average monkey would get about five marks.

So a student who scores only 5 marks knows nothing. The scale for these multiple-choice instruments really runs from about 5 marks to 25 marks.

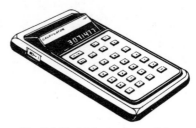

Fig. 5–1 Useful, but not essential

IN THE MULTIPLE-CHOICE INSTRUMENTS '5' IS '0'

5.3. Cumulative-number curves

We can take the mean ('average') mark, say, 18 marks, for a group of students. This is useful, but does not tell us if all our students got 18 marks, or if some students got 25 marks and others 5 marks. We can count how many students got less than 10, or more than 20 marks. This is useful. Even more useful is to draw cumulative-number curves.

You will already understand the histograms ('Pictures') A, C, E, and G on the left of Guide 5–2. The cumulative-number curves on the right of this figure are only these histograms drawn in another way. The cumulative number for a particular mark, *is the number of students who get that mark added to the number of students who get less than that mark.* Let us take Pictures E and F as an example. One student got 5 marks, 2 students got 10 marks, 5 got 15 marks, and 2 students got 20 marks. At 20 marks the cumulative number is $1 + 2 + 5 + 2 = 10$. Ten students got 20 marks or less. The cumulative-number curve is the line that joins up several cumulative numbers.

The multiple-choice instruments are out of 25 marks, so we write 0 to 25 along the bottom of each graph. We write the number of students up the side, say, 0 to 38 if there are 38 students in the class. In Guide 5–2 there are 10 students in each class, so we write 0 to 10 students up the side of each graph.

No student can get less than 0 marks, so the *cumulative-number curve always starts in the bottom-left-hand corner* of the graph. All students get 25 marks or less, *so the curve always ends in the top-right-hand corner.*

What does the cumulative number curve look like if all the students score 0? Picture A shows the histogram for this. All the students score 0, so the cumulative-number curve in Picture B goes up the left-hand edge of the graph and then along the top.

What does the cumulative-number curve look like if all the students score 25? Picture C shows the histogram for this, and Picture D the cumulative number curve for it. No student scores anything until we get to 25, so the curve stays along the bottom until we get to 25, and then it goes up the right-hand edge of the graph.

Curves B and D show the highest and lowest possible cumulative-number curves. What does the curve look like for ordinary middle range scores? Picture E shows the

scores of 10 students. One student got 5 marks, 2 got 10 marks, five got 15 marks, and 2 got 20 marks. Curve F shows that one student got 5 marks or less, 3 students got 10 marks or less, and 8 students got 15 marks or less. All 10 students got 20 marks or less.

Pictures G and H show the scores of two groups of 10 students. There are 10 'circle students' and 10 'triangle students'. You can see from Picture G that most triangle students score better than most circle students, but that some circles are better than some triangles. Picture H shows that the cumulative-number curves for the triangles and circles are widely separated—*the bigger the space between two cumulative-number curves the bigger the difference between the groups of students.* We can use this separation to find out if there is a significant (more than by chance) difference between two groups of students (Guide 5.4).

Picture B shows the worst possible cumulative-number curve. Picture D shows the best possible curve. Pictures F and H show curves in the middle, not very good or very bad. As *cumulative-number curves get better, they go from the top left to the bottom right in the direction shown by the arrow in Picture H.* If there are two cumulative-number curves in the same graph, you can easily see which is better unless they are very close together. You can also see how many students score less than 10 or more than 20 marks.

Comparing two groups of students of unequal size is sometimes easier if we change cumulative numbers into **cumulative percentages.** We can then use a scale from 0 to 100 per cent up the left-hand side of the graph.

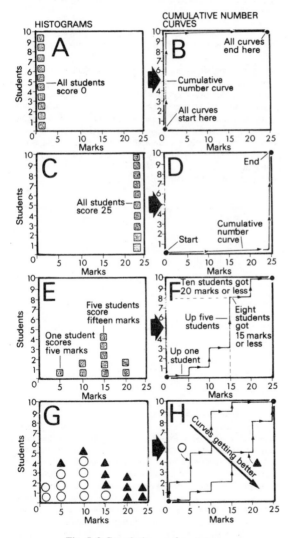

Fig. 5-2 Cumulative-number curves

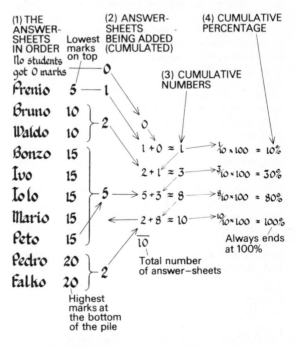

Fig. 5-3 Cumulative numbers and percentages

29

CUMULATIVE NUMBERS

Follow these steps in Guide 5–3.

(1) Correct the answer-sheets. Add up the total right answers on each sheet. Arrange the answer-sheets in order with the lowest score on top, and the highest score on the bottom of the pile.

(2) Count the number of sheets with each score. For example, in Guide 5–3 there is one student with five marks, two students with ten marks, five students with 15 marks, and two students with 20 marks. Write down the number of answer-sheets with each score.

(3) The number of students with the lowest score is your first cumulative number. Write it down. In Guide 5–3 nobody got zero marks. One student got 5 marks, so the first cumulative number is 1. Add this to the number of students with the next lowest score (2 students). This is your next cumulative number. Go on doing this down to the bottom of the pile.

(4) This is your list of cumulative numbers.

CUMULATIVE PERCENTAGES

(5) Count the total number of answer-sheets.

Divide each cumulative number (Step 4 above) by the total number of answer-sheets and (10 in Guide 5–3) multiply it by 100. This is the cumulative percentage.

PLOTTING CURVES FOR CUMULATIVE NUMBERS OR PERCENTAGES

Take a piece of graph paper, or use Guide 5–6.

Write the marks along the bottom from 0 to 25.

Write the number of students up the left-hand side.

What was the lowest mark? How many students got it? Say, no students got 0 marks and one student got 5 as in Picture F, Guide 5–2. Start at 0. Draw a line along the bottom from 0 to 5. Go up one student. Then go along to the next mark and then upwards again for the number of students (2 students) who got it. Do this until you have plotted all the marks. The line will end in the top-right-hand corner at the highest marks and the total number of students (or 100 per cent for cumulative percentages).

Remember, cumulative-number curves always start at the bottom-left-hand corner (0 marks, 0 students) and end at the top-right-hand corner (highest possible marks, total students). As we describe them here, they are always in steps, and are never sloping or rounded.

We can draw the average (mean) cumulative number curve for the class of monkeys described in Guide 5.2. This is the cumulative-number curve, or '0' curve, for students who know nothing. It is shown in Guide 5–5.

5.4. Is there a significant difference between the pretest and the postest?

Say, we gave the students the pretest multiple-choice instrument DIARRHOEA A, and we have the marks for this. The students studied the diarrhoea chapter over the weekend. Then the next week we gave them the postest, DIARRHOEA C. The marks for the postest are higher, but are they really (significantly) higher? Or are the

marks only higher by chance? We can easily find out. We can also use the same method to find out if the scores of two groups of workers are significantly different.

Before you begin, you must understand **proportions**. Proportions go from 0 to 1 in the same way that percentages go from 0 to 100 per cent. A proportion of 0·5 corresponds to 50 per cent.

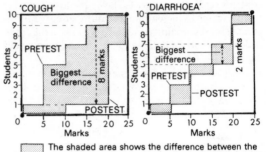

The shaded area shows the difference between the cumulative-number curves for the pretests and postests

Fig. 5–4 Cumulative number curves for pretests and postests—the biggest difference. Here are the cumulative-number curves for the pre- and postests for two chapters in the manual—'COUGH' and 'DIARRHOEA'. In 'COUGH' the pretest and postest curves are widely separated and the biggest difference is 8 marks. The proportion difference is 8 ÷ 10 = 0·8. For ten students in both groups the test number is 0.61, so the postest marks are significantly better. For 'DIARRHOEA' the proportion difference is 2 ÷ 10 = 0·2, so the postest marks are not significantly different

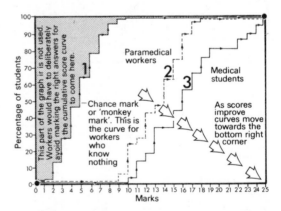

Fig. 5–5 Here are three cumulative score curves for one of the multiple-choice instruments—'MCQs EASY'. Curve 1 is the curve you would expect if workers knew nothing. It is the chance curve or 'monkey curve' (Guide 5.2). Curve 2 is from a group of 30 paramedical workers. Curve 3 is from a group of 21 medical students during their community medicine course. Only two of the students had done the paediatric part of the curriculum. The medical students look better, but the groups are small. Unfortunately there is no convenient graphical way to find out if the difference between unequal groups is significant. MCQs EASY contains some of the easiest and most important questions we could make, so these are not good scores.

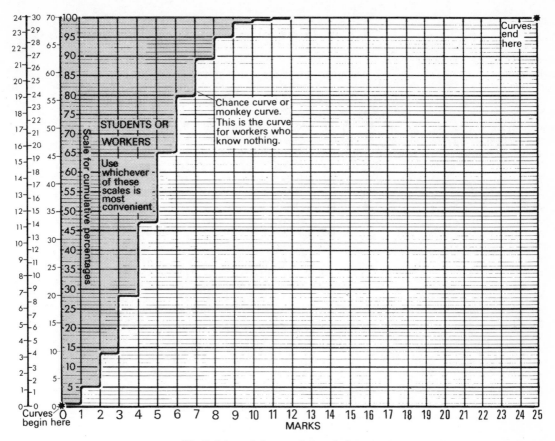

Fig. 5-6 A graph for cumulative number curves

The first thing we do is to calculate the cumulative numbers for the pretest and the postest. Then we draw the cumulative number curves for the pretest and the postest on the same piece of paper. We measure the biggest difference in students between the two curves. We then divide the biggest difference by the total number of students in the class. This gives us a number called the **proportion difference.** If the proportion difference is *bigger* than the **test number** in Table 5:1, the pretest and the postest marks are significantly different. If the proportion difference is *smaller* than the test number, the pretest and the postest marks are not significantly different. We will not explain the test numbers in Table 5:1 any more, except to say that they are a way of making the calculation easier.

SIGNIFICANT DIFFERENCE BY DRAWING— NUMBERS OF STUDENTS EQUAL CUMULATIVE NUMBERS

(1) Draw the cumulative-number curves for the pretest and the postest on same piece of squared paper.

(2) Find the biggest difference in students (or workers) vertically between the two curves.

(3) Divide the biggest difference by the total number of students. This will give you the proportion difference. For 'COUGH' in Guide 5–4 it is 8 divided by 10 = 0.8. To find the test number in Table 5:1 you must know the numbers of students or workers in each group (or in pretest and postest). In this example there are 10 students in both the pre- and postest, so the test number is 0.61.

In our example the proportion difference, 0.8, is bigger than the test number, 0.61 so the pre- and postests are significantly different.

CUMULATIVE PERCENTAGES

Draw cumulative percentage curves. Find the biggest percentage difference between the two curves, say, 20 per cent. Change this back into students by multiplying it by the total number of students, say, 30, and dividing by 100. 20 × 30 divided by 100 = 6 students. This is the biggest difference in Step (2) above. Go to Step 3 above.

THIS IS A VERY EASY METHOD— TRY IT!

31

TABLE 5.1

The test number

Number in second group	Number of workers in first group																			
	5	**10**	**15**	**20**	**25**	**30**	**35**	**40**	**45**	**50**	**55**	**60**	**65**	**70**	**75**	**80**	**85**	**90**	**95**	**100**
5	0·86	0·74	0·70	0·68	0·67	0·66	0·65	0·65	0·64	0·64	0·63	0·63	0·63	0·63	0·63	0·63	0·63	0·62	0·62	0·62
10		0·61	0·55	0·53	0·51	0·50	0·49	0·49	0·48	0·47	0·47	0·46	0·46	0·46	0·46	0·46	0·45	0·45	0·45	0·45
15			0·50	0·46	0·44	0·43	0·42	0·41	0·41	0·40	0·40	0·39	0·39	0·39	0·38	0·38	0·38	0·38	0·38	0·38
20				0·43	0·41	0·39	0·38	0·37	0·37	0·36	0·36	0·35	0·35	0·34	0·34	0·34	0·34	0·34	0·33	0·33
25					0·38	0·37	0·36	0·35	0·34	0·33	0·33	0·32	0·32	0·32	0·31	0·31	0·31	0·31	0·31	0·30
30						0·35	0·34	0·33	0·32	0·31	0·31	0·30	0·30	0·30	0·29	0·29	0·29	0·29	0·28	0·28
35							0·33	0·31	0·31	0·30	0·29	0·29	0·29	0·28	0·28	0·28	0·27	0·27	0·27	0·27
40								0·30	0·30	0·29	0·28	0·28	0·27	0·27	0·27	0·26	0·26	0·26	0·26	0·25
45									0·29	0·28	0·27	0·27	0·26	0·26	0·26	0·25	0·25	0·25	0·25	0·24
50										0·27	0·27	0·26	0·26	0·25	0·25	0·25	0·24	0·24	0·24	0·24
55											0·26	0·25	0·25	0·25	0·24	0·24	0·24	0·23	0·23	0·23
60												0·25	0·24	0·24	0·24	0·23	0·23	0·23	0·22	0·22
65													0·24	0·23	0·23	0·23	0·22	0·22	0·22	0·22
70														0·23	0·23	0·22	0·22	0·22	0·21	0·21
75															0·22	0·22	0·22	0·21	0·21	0·21
80																0·22	0·21	0·21	0·21	0·20
85																	0·21	0·21	0·20	0·20
90																		0·20	0·20	0·20
95																			0·20	0·19
100																				0·19

If you do not want to draw cumulative score curves, you can calculate the biggest difference like this.

SIGNIFICANT DIFFERENCE BY CALCULATION—NUMBERS OF STUDENTS EQUAL

Calculate the cumulative numbers for the pre- and postests—see Guide 5.3.

Arrange these in order and subtract the pretest cumulative numbers from the postest cumulative numbers. Don't worry if the result is negative. Find the biggest difference and calculate the proportion difference as before.

EXAMPLE. Here are cumulative numbers for two groups of students, the 'circles' and the 'triangles' in Guide 5–2, Picture H.

Score in marks	0	5	10	15	20	25
Cumulative number of circle students	2	5	9	10	10	10
Cumulative number of triangle students	0	1	2	5	8	10
Difference in students	2	4	7	5	2	0

Number of students 10. Biggest difference 7 students.

Proportion difference = biggest difference divided by 10.

7 divided by 10 = 0·7.

In Table 5:1 the number for 10 students in both groups is 0·61. The proportion difference is greater than the number in the table, so the scores of the 'circles' and the 'triangles' are really different.

If the two groups are *not* equal, you can make both groups equal to the smaller group, choose the number in Table 5:1 from this, and use the method we have given above. For example, if there are 16 workers in one group and 15 in another, you can use the number in the table for only 15 workers. Better, you can use the numbers in both groups and calculate by the method below. Unfortunately, there is no easy way of finding the significant difference by drawing when groups are unequal.

SIGNIFICANT DIFFERENCE BY CALCULATION—NUMBERS OF STUDENTS DIFFERENT

For each group work out the cumulative numbers as before. Divide the cumulative number by the total number of workers. This gives the cumulative proportion. For example, 4 workers divided by a total of 14 workers gives a cumulative proportion of 0·29. Here are two districts as a further example.

EXAMPLE. District Sidoardjo, with a total of 14 workers.

Score in marks	6	8	11	16	20	22
Cumulative number of workers	4	7	9	10	12	14
Cumulative proportion	0·29	0·5	0·64	0·71	0·86	1·0

District Bangkalan, total 20 workers

Score in marks	6	7	8	12	16
Cumulative number of workers	3	8	12	16	20
Cumulative proportion	0·15	0·40	0·60	0·80	1·0

Now for each score find the difference between the cumulative proportions from the two districts.

Score	6	7	8	11	12	16	20	22 marks
Sidoardjo	0·29	0·29	0·55	0·64	0·64	0·71	0·85	1·0 proportion
Bangkalan	0·15	0·40	0·60	0·60	0·80	1·00	1·00	1·0 proportion
Difference	0·14	0·11	0·05	0·04	0·16	0·29	0·15	0·0 difference

Note that in Sidoardjo there are no workers with seven marks, so at seven marks, the cumulative proportion is still the same as it was at six marks. It was 0·29 at 6 marks, so 0·29 is the figure that we use for 7 marks also. There are several other 'gaps' which are filled in the same way. For example, there is no Bankalan figure for 11 marks, so we use the same figure (0·60) as for 8 marks.

The biggest difference is 0·29. Find the test number in the table. There is no test number in the table for groups of 20 and 14, but there is a test number for groups of 20 and 15, so we look for this. It is 0·46. The biggest difference (0·29) is less than the test number (0·46) so the workers in these two districts are *not* significantly different.

Note. This is the Kolmogorov–Smirnov or KS method [7]. It is non-parametric, that is it does not assume that the marks follow any regular distribution, such as the normal distribution. This is useful because the results with these instruments are often not normal and are heavily skewed. The KS test is however, less powerful than the commonly used parametric methods employing the standard deviation etc. That is there must be a bigger difference between two sets of scores before the KS test will declare it significant. The KS test is probably the only test which is sufficiently simple for the uses we describe.

The material for this chapter was kindly given to us by Dr Michael Luck of Aston University.

TEACH A CLERK TO ANALYSE THE MARKS

6 Learning and relearning primary child care

'To teach if we are called upon, to be taught if we are fortunate.'
Kurt Waldheim, U.N. Secretary
General, from his message on *Voyager I*

6.1. 'How can I teach all this; I don't know it myself?'

The microplan can be used to train new workers, or to retrain older ones. Most of this chapter describes the use of the microplan in training schools. Guide 6.7 describes retraining.

The first thought of many teachers on seeing the workers' manual will be that they don't know it themselves. To which we answer—Don't worry, the manual and the test instruments are designed for the student to teach himself. The microplan is a modern approach to primary child care and we expect that many things in it will be new to many teachers. *Learn the manual with your students.*

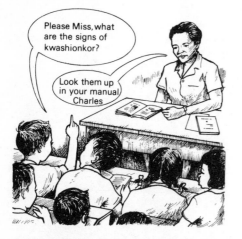

Fig. 6-1 Don't be ashamed if you do not know the answer

'It is not in the curriculum', or 'There is not room in the curriculum', some readers will say. To which the answer is that, if the students are later going to have to care for children without a doctor to refer to, there is nothing more important for them to know than the contents of the workers' manual. Somehow time must be found for it. If, for example, there is too much anatomy in the curricu-

lum, remove it to find time for primary child care. When curricula are planned on a national scale they can incorporate this microplan, and any other relevant ones that may subsequently become available. Microplans should determine the curricula, not vice versa.

The purpose of the microplan is to improve the competence of all students who are being trained to provide primary child care. It should be particularly useful to medical assistants and registered nurses. It should also be useful to enrolled nurses, particularly enrolled community nurses. Some of them may however find its language difficult.

Teaching the microplan may be difficult in schools where the things students read about and see done differ widely, and where authority may not favour them. Teachers facing this difficulty have our sympathies.

MICROPLANS SHOULD DETERMINE THE CURRICULA, NOT THE OTHER WAY ROUND

6.2. The educational objectives of the microplan

Our educational objectives tell us what a worker should know or be able to do at the end of his training. For example, 'The worker must be able to put up a nasogastric drip.' These objectives must be relevant (the task he is to do must be one that the health service requires), they must be behaviourally defined (they must be described in terms of what we can see a worker doing), and we must be able to measure them. If we are going to measure them, we must define them completely. For example, it is not enough to say that 'he must be able to describe acute inflammation'. We must also say exactly what he is to describe about it. If we do this, we repeat what is in the workers' manual.

Fortunately, a microplan makes a separate detailed list of educational objectives largely unnecessary. Everything that a worker needs to do or know about child care is defined in detail in the workers' manual. This contains nothing unnecessary, so the 'knowing' (cognitive) objectives of the microplan are, ideally, to know the whole manual. If there is not enough time for this, he should know its most important parts. We can find out if a student has reached these objectives by testing him with the multiple-choice instruments. Even more important, he must be able to look up what he does not know. We can easily measure if he reached this objective. We can see if he gets good scores with the SICK CHILDREN instruments with his manual open. The 'doing' (psychomotor) objectives of the microplan are to be able to do everything in it. Unfortunately, we can only do this in part. Booklet B contains check-lists for all the skills we can easily measure.

When the course starts discuss its objectives with the students. Explain which chapters you will cover and what the pass levels are. Tell them which skills they must learn. Let them fill in their scores for the multiple-choice instruments on the page provided at the end of the manual. Ask them to keep a record of their scores with the check-lists.

DISCUSS THE COURSE OBJECTIVES WITH THE STUDENTS

6.3. Using the test instruments

Cutting up copies of the Guide. This book is made so that it can be cut up and the three booklets separated from it. This wastes the first part of the book, but this is quite small. If possible, have three booklets (from one guide) for use by each student or worker. If necessary, and this is not so good, one guide can be split between three students, so that they have one booklet at a time and exchange it with one another. Cut the guide with a knife between the coloured pages separating the booklets. Staple the pages in the booklets to hold them together. If possible, make them a strong cover. Keep these booklets for use in next year's class. *If you only have one copy of this guide, you can cut the booklets into groups of two or three pages, or even single pages, and distribute these among the class.*

Can they use the manual? Students and workers must be able to do two things. First, they must be able to read and understand the manual. Secondly, they must be able to use the index and cross references, etc. We can measure how well they can do both these things. If workers can understand the manual, but are not good at using it, we can easily teach them. But if they cannot read it well enough, they will have to be taught to read. This is much more difficult.

There are several instruments to test reading ability, or the ability to use the manual, or both of them together. Do the following pretests when you first see the students. They will quickly tell you which the good students are, and if the class can use the manual.

Instrument—READING PRETEST (Booklet A). This is an example of a Cloze test [8]. *People who can read a piece of text easily can guess words that are missing.* If we measure how good they are at guessing missing words, we know how good they are at reading. In a Cloze test a few paragraphs from a book are written out with every seventh word missing (or some other multiple). If a worker can guess more than 50 per cent of the missing words he can easily understand the book. If he can guess between 36 per cent and 50 per cent of them he will only be able to understand it with difficulty. But if he can only guess less than 36 per cent of the words, he cannot understand the book without help. He may however be able to understand some words in it. This READING PRETEST is useful for deciding how well a group of workers can read the manual. It will also tell you which of your workers cannot read the manual well enough. The READING PRETEST is *not* intended to be a test of knowledge. So *the reader need not have read the test paragraphs in the manual before he does it.* Cloze tests like this are easy and objective. You can make them for other books by typing out a few paragraphs with every seventh word missing. You can also use a READING PRETEST to help choose trainees who can read.

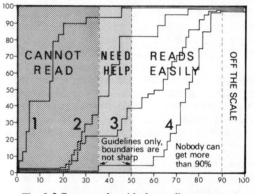

Fig. 6–2 Some results with the reading pretest.

All cumulative score curves are from Cloze tests with Sections 9.1 and 9.2 of the Indonesian experimental edition of the workers' manual. Each curve shows one group of workers only and similar results may not be found elsewhere.
  1. Trainee community health workers, Surabaya.
  2. Auxiliaries (PKE) in service in East Java.
  3. Paramedical workers (Bidans and PKC), East Java.
  4. Medical students, Surabaya.
The increasing reading skills of successive groups of workers is well seen. The community health workers are almost completely illiterate and cannot use the manual. Almost all the medical students read it easily.

The READING PRETEST contains 50 missing words. So count the right answers and double them to get the percentage right. Count only the words which are exactly right. It is taken from Section 9.1 of the manual.

These are the right answers—1 from, 2 in, 3 If, 4 few, 5 of, 6 Section, 7 stools, 8 sometimes, 9 stools, 10 passes, 11 Sometimes, 12 diarrhoea, 13 green, 14 passed, 15 does, 16 Diarrhoea, 17 malnutrition, 18 often, 19 cause, 20 are, 21 But, 22 can, 23 diarrhoea, 24 gut, 25 healthy, 26 on, 27 has, 28 the, 29 meets, 30 They, 31 the, 32 mother, 33 Some, 34 digesting, 35 the, 36 grows, 37 in, 38 in, 39 faeces, 40 can, 41 because, 42 to, 43 body, 44 he, 45 and, 46 micro-organisms, 47 harm, 48 children, 49 children, 50 every.

IF NECESSARY, TEACH THE STUDENTS HOW TO USE AN INDEX

DIFFICULT WORDS TESTS (Booklets A, B, and C). The READING PRETEST is useful for testing how well workers understand the manual, but it does not specifically measure how well they understand the more difficult words. We can do this with the DIFFICULT WORDS PRETESTS A, B, and C. These tests are also useful for teaching the vocabulary. So if your students do not know the vocabulary, test and teach them again and again, until they do know it.

MATHS PRETEST (Booklet A). The manual contains tables to make doses easy (Manual 3–12 to 3–17). But some simple maths is often necessary. This pretest measures if a worker can do the maths that the microplan needs. It also measures if he can use the scales on syringes, thermometers, and balances, etc. The questions vary, and some are more difficult, such as doses calculated from mg/kg/day. Because such calculations are too difficult for most primary care workers, it is fortunate that they are seldom necessary. Because the questions vary, analyse them carefully by the method in Guide 3–6. What kinds of calculations can your workers do?

MANUAL POSTEST (Booklet C). Some workers can understand the workers' manual but cannot use it because they cannot use an index, or find the references. The instructions for using it are described in Section 1.4 of the manual and again at the beginning of the index. Teach workers how to use the manual, and then test them with this instrument a few days later.

THE MANUAL POSTEST IS THE MOST IMPORTANT INSTRUMENT

SICK CHILDREN INSTRUMENTS (Booklet B). Health workers should be able to look up something in a manual. We can easily measure how well they can do this by using multiple-choice questions which are done with an open manual. You can use any of the SICK CHILDREN instruments to measure this. With an open manual most people with a university education, but without any medical training, get about 90 per cent of these questions right, taking about three minutes for each of them. Junior workers take much longer. If students get good scores with the SICK CHILDREN instruments, the following instruments will not be necessary—the READING PRETEST, the DIFFICULT WORDS PRETEST, and many of the questions in the MANUAL POSTEST.

IF THE MANUAL IS TOO LONG, USE THE PARTS YOU WANT

6.4. Learning the microplan in a training school

Start by explaining how to use the manual. This will take at least an hour. A complete course on the microplan will probably take about six months at the rate of a chapter a week. The longer chapters will take more than a week, whereas two of the shorter ones might be done in the same week. Go through the manual following the chapters in the order given in Manual 1.4—'How to learn.' This lists the more important chapters. Do these thoroughly. Don't worry if you don't reach the end of the manual. If each student owns a manual and can use it, you have achieved your major educational objective. If the students have some secondary education, 20 hours teaching will probably be enough to make them thoroughly familiar with the use of the manual, and its more important chapters.

TEACH THE STUDENTS TO TEACH THEMSELVES

Each student must have his own copy of the manual and take it away with him at the end of the course. They must be taught to use it, because most students will not learn how to use it by themselves. If the students are going to learn efficiently the school must have one set of test booklets A, B, and C for each student. *Cut these from extra copies of this guide.* Staple the cut pages. Keep the A and C booklets yourself for the pretests and postests. Give them out at the beginning of a lesson and collect them at the end. Give one Booklet B to each student—to keep during the course only. Ask students to sign for them. Collect all these B booklets at the end of the course and give them out again next year. These booklets save the need for much photocopying, typing, and stencilling. All tests are answered, either on the special answer-sheets, or on ordinary paper, so there is no need for students to write on the booklets. If they are looked after carefully they can be used again many times.

ONE STUDENT ONE MANUAL

At the beginning of the course do the READING and MATHS PRETESTS to find out how well the students can read their manuals, and if they know enough maths to work out doses.

Do the MANUAL POSTEST early, soon after you have taught the students how to use the manual. It is very useful for teaching students how to use the manual. Analyse the students' answers by the method in Guide 3.6. This will show you where they have difficulty.

At the end of the course do the OVERALL POSTEST and the postests for the WEIGHT CHART and the DOSES.

Make the best use of the SICK CHILDREN instruments. There are 18 of these. Tell the students to do them with their manual *open,* either alone or in pairs. Ask them to look for the *presenting symptoms* in each question, and then to find these in the index. Tell them to go from the index to the right section in the manual. Another way of doing the questions is to look up each answer in turn until you find the right one. This is much less like real life, so discourage the students from doing the questions this way.

Some students have never used an index, or even owned a book. When they start they may take a quarter of an hour over each question. To begin with, they will find the 'matching' questions difficult. If necessary, at the beginning of the course, ask all the students questions in class and let them all look up the answer in their manuals. Show them some questions on the overhead projector, and discuss these. Use some of the questions in the SICK CHILDREN instruments to play the 'clinic game' described in Guide 3.8.

LEARNING THE MICROPLAN IN CLASS

If the manual describes some diseases that the students will never see, such as vitamin A deficiency, for example, ask them to cross these diseases out. Go through the manual with them. Do the same with the multiple-choice questions. If possible insert new questions or new answers.

Choose a few objectives before each class and try to reach them. Try hard to prevent them teaching what is not relevant.

If doctors from outside the school come and teach, give them a manual and make sure they know what the objectives of the microplan are.

If class time is short, ask students to do most of the multiple-choice questions out of class. Use class time for discussing the answers.

If students have manuals don't copy the manual onto the blackboard. Don't teach them what they can easily look up.

Follow every multiple-choice instrument with time for discussion.

Don't discourage students with low scores—rising scores are what matter.

6.5. Learning the microplan in clinics

If possible, each training school should have a model health centre in which its students can work and learn.

Unfortunately, there are many schools where students qualify without having seen all the cases they should recognize later. Encourage students to see as many cases as they can. Clinics and out-patient departments are better than wards, because these contain the kind of cases the students will later have to care for. If, however, there are important cases in the wards, such as children with severe insuction, make sure all the students see them.

IF THERE ARE GOOD TEACHING CASES IN THE WARDS, LET ALL THE STUDENTS SEE THEM

LEARNING THE MICROPLAN IN CLINICS

Let one or two students sit with doctors or nurses examining children in a health centre or out-patient department. Don't send them out on their own unsupervised until late in their training. Especially don't let them learn bad habits from poorly trained workers.

Ask them to use some of the instruments in Chapter 4 of the Guide. Students can apply these instruments in pairs and report their results to the class.

CLINICS AND HOMES ARE THE BEST PLACE TO LEARN PRIMARY CARE

Because real-life experience may be so difficult to get, schools must use role play and simulation. Here is one example.

ROLE PLAY IN THE USE OF A 'CARING FOR ...' SECTION

Divide the class into pairs. Ask one student in each pair to choose a disease and to note down from his manual its signs and symptoms. He can play the part of the sick older child. Or he can be the mother of a sick child, the child himself being a model, a student, or imaginary. Tell another student to use his manual to question the 'mother' of the sick child, and find the right diagnosis and treatment.

6.6. Organizing a skills lab

If students are not going to practise their skills in a clinic, they need somewhere else to practise them. That place is called a 'skills lab'. It can be a special room, but it need only be a cupboard where the equipment can be kept.

The skills check-lists are described in Guide 4.5. Students can learn and practise many of these skills on themselves, on a model, or on a normal child if one can be persuaded to co-operate. Students can also act (simulate) the procedures using their imaginations to supply what is not in the class-room. When a student is imagining something, ask him to say what he is doing, for example, '... now I am putting a 1 cm length of ointment on to the child's lower lid ...'. When the skills check-list says

' ... the worker must be able to explain to a mother ...', ask one of the students to act the part of the mother. Often, the time between one event and the next will have to be imaginary. The real thing is much better than trying to imagine it, so provide the right equipment if possible. The special equipment for child care is listed in Table 3:2 of the manual. Every training school should have at least one complete set. Some extra bowls and trays, etc. will also be needed.

A SKILLS LAB

Use the skills instruments in Booklet B.

Get *all* the equipment necessary and put it in a special room or cupboard.

Explain to the students that they must practise these tasks on each other, either in class time, or in their own time. One student should do the task while another student uses the check-list. Tell them that they may be examined on any of these skills at their final examination.

Teach them to put back the equipment when they have finished.

6.7. Relearning

If we are going to improve the quality and coverage of our services we must retrain our workers, and ourselves. Fortunately, we can do both of these things at the same time. Much retraining is 'on the job', it is part of implementing the microplan in a health centre and is described in Guide 7.8. Here we describe retraining groups of workers.

Usually, very little time is available for retraining. Workers being retrained are older, less literate, and more experienced than students in training schools. They may have bad habits and have more 'face to save' than students. Their experience may have given them many questions they want answers for. Because time is so short, use it in the best possible way. There will only be time to reach a few very important educational objectives. Make *these objectives from the services diagnosis* (Guide 7.3). Are weight charts to be introduced in the district? If they are, teach about them. Are workers treating diarrhoea in the best way? If they are not, teach about it.

Here is an instrument called 'Group Teaching', which you can apply to yourself, or another person can apply to you. The most important point is the first one—to teach so as to *change* what workers do.

INSTRUMENT—GROUP TEACHING (Particularly for relearning)

Before the lesson did I make a short list of educational objectives based on the service diagnosis (Guide 7.3)—the things I wanted the workers to do (or not do) as the result of my teaching?

Did I make sure that the workers could use the manual (as shown by the MANUAL POSTEST) and so teach themselves?

Did I stress a few important points of practice? (Or spend too much time on unimportant anatomy, etc.?)

Did I stay inside the microplan where possible? (Or did I introduce much knowledge of my own to impress the workers with how much I knew?)

Did I let the workers make notes of new material only? (Or did I dictate what was already in the manual?)

Did I forget the rarities? (Or did I teach about niclosamide, when tapeworms are very rare in the district?)

Did I explain the material in the manual with local examples, local beliefs, etc.?

Did I spend too much time doing multiple-choice questions, which workers could have done in their own time?

Could everyone hear what I said?

Could everyone see what I wrote on the blackboard?

Did I look at the class while I was teaching, or did I look at the blackboard or the ceiling?

Did I use any teaching aids other than the blackboard, or do any demonstrations, or get workers to actually do things?

Did I have any irritating mannerisms while I was teaching?

Did I use any evaluation instruments to find out how successful I had been in teaching?

Did I talk for 20 minutes and leave plenty of time for answering questions? (Or did I talk for a whole hour?)

START BY MAKING YOUR EDUCATIONAL OBJECTIVES FROM THE SERVICE DIAGNOSIS

---

7 Implementing the microplan

'There are no bad soldiers, there are only bad officers.'
Old army saying

7.1. Levels of implementation

Many people have a part to play in implementing this microplan and so *improving the quality and coverage of primary child care*. We hope that ministers of health will give it their blessing, and that sweepers in clinics, together with everyone in between, will play their part. It needs to be implemented at several levels—in a ministry of health, and through it in the regions, districts, and health centres.

In the previous chapter we described how a microplan can be used in training schools to form new workers. In this one we describe how it can be implemented in districts and health centres. We shall say little about the task of a ministry of health, or about the regions. The job of a ministry of health is to adapt the microplan to the country, to suggest national targets, such as, for example, to provide a weight chart for every child, to print enough manuals, to adapt and produce many sets of visual aids, to arrange the necessary finance, to make sure that the drugs and equipment in the microplan are available and match these in the government stores list (if there is one), and to arrange for the manufacture or import of everything necessary (Manual 3:1, 3:2). A ministry can also require that the microplan be used in *all* appropriate training schools and set minimum pass levels for the test instruments. The task of the regional headquarters is to hold a meeting to discuss the implementation of the microplan with district medical officers.

However even if there is no national, regional, or district programme, you can still implement the microplan in your health centre. It may not fit the country perfectly, and you may not be able to get all the equipment, but it may still be very useful.

The effect this microplan has on improving quality of care and coverage depends almost completely on ourselves as managers—how much *we* want to improve primary child care, and how hard *we* work. Like most sayings, the saying at the top of this page is only partly true—managers (officers) train and lead the workers (soldiers). If our workers are not good we must blame ourselves. If we want to, we can do something with this microplan. We can teach, lead, and encourage our workers to give better care. The most important of us are the doctors and senior nurses who are with the workers every day.

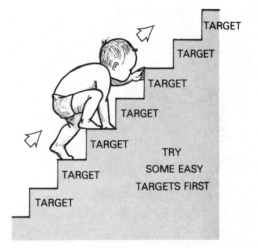

Fig. 7-1 Quality improves as each target is reached

**MANAGERS DETERMINE
THE QUALITY OF PRIMARY CARE**

7.2. A six-months implementation programme

At one extreme the implementation of a microplan can be very thorough. At the other extreme it might merely be the issue of manuals. Giving out manuals might improve knowledge, but it is unlikely to improve significantly the way children are cared for. Here we shall take the middle way, where you, as a district medical officer, have some time and money for the microplan, but not enough to reach every target. We will assume that you have a few months, but you may be able to do much in a few weeks, or even days.

Improved care is most likely to result from ALL workers and managers choosing and reaching targets *together*. Some targets should be decided by the ministry of health and be nationwide. But most targets should be decided as low as possible in the staff pyramid with full worker participation. These targets should be recorded on the health centre notice board, and reported to district headquarters. This target setting needs good management, much carefully guided group discussion, and plenty of teaching. Teaching is required to teach the workers what targets they might reach, and *why* it is so important to reach them.

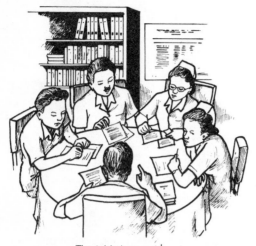

The table is round !

Fig. 7-2 Workers and managers decide targets together

WORKERS AND MANAGERS SHOULD CHOOSE TARGETS TOGETHER
TARGETS SHOULD BE RECORDED AND REPORTED

Fit the microplan into other steps in health centre programming. Implement it as an upgrading activity lasting six months or a year. *Begin and end the programme with a meeting for all the managers in the district.* Managers and workers often welcome new knowledge and new practices, and the programme will probably be greeted with great enthusiasm. The fact that there is a programme at all will improve their morale. Try to upgrade and retrain *everyone* in the district who provides any kind of primary child care. If possible, this should gradually include traditional practitioners and 'needlemen'.

We base our description on the experience of implementing the microplan in several districts in Indonesia at a time when its components were much less well developed than they are now. In Indonesia one district medical officer (dokabu) is responsible for about 500 000 people and has 5–10 doctors, 15 health centres, and about 50 nurses, male and female, working under him. *Districts with other staff patterns will need to implement the microplan in a different way.*

7.3. What are the faults of our services? The Service Diagnosis

Your district will have some services already. The purpose of implementing the microplan is to improve them. Before you can do this, find out in detail what the faults of your services are. Diagnose what is wrong with them, or make the *service diagnosis*.

A clinical diagnosis tells us why a patient is not healthy. A service diagnosis tells us in what ways a health unit, such as a children's clinic, is not giving the kind of care it reasonably could, which is the care described in the workers' manual. You can make a service diagnosis by measuring your services and your workers against as many as possible of the instruments and targets provided in this guide. When you have done this you will have found the quality profile of your services (Guide 2.8). There are workers' targets for knowledge and skill and joint targets (all in Booklet B). There are also managers' targets (Guide 2.5). There are 180 targets altogether, so don't be overcome by them. Try some of the joint targets first, because you can more easily find if you have reached them or not. You will soon see where your services already reach these targets, and where they fall below them.

CHECK YOUR SERVICES AGAINST THE JOINT TARGETS FIRST

A service diagnosis, a clinical diagnosis, and a community diagnosis are the same in several ways. They all begin with the search for information. For all of them we need to know how serious diseases are as causes of death or disability. All require that we find out what people's beliefs and attitudes are—those of the staff, the patient, or the community. Manageability, or what can be done, is important to all of them. But they are different in other ways. A clinical diagnosis concerns one child only whereas a service diagnosis and a community diagnosis concern many children. Also, many sick children recover without treatment. 'Sick' services seldom do.

As health workers we can only cure some diseases. As managers we can only cure some of the faults of our services. For example, we may be unable to get more drugs for our clinics, or pay our staff more. But we can teach them to give safe injections and make sure they discourage bottle feeding. The 'manageability' of the faults of our services—what we can do about them—is thus a specially important part of a service diagnosis.

7.4. Choosing priority targets

Your service diagnosis will show you the faults of your services. Now choose which targets you want to try to reach, and decide how important each one is. When you choose your priorities, ask yourselves these questions.

(1) How important for death and disability is each

target? This depends partly on how common (prevalent) each disease is in your district.

(2) How easily can I reach each target? What can I do about it? (How manageable is it?) Positive targets will probably be easier to reach than negative targets.

(3) How important does the community think each target is? Ask the community leaders.

(4) How important do the workers think each target is? Ask them.

Weight each of the four questions by giving them 'plusses' from '0' to '+ + + +', as in Table 2:2 in the Manual. Multiply these plusses to get a score. The answers to these four questions will vary greatly from one district to another, so will priorities. Some common priority targets will probably be to encourage breast-feeding, to use glucose–salt solution, to give a weight chart to every child, and to diagnose and manage TB and other lower respiratory infections correctly. The targets that we suggest are specially important have a star put beside them.

Targets concern everyone who provides health care. So, everyone should play a part in choosing them—district medical officers, senior nurses, midwives and workers. Choose your own priorities first, discuss them with the workers and alter them if necessary. But, what if the different levels of staff do not agree? Managers' targets are for managers only, so there is no difficulty here. We suggest that, if there is a disagreement over workers' targets, the workers decide, because, unless they themselves decide, they will probably not work hard to reach them. The job of the manager here is to show which targets are important and which targets they might reach. Sharing targets in this way will be new to many health services. If well managed, shared targets may also be very effective.

TRY THE EASY TARGETS FIRST

7.5. Changed attitudes through group discussion

The purpose of the microplan is to *change* services—and make them better. If we can change what people think—their attitudes—we can change what they do, and so improve the services they give. Obtaining this change in attitudes is the first step. Our major resource for improved services is the staff we have already. Changing what they think and do may greatly improve services—even though there are no other inputs. Changed attitudes and improved services are more likely if everyone meets together, discusses together, works together, and changes together.

Implementing the microplan involves a change in knowledge, attitude, and practice by both workers and managers. The managers need discussions at district headquarters. The workers need discussions in the health centres, or in larger groups. Since most people can easily

talk much and achieve little, these discussions need to be guided carefully so that they reach objectives and make good use of the time available.

How you can find and pay for the necessary time for group discussions depends on local circumstances. Sometimes, an empty school can be used during the holidays. Weekly group meetings in the health centres can be used, but this is not likely to be enough. Residential meetings lasting a weekend, a week, or even a fortnight are better. Although small groups of a few people can gather for discussion, in a health centre for example, it is better for 20–40 people to meet for several days. Large groups more easily generate the enthusiasm and a togetherness which is necessary for changes in attitude and practice. These larger meetings also provide an opportunity for group teaching (Guide 6.7). Group meetings have the added benefit of reducing any tensions there may be between groups of workers, medical assistants, and midwives, for example.

THE PURPOSE OF A MICROPLAN IS TO CHANGE SERVICES SO AS TO IMPROVE THEM

7.6. Implementation in a district—the district medical officer

Begin by making a programme with a check-list of the steps you need to take. We deliberately do not suggest a time scale, because this is likely to vary so much. Obtaining funds and ordering the necessary equipment may have to take place a year or more before the rest of the programme. The issue of new equipment at the start of the implementation programme helps to make workers believe that managers really are keen to improve services. Make the best use of whatever time and money there is. If money and time are scarce, can it be reallocated to primary child care from something which is less important? The biggest cost is likely to be that of gathering people for group meetings, and accommodating them if meetings last longer than a day. This may be more economically done in several outlying places rather than in a single central one.

Start and finish with a district meeting. These will probably be the high-points of the programme. Prepare for the first meeting carefully and start all at once 'with a bang'. Don't make the programme a burden. Make it enjoyable. Where possible run a competition between staff and between clinics. Let everyone know the test results and let workers compete with themselves.

GETTING READY—THE TASK OF THE DISTRICT MEDICAL OFFICER

ADMINISTRATIVE STEPS. **Either implement the microplan yourself, or delegate it to someone else.**

Discuss the idea with community leaders. Find out their

priorities, and enlist their help. Lend them a copy of the manual and this guide. Show them its opening message to the community leader.

If necessary, obtain permission from provinical headquarters.

Obtain the necessary funds.

Make a quick survey to see what drugs or equipment in the microplan (Manual 3:1, and 3:2) it would be useful to introduce, such as auriscopes. If possible, order anything which is lacking. Try to issue this at the first district meeting.

Print enough weight charts. If necessary, use paper ones (Guide 8.7b).

Order one manual for each worker, and plenty of copies of this guide, so that each worker can borrow a booklet of questions. If possible, obtain visual aids. Order or make overlays, stencils for answer-sheets, and self-correcting ink. Each health centre will want a copy of the nutrition manual [1] and the laboratory manual [2]. Where necessary, the booklets of questions can be used by several workers. The booklets and the visual aids can be used by different districts or clinics in rotation, since they are less necessary once an implementation programme is over. They are however a useful possession, and every district should have a set.

Inform the key managerial staff, both doctors and nurses. Try to make it their programme. Give them a copy of this guide, and a workers manual. *Try* to make sure they have read most of both of them before the first district meeting. Unless they have read the manual, they cannot teach the workers. Get them to start thinking about targets and priorities.

Decide when the first meeting will be and whom to invite.

If appropriate, book the necessary residential accommodation.

THE DISTRICT MEDICAL OFFICER'S SERVICE DIAGNO-SIS. Start to make a service diagnosis (Guide 7.3) yourself. This will show where the care your staff give now falls below that defined in the microplan. It will also show you the kind of targets that are necessary and possible. You will not be able to use all the many instruments and targets we give, so choose the more important ones. Test a sample of workers with some of the instruments.

ONE WORKER ONE MANUAL

7.7. The first district meeting for health-centre managers

The microplan is likely to cause much discussion at the first meeting. If the doctors from the local medical school spend too long discussing details from the manual, there will not be enough time to discuss other parts of the programme. So if the manual is likely to need much discussion, arrange that this takes place in smaller groups before the first meeting. There may be subjects on which the manual differs from local practice. Try to resolve these differences before the first meeting. For example, don't waste time discussing such matters as whether a newborn baby should be bathed or not, or what the role of the vernix caseosa is. Try to steer discussion away from such details towards more important matters.

At the end of the first meeting the managers from each health centre *must* know what they are to do. One day is not enough, and at least three days may be needed. Discuss possible targets, but make no firm decisions, leave these to group decision in the health centres.

AT THE END OF THE FIRST MEETING THE MANAGERS FROM EACH HEALTH CENTRE MUST KNOW WHAT THEY ARE TO DO

FIRST DISTRICT MEETING—PREPARATION.

OBJECTIVES. At the end of this meeting the manager should:

– be able to implement the microplan in his (her) own health centre.

– be able to obtain the necessary equipment and supplies.

– know the date by which health-centre targets must be reported to the district headquarters, and the date of the second meeting at the end of the implementation programme.

– have read the managers' guide and the manual and understood their local interpretations.

ADMINISTRATION. The largest useful size for the meeting is 40 people. Ask all the doctors and senior nurses from the health centres and as many of the workers as there is room for. There should be at least one person from every unit. Invite a few community leaders and let the most senior leader open the meeting.

Ask everyone to bring their guides and manuals. Try to make sure that these have been at least partly read before the meeting.

Invite the doctor in charge of the children's ward in the district hospital. Let him briefly present the priorities for primary child care as he sees them.

Discuss quality of care and the service diagnosis. Present any data you have on the service diagnosis. Present this on flip charts, an overhead projector, or a blackboard. Break up into small groups and discuss possible targets. When groups convene present your targets and let the groups present theirs. Discuss how they might be implemented.

Demonstrate the overlay and the self-correcting answer-sheets, and make sure that managers know how to use them, can make them, and have the right materials. Give them a few sheets of squared paper (Guide 5.4).

Demonstrate all new procedures, such as the use of a nasogastric tube.

Issue any new equipment that may be available.

7.8. Implementation in a health centre—the health-centre doctor

After the district meeting managers return to their own health centres to implement the microplan. *The targets they and their workers decide on are the important ones.* Health centre meetings will probably have to take place in small groups at convenient times during the working week. If the regular weekly meeting is the only time you have, use it. If possible, gather workers together residentially in larger groups for a longer time. Before you teach a group, read Guide 6.7. If possible, a period of intensive teaching should be followed by continuous teaching, a little over a long time.

HEALTH CENTRE IMPLEMENTATION
THE TASK OF THE HEALTH-CENTRE DOCTOR

Explain the programme to the workers. Explain that they will learn more about medicine and will learn to give better care. They will probably have to change some of the things they do. They will probably have little to say at first, but after a few meetings they will have many questions to ask.

Tell the village leaders about the programme and get their support.

Make a *detailed* service diagnosis for the health centre. Use as many of the instruments and targets as you can.

Sit with your workers, watch carefully what they do. Apply the 15 POINTS instrument (Guide 4.14). What is on their tables? What equipment are they using? Are mothers seated while their children are examined? Are children examined naked? Are sterile spatulae used? etc. etc. Fill in what you find on the dotted line provided for each target.

Apply the special set of pretests as soon as possible—the READING and MATHS pretests, and the OVERALL PRE-TEST. If possible, apply MCQs EASY, and MCQs VARIED. If there is not time to do these in working hours, let workers take them home. Explain that low scores are no disgrace and will not be punished.

Make a time budget and decide how much time you have and how you are going to spend it.

Decide on your own targets and priorities.

Give each worker a manual. Explain the idea of targets to them. Ask them to read as much of the manual as they can and to list the targets they would like to reach.

Leave them a few weeks to read part of the manual.

Call them together and ask them to present their targets. Present your targets. Discuss these with them. If possible choose targets from the whole manual. If this is not possible, choose targets from a few chapters only. Agree about the targets and about when they are to be reached. Send the list of targets to the district headquarters by the chosen date. Put the list of targets on the notice board and cross them off as you reach them.

Work with the workers to achieve as many of the targets as possible.

Encourage workers to learn from the manual. Apply the MANUAL POSTEST early, soon after you have explained the manual. Use it as a teaching aid. Teach them to use the

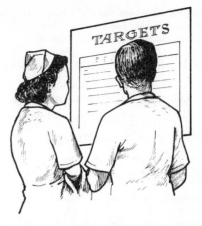

Fig. 7–3 Put your targets on the notice **board**

index. Lend each of them a copy of Booklet B. Give them a supply of answer-sheets, and explain how to use the alkaline ink. Don't start at the beginning of the book. Start at the most important chapters (Cough, Diarrhoea, etc.). Often it is convenient to apply the postest for one chapter (Booklet C) at the same time as the pretest (Booklet A) for the next. If this is not possible, arrange for the workers to teach and test themselves ('distance teaching').

Whenever you examine a case, be sure that a worker is present to watch and learn.

Make sure any new equipment is used, and that a new auriscope, for example, does not just stay in a cupboard.

If possible, borrow a projector, show the visual aids, and discuss them.

Revise your standing orders and make sure that all workers from the sweepers upwards know what they should do.

CAN THEY USE THE INDEX?

After six or nine months it will be time for evaluation. Do this first in the health centres, then at the district headquarters.

HEALTH CENTRE EVALUATION

Do another survey using the same instruments that were used for the service diagnosis. Apply the *OVERALL POS-TEST* and the *WEIGHT CHART POSTEST*.

Give a small prize to the worker with the most well thumbed manual.

What targets have been reached?

Plot cumulative score curves. Put pre- and postests on the same graph. Average the pretests for some or all of the multiple-choice instruments. Compare them with the postests. Use the methods in Guide 5.4 to see if there has been any significant change.

What targets have not been reached, but might be reached during the next few months? What extra targets have been reached that had not been listed?

7.9. The final district meeting—evaluation

Finally there is the last district meeting, which sums up and closes the immediate implementation of the microplan.

LAST DISTRICT MEETING—EVALUATION

Ask a community leader to preside.

Invite all the managers, and as many of the workers as possible.

Ask representatives of each health centre to present their achievements.

If appropriate, present a small prize to the best worker, the best manager, and the best health centre.

Remind the meeting that although they have achieved something, there is much more to be done. Improving child care does not stop here.

Some targets will have been reached and others not. Probably only a few of the workers will have shown themselves to be microplan competent. Some workers may not have been retrained. Perhaps coverage is so low that ten times as many workers are needed. If government cannot train workers quickly enough, can community health workers be trained to help? Another programme may be needed to reach more targets, or perhaps the next priority will be a different microplan, such as maternal care. Don't let the quality of care fall back when the programme ends. For example, if you have started to supply weight charts, make sure the supply continues.

DON'T LET QUALITY OF CARE DETERIORATE WHEN THE PROGRAMME ENDS

7.10. Some problems

Implementation produces many problems. Here are suggestions for some of them.

SOME PROBLEMS

The manual does not fit local conditions. **Go through the manual and the multiple-choice questions, with the group, and cross out what does not apply. Or make a handout describing the necessary modifications.**

Some workers have very low marks. **Older workers are especially likely to get low marks. They may have difficulty reading the multiple-choice questions. The READING PRETESTS will show up these weak readers. Questioning may show that they know more than their marks suggest. They may need careful personal teaching. If, however, they are likely to be dangerous to their patients, move them to other jobs.**

IMPROVED QUALITY OF CARE DEPENDS MOSTLY ON ONE THING— HARD WORK

---

8 A look at the workers' manual

'It all looks so good on paper, but oh dear, you should see the reality!'

Anon

8.1. Introduction

Many chapters of the workers' manual require comment from the point of view of the teacher or manager. The targets for each chapter are in other parts of the guide, so here we will discuss only some of the technologies, the problems concerning them and also methods of teaching. *The section numbers in this chapter correspond to the chapters in the workers' manual.*

The microplan requires very little anatomy and physiology and many students will know it already. If the curriculum contains too much anatomy, remove it.

ANATOMY
Most of the anatomy required by the microplan can be seen or felt on the body. Ask students to name the parts of their own bodies. Ask them to examine one another's ears, throat, and eyes.

8.2a. Disease in the child and the community

The manual contains just enough explanatory knowledge to make the tasks that a worker has to do seem reasonable to him. For example, unless he understands how an acute skin infection can cause septicaemia, he will not understand why he has to treat it so urgently.

DISEASE IN THE CHILD
Use a microscope to show students red cells, pus cells, and some of the organisms that cause disease in children. Most laboratories can make films of Gram positive cocci and tubercle bacilli.

8.2b. Beliefs and customs

There are so many beliefs and customs about disease that the manual can only give a few examples. But nothing is more important for a child than what his parents think about why he is ill, and how they manage him.

BELIEFS AND CUSTOMS
Here are three exercises which you can give students or workers for later discussion as a group.

Ask workers to list as many local beliefs and customs as they can and to decide whether these are good, bad, harmless, or uncertain.

Ask them to record in a notebook the beliefs and customs they meet during a month's work in the clinic. They can also ask their own relatives.

'Mothers' diagnoses'. Ask the mothers of sick children (a) what they think their children's diseases are, (b) what caused them, (c) what can cure them, and (d) where they learned this. Any diseases can be studied in the way. Some important ones are kwashiorkor, TB, diarrhoea, and fits.

8.2c. The community diagnosis

The manual describes a simple way of making the community diagnosis that can be used for group discussion (Manual 2.10). 'Measurements' are made with 'plusses' which are subjective and inexact. They are however rapid, and practical enough to make workers or students begin to think about the importance of disease to the community and its manageability. This is all that is necessary. More exact measurement is beyond the microplan. 'Plusses' are multiplied not added, so that zero in any category makes a zero product. Multiplying also results in a higher product when the plusses are evenly spread between categories.

THE COMMUNITY DIAGNOSIS
Hold a meeting with the workers. Before the meeting ask patients, laymen, or village leaders to list the diseases which they think are most important.

Ideally, data for the 'how common' column should be collected by simple survey. If you cannot do this get it from clinic records, or from the personal experience of the participants.

Some information for the 'how serious' column may also be obtainable from the clinic records. Probably it will again have to come from personal experience.

Guide the workers in discussing ideas on 'manageability'.

Make the community diagnosis on a blackboard and record it on the wall of a clinic or training school. Bring it up to date when necessary.

8.2d. Health education

The manual says much about personal health education, but little about group health education, because this is described in great detail in the nutrition manual [3], and is similar for child care. The only difference is that different behaviour changes are needed. Some of these are listed (Manual 2.12). The educational diagnosis described below follows that in Section 10.1 of the nutrition manual.

THE EDUCATIONAL DIAGNOSIS FOR CHILD HEALTH

After workers have made the community diagnosis ask them to list the behaviour changes the community needs. Write these in a column on the blackboard. In a second column show the importance of these as 'plusses'. In a third column try to judge whether changes will be easy or difficult. Workers familiar with the community may be able to estimate this. Multiply out the plusses as described in Section 2.10 of the manual. Use the resulting score for setting priorities in your health education plan.

Write out lessons for each behaviour change, give each lesson a name, and state the 'wants' to which it can be linked. Make the visual aids for it, and list some questions for evaluating it.

8.2e. Health *with* the people

Nothing is more important than the involvement of the community in their own health care. The way the community is involved will vary greatly from district to district. We think the emphasis should be, health *with* the people, rather than health *by* the people, since they cannot provide health services themselves. Leading, organizing, and teaching the community, and especially its leaders, to care for itself is our greatest challenge as managers. Can we persuade the community's leaders that they have a part to play in caring for its children? Who are its leaders? Are its nominal (obvious) leaders its most important ones, or are there other people who are the community's real leaders? Can we help the community to find out and express its needs? Can we teach the community to use its resources, human and material, to provide care for itself—especially for its least fortunate members? We list a few community targets (Guide 2.5). Only imagination and much hard work will convert them into child care.

OUR GREATEST CHALLENGE—
HELPING THE COMMUNITY
TO HELP ITSELF

8.3a. Drugs

Clinics need at least fifty drugs and expendable supplies —the 'important 50' discussed in Manual 3.7. Clinics also need at least 20 important items of equipment (Manual 3.50). Lack of any one of these will lower the quality of care. We discuss the cost of drugs in Guide 9.1. This depends partly on how they are bought. Drugs are much cheaper when they are bought under their generic names, such as chloramphenicol, for example, rather than as

proprietary preparations, such as 'Chloromycetin'. With one exception, 'Aspirin', only generic names are given in the drug list. Educating the staff to use generic names may be difficult.

There may be some drugs that should *not* be used. These will vary from country to country. We list only a selection of them among the joint targets in Booklet B.

Benzyl penicillin is the best kind of penicillin for newborn babies and is useful for severe infections, particularly meningitis and osteomyelitis. If it is not available, procaine penicillin can be used instead. **Benethamine** or **benzathine penicillin** are useful because a single injection cures many acute infections. Thus a mother need not bring her child for daily injections. These penicillins are more expensive than procaine penicillin, but their cost has recently fallen, so they are now more competitive.

Ampicillin. This is included because it is very useful and has recently become cheaper.

Chloramphenicol is a cheap and effective broad spectrum antibiotic. Its dangers have probably been overestimated. We have therefore included it and have given repeated warnings that it is *not* to be used for mild infections.

Great difficulty was experienced in trying to make simple instructions for the use of antibiotics appear rational to primary care workers. The terms 'antimicrobial' and 'antibiotic' were both found necessary and have been given limited definitions (Manual 3.11). The different kinds of organism, bacteria, etc. are briefly explained and their susceptibility to the common antibiotics discussed.

Since this version of the microplan is primarily intended for sub-Saharan Africa a compound tablet of **isoniazid** and **thiacetazone** has been included. Thiacetazone is not suitable for use in some parts of South-East Asia where it is said to cause too many side effects.

The management of malaria described in the manual is that suited to areas where *P. falciparum* is holoendemic. The manual emphasizes the diagnosis and treatment of cerebral malaria. It tells the worker to give **chloroquine** to every child with a fever as well as any other drugs he needs. It does not describe the radical cure of other kinds of malaria with an 8-amino quinoline, such as **primaquine**. In cases of infection with other species than *P. falciparum* other regimes are necessary.

Opinions differ about the place of chloroquine versus intravenous **quinine** in the treatment of severe malaria, especially cerebral malaria. So the microplan includes both drugs. The ampoules of quinine in Manual 3:1 contain 60 mg in each ml, compared with the BP strength of 300 mg in 1 ml. This weaker solution makes children's doses easier. The manual advises that chloroquine be given *subcutaneously* rather than intramuscularly, since it is absorbed more slowly after a subcutaneous injection. By this route toxic reactions, particularly death, are less likely. There are however differences of opinion on this point. Where chloroquine resistance occurs workers may have to give sulphadoxine with pyrimethamine instead, or intravenous quinine. **Pyrimethamine** resistance is now so widespread, and so easily induced that its place in the drug list may not be justified.

Emetine is cheaper than metronidazole, but it is less convenient, because it has to be injected. It is not in the microplan. Give 1·0 mg/kg daily in two divided doses for one week. Don't give a second course for at least six weeks.

Tetrachlorethylene (TCE) is more toxic than **bephenium,** but only about a hundredth of its cost. The right dose is important.

Some firms now make **iron dextran** comparatively cheaply, thus making it practicable for clinic use. The simple dose formula in the manual makes its dosage easy.

The manual advises that **paracetamol** should replace **aspirin** for children because aspirin is more toxic. Paracetamol is however more expensive.

Paraldehyde is the safest drug for auxiliaries to use for treating fits. It is safer than **phenobarbitone** and cheaper than diazepam.

Promethazine serves as both an antihistamine and as a sedative. It is particularly useful as a cough suppressant and is most conveniently used as a syrup.

'Children's cough mixture' is important to the economy of the clinic (9.1), and may be cheaper if it is made in the clinic, as described in the manual.

Syrup of **ipecacuanha** is commonly used in Europe and North America. In communities where the common kinds of poisoning can be treated by making a child vomit, ipecacuanha should be available in clinics.

Water for injection. In small ampoules sterile water is comparatively expensive. In rubber-capped bottles of 100 ml or more it is cheaper, but more readily contaminated. If it is supplied in larger bottles, it should contain an antiseptic, and must *not* be used for reconstituting vaccines.

Hypochlorite should be more widely used (Manual 3.48). It is cheap and can be made locally by electrolysis of salt. It is safe, and when no longer active it changes into common salt. It is cheaper if purchased as a domestic bleach than in a strictly medicinal form. Choose a locally produced bleach that does not contain a detergent.

8.3b. Equipment

Where possible all equipment should be made locally. The largest item is a weighing scale. The hanging scale shown in Manual 5–3 is not necessarily the best one. Some clinics hang the child to be weighed in a small seat, a basket, or the cloth his mother uses to carry him. In some countries there are locally made beam balances which are very suitable for weighing children.

Nylon or polymethylpentene syringes should replace glass ones, because they do not break and can be autoclaved. Each clinic should have a stock of at least 30. A pressure cooker will hold about 60 2-ml syringes.

In many clinics great confusion results from the use of a mixture of Luer and Record fittings for syringes and needles. Clinics should use one or the other. *If possible the entire health service of a country should use Luer fittings only.*

STANDARDIZE ON LUER FITTINGS

8.4. Immunization

The WHO's expanded programme of immunization aims to supply vaccines to mobile teams and to static health units. The manual discusses only static units. It stresses that vaccine must be given *while it is still effective* and describes how this can be done. This is only possible if clinics have a satisfactory refrigerator. Front-opening domestic refrigerators of the kind used in temperate climates are under-powered and under-insulated for hot countries. A refrigerator for storing vaccine in the tropics should open from the top and have enough power and insulation. It should have a dial thermometer that can be read from the outside.

It is arguable as to whether a primary health worker need know about the various kinds of immunity—natural, active etc. This knowledge does however explain many necessary actions.

The manager's target that requires all vaccines to be available in a clinic every day is a difficult one (Guide 2.5) It is important because workers should immunize healthy and mildly ill children instead of giving them unnecessary drugs. If possible, the immunizations should be given by the workers who are caring for children clinically, and not by workers who do immunizations only.

We can stop measles, polio, and whooping cough spreading in a community by immunizing about 80 per cent of its children. These children give the whole community a 'herd immunity'. The 20 per cent of children who are not immunized are too few to let the organisms live in that community. So our target is to have 80 per cent of children immunized. Tuberculosis spreads from adults to children, and tetanus from animals to the soil and then to children. With these diseases there is no herd immunity among children, so our target should be to immunize 100 per cent of children. The best way to find out how many children have been immunized is to do a weight-chart survey (Guide 4.2), and tally the immunizations recorded on the weight charts. Another way is to find out how many people there are in the clinic area, and what the birth rate is (say 30 per 1000 per year, if you don't know). You can then calculate how many children are being born into the clinic area each year. The clinic's tally sheets (Manual 6–4) will tell you how many children you are immunizing each year. From this you can work out how many children you are immunizing completely or partly.

In some clinics workers teach mothers to bring an empty bottle with a lid, a cup and a spoon, clean diapers and a plastic bag for dirty ones. Apart from the bottles, the microplan contains no instructions for this.

8.5a. The ten steps

The manual divides the care of children into ten steps. This helps workers to care for children in an orderly way. It lays great stress on weighing a child and makes this the first step in caring for him. Special tests (the fourth step) are listed in the manual but are not discussed. These should be the subject of a separate laboratory microplan. Few things are more important for the quality of a child's care than measuring his haemoglobin, or looking for ova in his stools. Although an accurate diagnosis is often impossible in primary care, workers should try to make one (step five) and record it. This helps them to think about the children they are seeing.

Although management and treatment (steps six and seven) are often mixed, they have been carefully separated in the manual. Treatment consists of giving drugs and carrying out procedures. Since these are standardized, they are easily taught and evaluated. Management on the other hand is what is done with a child. Since it requires judgement and depends greatly on local conditions, it is more difficult to teach and evaluate. Multiple-choice questions are of little help, because they need a definite answer, whereas management decisions are usually opinions which need discussion. Management is best taught with real children in a real clinic, but role-play can be useful.

ROLE-PLAY FOR MANAGEMENT DECISIONS

Ask members of the class to act the parts of worker, mother, and child, and also whoever else is necessary, such as a grandmother or a doctor. Tell the class where the clinic is supposed to be, how far it is from a hospital, etc. Tell the 'mother' and the 'child' what their story is to be. Act this out and discuss with the class whether the health worker made the right management decision.

The longer clinical multiple-choice questions will be helpful in providing ideas for this role play. Put in more local details than these questions give.

The explanation (the eighth step) is repeatedly stressed because it is so often forgotten. To help workers remember it, an explanation follows every treatment given in the manual.

Family planning has been made the ninth step. This is a small compensation for having separated a mother from her child and made this microplan for children only. Even good child-care workers often omit any mention of family planning. It is scored for in the 15 POINTS instrument (Guide 4.14).

8.5b. Arranging the clinic

In a small clinic one worker has to do everything for every child. But in a big clinic with several workers there are many ways of arranging the work. Each worker could do all the ten steps for some children (Picture A, Guide 8–1).

This allows each worker to spend enough time with each child and his mother to get to know them, or a child can go along a 'conveyer belt' of workers who each take him through one or two steps only (Picture B). Like this no worker spends enough time with any child to get to know him.

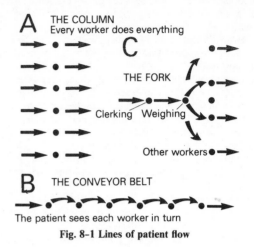

Fig. 8–1 Lines of patient flow

Ideally a child should be cared for by one worker only. However, this may be difficult to arrange, so compromise is usually necessary. A good compromise is for one worker to weigh all children, while the others do as much as possible for each child. We have called this pattern 'the fork' (Picture C). It also shows a clerk keeping the records.

If workers are to get to know the families they care for, they should see mothers and children together. If possible a mother and her child should be able to get any kind of care they need from the same worker. This may be difficult to arrange, but it is worth great effort to do so.

The manual defines integrated care as the ability of a clinic to provide well- and sick-child care, family planning, and maternity care on the same day in the same place. Thus mothers need only make one visit to the clinic instead of several. Integrated care does *not* mean that the clinic has to do more work, but merely that the work is arranged in a different way. Integrated care should be available six days a week. Mothers soon get to know when they can get care, and will come on any day.

We found integrated care more difficult to evaluate than we expected. What is announced on the clinic notice board, what is observed on a visit, and what is said in answer to a question are apt to differ. Also, there is every stage between completely integrated care and completely 'disintegrated' care.

8.6. Recording, reporting, and sterilizing

In most clinics much time is wasted in recording and reporting, so we have reduced it to the minimum. The child's mother keeps his weight chart and any continuation cards that might be necessary. The clinic keeps only a tally and a special-care register for those children who need it.

The quality-of-care score is an innovation. The targets chosen are those suited to one particular country. Elsewhere they might be quite different, and should anyway be changed sometimes. In Guide 9.2 we discuss the great potential value of reporting some of the quality-related targets as part of the routine reports sent in by health centres.

Trials have shown that small domestic pressure cookers are very useful in clinics. Their disadvantage is that they are too small to hold the family planning equipment.

8.7a. When should a child first be given porridge?

The workers' manual advises that a child should be given porridge for the first time when he is four months old. The foods a young child is given may not be clean and may cause diarrhoea, so it may be better for him not to be given porridge until he is six months old. If however he is given porridge too late, he is in danger from malnutrition. Finding the best compromise may not be easy either for the individual child or for the community. We need to weigh up the risks of failure to grow by not being given porridge early enough, and the risk of getting recurrent diarrhoea by having porridge too early.

8.7b. Weight charts

These became practical in the children's clinics of the developing world when Morley [9] devised a method which removed the need for health workers to calculate a child's age in months. Another of his innovations was to let mothers take their children's charts home in a plastic bag. *If the importance of keeping weight-charts is properly explained to mothers, only 1 per cent of the charts are lost.* Mothers lose fewer charts than are lost by most filing clerks in clinics. Also, if a mother keeps her child's weight-chart, she learns from it. Health workers can look at a child's chart when they visit him at home. Also, clerks need not waste time searching for it in their files each time the child visits the clinic. The use of weight-charts is thus a 'star target' (Guide 2.2) of the greatest importance.

WEIGHT CHARTS ARE ONE OF THE MOST USEFUL TECHNOLOGIES IN THE MICROPLAN

There are many kinds of weight-chart. The manual illustrates Morley's latest version. The graphs for the first three years of life are on the inside page and the graphs for next two years are on the outside. Its 'unisex' standards for boys and girls combined replace the older Harvard standards. Weight charts are recommended by WHO for international use [14].

Copies of the weight chart are available for relettering in a local language and local printing (TALC). If charts are going to withstand much handling during many attendances at the clinic, they should be on good quality card. This should not be less than 120 g (grams per square metre). If possible, use green ink on yellow card, because this matches the visual aids, such as the flannelgraph of the weight chart that is available from TALC. If you cannot afford to print on card, you can duplicate weight charts on paper, but this is not so good. A paper chart is however *much* better than nothing, and it is surprising how long some mothers will keep them. A good quality plastic bag is desirable. It should be about 3 cm longer than the folded card. In many clinics weight charts are very poorly used, so we have provided several instruments to measure the quality of their use (Guide 4.8 to 4.11, and the WEIGHT CHART POSTEST in Booklet C).

TEACHING ABOUT WEIGHT CHARTS
Use the large flannelgraph of a weight chart that can be obtained from TALC.

Cardboard charts are expensive to practise on, so let workers practise on paper ones. Stencils for these are obtainable from TALC.

EVERY CHILD MUST HAVE A WEIGHT CHART. IF YOU CANNOT AFFORD CARD, USE PAPER

8.7c. Nutrition education

If workers are going to change mothers' food practices they need a minimum of theoretical knowledge, they must know about local food habits and prices, and they must understand the family they are trying to educate. Unfortunately, many clinic staff have had little nutrition training, or they have been badly trained. So more nutrition teaching is an important part of implementing the microplan.

Breast-feeding is the 'first rule of good nutrition' (Manual 7.2). The manual takes the view that if a poorly nourished mother becomes pregnant, she should go on breast feeding. Her nutrition will not be improved if she goes on, but her child may die if she stops. In some districts almost all mothers breast-feed. In other places, especially towns, much hard work will be necessary to undo the harm done by the advertisements of the milk companies, and to restore breast-feeding. Start by trying to improve staff knowledge and attitudes. One way to do this is to organize a discussion about instrument BREAST- AND BOTTLE-FEEDING (Guide 4.7, Booklet A). This measures staff attitudes and provides a way of improving them. For a guide to discussing this instrument, see Manual 26.7 to 26.18.

8.8. Cough

Lower respiratory infections kill about as many children as diarrhoea. So workers must diagnose them early, and treat them adequately. The manual uses six signs to diagnose them—cyanosis, a moving nose, fast breathing, stridor, wheezing, and insuction. The respiratory rate is important, and a rate of over 60 is diagnosed as pneumonia. Little published evidence can be found for this, but it has the support of many experienced paediatricians. We do not describe the use of a stethoscope, because it is not necessary, and may cause confusion. Also there may be people who do not want a doctor's status symbol handed to a junior worker.

The manual diagnoses bronchiolitis on the criteria of wheezing and cyanosis in a child less than a year old, and treats it as if it were pneumonia. This prevents workers treating children of this age for asthma.

8.9. Diarrhoea

Glucose–salt solution has been the great recent advance in the treatment of all kinds of acute dehydrating diarrhoea, including cholera, provided a child is not too severely dehydrated and does not have other complications [10]. Packets of powder to make this fluid should be on sale in every village or delivered through health centres or village health workers, so that it becomes a widely used home remedy.

All primary care workers must have packets of glucose–salt powder, and be able to teach mothers how to use it. The prepared solutions should be kept covered in a cool place and left-overs should not be used.

For clinic use it would be conveninent if the powder for glucose–salt solution were available in large tins, or, in dry climates, in bags, and supplied with a scoop holding sufficient powder for one litre. Until now, however, it has not been marketed in this form. Most clinics will thus have to make glucose–salt solution from the raw materials. This is easier if a special plastic scoop available from TALC is used, as illustrated in Manual 9–10b. The fluid can be coloured and flavoured if this would make it more acceptable locally.

Mothers must make their oral rehydration fluids with sufficient accuracy. The great danger is that they make them too strong. Random samples prepared by mothers should be checked periodically for accuracy by arrangements with a biochemistry laboratory. The values aimed for in the mmol/l are sodium 90, chloride 80, potassium 20, bicarbonate 30, and glucose 110.

Mothers may have difficulty in measuring a litre of water, so a locally available litre-container should be found. Some clinics hire out plastic one-litre bottles which mothers return later.

If a dehydrated child is vomiting, or is too weak to drink, his life can often be saved by giving him glucose–salt solution through an intragastic drip (Manual 9.24). This is easy, the equipment can be used many times, and it does not require expensive intravenous fluids, so all workers should learn how to do it. The old drip sets and empty infusion bottles from a hospital can be used.

The manual describes another method of using glucose–salt solution to save the life of a child who is too weak to drink (Manual 9.24). In this method a child's mother lets the solution from a drip set fall drop by drop into his mouth, without using an intragastric tube. This may be useful since an intragastric tube may not be available, and his mother may not be able to manage it. Small volumes may also be given as sips from a spoon, particularly if there is vomiting.

The figures for intravenous fluid replacement treatment in the manual are deliberately cautious, and are advised for conditions where supervision may not always be perfect. Under better conditions of supervision, and with more experienced staff, the following dosage figures for children may be better—an initial replacement with 30 ml/kg of fluid during the first hour, followed by 70 ml/kg during the next five hours. This should be followed by reweighing and maintenance treatment.

8.12. Leprosy

The instructions in the manual include those taken from the report of the 1976 WHO Expert Committee on Leprosy. Particularly important recommendations include the starting of dapsone treatment at full dosage, and the treatment of lepromatous and borderline leprosy with dapsone and clofazimine combined.

8.15. Fits

The manual takes a radical approach to meningitis. It holds that any child with a fit should have a lumbar puncture, unless he is a known epileptic and has no fever at the time of the fit. This is good practice, and is easy. Lumbar punctures are commonly done by auxiliaries in several parts of the world. However, the manual gives strict warning that lumbar puncture should only be done by workers who have been carefully trained. It also gives detailed instructions for deciding when lumbar puncture is essential and when it is not. Since, under primary care conditions, the danger of an implantation dermoid, from the use of a needle without a stylet, is probably less than that of meningitis from a dirty needle, the manual advises the use of sterile disposable needles. These are very sharp, and very convenient.

The treatment for meningitis which is given in the manual is not ideal. It is described because it uses drugs already listed for other diseases. If the large doses of penicillin advised in the manual (600 mg of benzyl penicillin 3-hourly) are too expensive, smaller doses can be given, but are not so effective. If possible, chloramphenicol should be given intravenously or intramuscularly for the first two days, or until the child improves, after which it can be given orally, or by tube. In children under 2 months old kanamycin (7·5 mg/kg intramuscularly 12-hourly) should replace chloramphenicol. Gentamycin can also be used.

8.17. Ears

Chronically discharging ears are common. An important task of primary care workers is to prevent them by treating otitis media early and correctly. There is a school of thought which believes that primary care workers can give antibiotics on suitable indication without examining a child's ears. China's barefoot doctors are said to do this. The manual takes the view that examining the ear-drum is important in any child with fever, however difficult it may be. Adult ear-drums are easier to see, so workers should practise on them.

There is considerable difference of opinion about the importance of myringotomy compared with the administration of antibiotics alone in the treatment of acute otitis media. ENT surgeons usually like myringotomy and paediatricians antibiotics. The manual sides with the latter and does not mention myringotomy.

Opinions differ on the safety of allowing auxiliaries to remove foreign bodies from ears using a bent paperclip as a hook (Manual 17–12).

8.18. Mouth and throat

The microplan assumes a high prevalence of tetanus, considers immune globulin too expensive, and, with some hesitation, describes the use of tetanus antitoxin. The management of tetanus is based on the paper by Patricia Bradley [11]. It is generally thought that tetanus can be treated only in hospital, and that children with neonatal tetanus always die unless they are treated there. Working in a very poor community in Bangladesh, she used out-patient treatment to save the lives of half her cases of tetanus, about half of whom were neonates. For the initial sedation she used chlorpromazine (4 mg/kg, maximum 25 mg) whereas the manual uses paraldehyde.

8.22. Anaemia and jaundice

One of the greatest deficiencies in the technology available for primary care is a satisfactory method for measuring haemoglobin. Sahli's method is better than nothing, but it is not accurate enough or easy enough. All other methods are too expensive. We have written this chapter in the hope that a suitable device will shortly become available. The causes of anaemia differ in different places, so, when this microplan is adapted, this is one of the most likely chapters to require alteration.

The manual refers frequently to 'children's iron mixture'. This is Ferrous Sulphate Mixture Paediatric BPC. It contains ferrous sulphate 60 mg, ascorbic acid (vitamin C) 5 mg, orange syrup 0·5 ml, chloroform water double strength 2·5 ml, and cooled boiled water to 5 ml. Vitamin C helps the iron to be absorbed. You can make this mixture with vitamin C tablets. There are other things in the tablets and these sink to the bottom of the mixture. Trials of this mixture have been limited, but it promises to be very valuable.

8.23. Urinary and genital symptoms

Gonorrhoea is becoming more common in many countries in the world. Children are often infected where standards of domestic hygiene are low, and health workers should look out for them. Because there are no alternative drugs which are cheap enough, no alternative treatment is given for penicillinase-producing gonococci.

8.24. Not walking or talking

After the diseases caused by malnutrition and infection, the backward child is the next most important problem in primary child care. The manual includes Down's syndrome, cerebral palsy, and with somewhat less justification, sporadic cretinism. Even so this is treatable and some auxiliaries do diagnose it. To avoid confusion between sporadic and endemic cretinism, the manual uses the more modern term 'iodine embryopathy' for endemic cretinism, and describes its prevention with iodized oil in areas where the iodization of salt is not practicable. Iodine embryopathy is seen in some areas only, but where it is seen, it is likely to be a major public health problem.

8.26. The newborn baby

The manual places great emphasis on establishing breast-feeding and discouraging bottle-feeding. Only the most minimal account of artificial feeding is given, since it is covered completely in the nutrition manual [3].

Two starred targets are that workers should be able to express breast milk and be able to tube-feed a baby who is too weak to suck. Workers must have suitable polythene tube for this (Manual 3:1).

Another important target is that workers should be able to recognize and treat septicaemia in babies. This is comparatively common and is not recognized often enough. Penicillin with streptomycin or ampicillin are the drugs described for its treatment. They are not necessarily the best drugs, but they are the only ones likely to be available for primary care.

9 Some other aspects of microplanning

'It is fascinating to see how much detail you have put into something which we have been looking at from another angle. It is precisely this need for microplanning which we also have identified.'
  Dr Susan Cole-King, a colleague writing from Ghana

9.1. Can primary child care be cheap enough?

If *all* the children in poor communities are to get primary care, it must be cheap. In Guide 7.6 we discuss briefly the costs of implementing the microplan. Here we discuss its running costs.

The two most expensive parts of primary care are the salaries of the workers who provide it, and the cost of the drugs they use. If salaries are going to be cheap, care must be given by many junior workers on low salaries, supervised by a few more highly paid managers. Let us say an enrolled community nurse earns $1000 a year and sees 40 children a day for 25 days a month. The cost of seeing each child will be about 8 cents.

The cost of drugs for primary child care depends on how we use them. If most children coming to a clinic get an antibiotic, costs will be higher. Cough mixture costs almost nothing. So, if many children are given cough mixture only, average costs will be lower. Cough mixture and other cheap placebos, such as yeast tablets, are important for keeping drug costs low.

The cost of drugs depends partly on how we buy them. Guide 9–1 shows the cost of treating an 11 kg child with a course of the more common drugs at prices charged by UNICEF in 1976. Anyone who buys drugs in large enough quantities can buy them at these prices. If we leave out ampicillin, the syrups, and drugs for TB and leprosy, since few children need them, the average cost of a course of the remaining drugs is about 10 cents. Some children may need more than one drug, but others will need no drugs or cough mixture only. 10 cents may be less than the price of the transport that brought the child to the clinic.

The stars in Guide 9–1 show the cost of some of these drugs when they were bought at a typical retail pharmacy in a developing country in 1977. To make these prices more comparable,10 per cent has been added to the UNICEF costs for one year's inflation between 1976 and 1977, and another 10 per cent for distribution costs. Twenty per cent has been taken off the retail pharmacy prices as a discount for bulk purchases. Some drugs are cheaper in the pharmacy, probably because of errors in accounting. Drugs from the pharmacy still average 160 per cent more. So the cost of drugs depends greatly on how and where they are bought.

There are other costs, but these are small compared to drugs and salaries. Let us allow 10 cents for staff, 10 cents for drugs, and 5 cents for other costs. The total is 25 cents per visit. Many countries have only $1 per head per year to spend on the health of each of their people. This would buy four visits for primary child care. But $1 will only buy four visits if care is given by junior staff on salaries the community can afford, if they see many children each day, and if drugs are bought cheaply.

9.2. On educational theory

In its publication [12] WHO has advocated that educational objectives should be defined, measurable, and detailed; that there should be a pretest at the beginning of a period of instruction, a postest at its end; and tests in between which the students can use to teach and test themselves [12]. As you see, we have followed this theory to the letter and spent a year making the multiple-choice instruments alone. This is not that we are sure that such rigour is useful, but consider that it is worth the experiment, particularly since the instruments are probably more useful as teaching aids than they are for evaluation. One thing is certain, under the conditions for which this microplan was designed, the multiple-choice instruments necessary for such rigour have to be provided for the teacher, because he cannot make enough good ones himself. The average teacher does very well if he produces 25 reasonable questions at the end of a term. But even when provided with more than two thousand questions, how many are practical in the average auxiliary training school? How much time can, or should, the students spend doing them? At 20 minutes an instrument (the absolute minimum) at least 30 hours is needed. Is this the best way of using such time? So far the largest number of these instruments ever done by the same class has been 30, which were all that were available at the time. We look forward to hearing from the schools

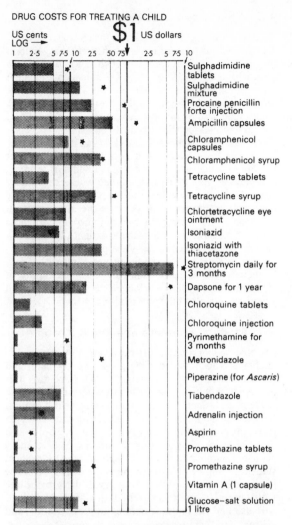

DRUG COSTS FOR TREATING A CHILD

US cents
LOG → $1 US dollars

1 2·5 5 7·5 10 25 50 75 2·5 5 7·5 10

Sulphadimidine tablets
Sulphadimidine mixture
Procaine penicillin forte injection
Ampicillin capsules
Chloramphenicol capsules
Chloramphenicol syrup
Tetracycline tablets
Tetracycline syrup
Chlortetracycline eye ointment
Isoniazid
Isoniazid with thiacetazone
Streptomycin daily for 3 months
Dapsone for 1 year
Chloroquine tablets
Chloroquine injection
Pyrimethamine for 3 months
Metronidazole
Piperazine (for *Ascaris*)
Tiabendazole
Adrenalin injection
Aspirin
Promethazine tablets
Promethazine syrup
Vitamin A (1 capsule)
Glucose–salt solution 1 litre

Fig. 9-1 This shows the costs in US of giving an 11 kg child the shortest course of the drugs shown in the workers manual (3–12 to 3–17). Data from UNICEF 1976 catalogue. Stars show retail 1977 prices in one developing country pharmacy after deducting 10 per cent for a year's inflation, 10 per cent for transport and 20 per cent discount for bulk purchase. Note that this is a logarithmic scale.

who use them, if this approach is indeed wise—and *practical?*

9.3. Using the health information system to promote quality of care

Health information systems (recording and reporting systems) usually report only sickness and death. They could also report targets for quality and coverage. If, as managers, we had to report these targets we might try harder to reach them. A selection of the targets we give could be reported, say, every six months. These could either be reported individually, or they could be combined into a 'quality score' like that in Section 6.8 of the workers' manual. Coverage could be reported as the percentage of the children in the community with a weight chart. The targets chosen for national reporting must be *practical,* and they should be changed from time to time. We understand that the ministry of health in Indonesia intends to include the reporting of some targets in its health information system. We hope that other countries will follow.

Reporting quality and coverage targets in this way would help to make managers try to reach them. It could be a powerful component of the microplan.

9.4. Job descriptions

The manual is written for the 'primary care worker', and not for any special kind of worker. This has made the microplan more useful, but it cuts across usual ideas about job descriptions. When we began we thought that job descriptions would form a useful component of the microplan. As we worked we changed our minds. We now think that microplans should be part of a job description.

A job description has two parts. Firstly there are a worker's *technical* tasks, such as diagnosing measles, expressing breast milk, or putting up a scalp vein drip. These are the same all over the world and change little. Secondly, there are the *administrative* parts of his job, such as his daily work routines, and a statement of who he is to supervise, or who is to supervise him. These administrative matters depend on the local situation and may need changing often. Job descriptions are thus a mixture of two different things.

Detailed job descriptions are difficult to make. If they are made and kept to they may prevent the necessary changes. It is too easy for a worker to say 'But it's not my job'. One experienced administrator said that *detailed* job descriptions are a sign that something is wrong with an organization. They are a bureaucratic attempt to get good working routines. A good team spirit makes them less necessary, because in a good team workers do the jobs that need doing. *We think that the detailed technical parts of a health worker's job description are best described in terms of microplans,* and that the administrative parts of it should be specified more loosely, so that they can be determined by local needs, and defined by local standing orders. A midwife, for example, might be expected to employ the technology in this microplan and one on mother care. The administrative parts of her job would be described in standing orders.

9.5. Language

A worker can only use the manual if he can understand it, so the manual must be easily understood. Two kinds of reader need an easy manual. The first is the worker reading an English manual when English is his second language. The second is the less educated worker who is reading the manual in his own language after it has been translated from English. This translation will be easier to understand if it has been made from easy English. For both these reasons we have tried to make the English in the workers' manual as easy as possible. It is written in a special kind of easy English which others have referred to as 'manualese'. This has its own small vocabulary, and no sentences (except lists) are over 20 words. There are few passives, and very few idioms, etc. Guide 9–2 shows the results of a Cloze test (Guide 6.3), like the READING PRETEST on two Indonesian passages translated from the same English passage in the manual. (1) was translated into Indonesian from an early version of the English manual; (2) translated into Indonesian from the same passage of the manual after it had been further simplified into English 'manualese'. You will see the workers got higher scores when the translation was made from 'manualese'.

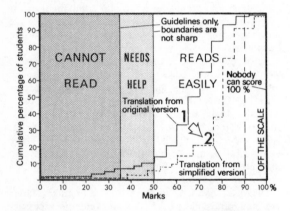

Fig. 9–2. How simplifying a text improves its readability after translation. Section 4.2 of the manual was translated into Indonesian, (1) from an early version of the English manual, and (2) after it had been further simplified into 'manualese'. Cloze tests were made from each version and given to 114 trainee midwife tutors, and trainee midwives. Simplification of the text has produced a significant improvement in their scores.

These workers could mostly 'read easily' anyway. Much more useful would be the improvement that might be expected to take place after simplification for workers in the 'cannot read', and 'needs help' range.

The 'manualese' of the workers' manual is useful, but is not perfect. We hope to improve on it in later editions. Because junior health workers need easily understood manuals, all languages need their own kind of 'manualese'.

**ALL LANGUAGES NEED
A 'MANUALESE'**

9.6. What is the best kind of algorithm?

There is a 'Caring for ...' section at the end of Chapters 8, 9, 10, etc. of the manual. These are the steps that a worker should follow to solve a problem, such as how to care for a child with a cough. These sets of problem-solving steps are called algorithms. An algorithm is a set of rules for getting a specific output (a diagnosis) from a specific input (signs and symptons). The workers' manual uses one way of making these clinical algorithms. There are other ways, such as those of Essex [13] and Hirschorn [10]. We do not know which of these is best and under what conditions. One may be best with students in training, and another may be best for trained workers in a busy clinic. The time available for seeing patients may be very important in determining which is the most practical algorithm. This microplan was designed in Indonesia where there is plenty of time to see patients, because few patients come to the clinics. When patients must be seen in three minutes or less, the Essex type of algorithm may be better. We hope to compare different kinds of algorithm, and will be delighted to collaborate with anyone wanting to take part in these trials.

9.7. Medical students and the microplan

The first task of a university department of community medicine is to organize some good primary care, and teach students how to manage it. We hope that this microplan will be useful for both these things.

Medical students are often sent to visit health centres, but they sometimes do not know what to do when they get there. Applying the instruments in the microplan is a useful exercise in measuring the quality of care and a good background to discussions about it. Any medical student should be able to use the manual even before he has done his course in paediatrics. It will also provide him with a useful introduction to child care. Medical students will also find the multiple-choice questions useful—and get many of them wrong.

9.8. Adapting the microplan

The more perfectly adapted a microplan is to a country, the more useful will it be in improving its primary child care. This version fits no country perfectly. If it is to fit better, it will need to be carefully adapted to local conditions, and if necessary translated. Adaptation and translation is to be without royalty or credit, and can be done by governments, or by voluntary agencies. WHO and UNICEF will be delighted to consider requests for assistance.

Any part of either the manual or the guide may be used in any way which might be useful, but adaptation of the system as a whole is only possible within certain limits. For example, any disease or most technologies could be added or deleted without difficulty, but to remove the possibility of the worker giving injections would virtually destroy the microplan.

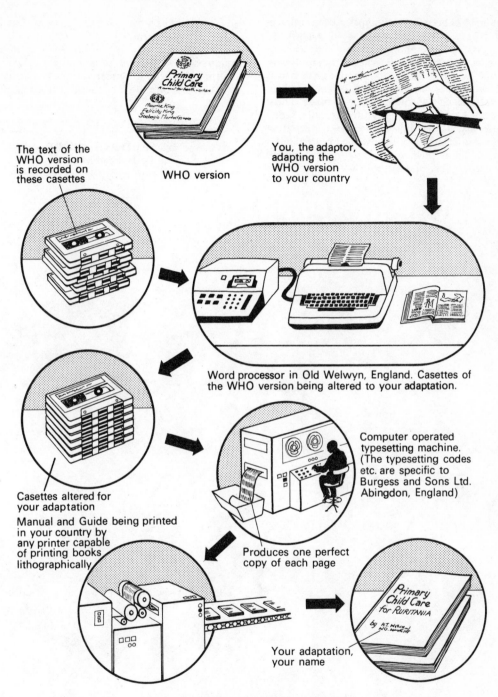

The text of the WHO version is recorded on these casettes

WHO version

You, the adaptor, adapting the WHO version to your country

Word processor in Old Welwyn, England. Casettes of the WHO version being altered to your adaptation.

Casettes altered for your adaptation

Manual and Guide being printed in your country by any printer capable of printing books lithographically

Computer operated typesetting machine. (The typesetting codes etc. are specific to Burgess and Sons Ltd. Abingdon, England)

Produces one perfect copy of each page

Your adaptation, your name

Fig. 9–3 Adapting the microplan in English

This edition has been optically typeset from 'Infotec' computer type cassettes. Adaptations in English or further English editions can easily be made by altering these cassettes on a special typewriter without retyping the parts that require no changes. We hope that there will also be 'master tapes' in other major languages, from which country specific adaptations can be made. These adapted tapes could then be re-edited in later years, where necessary. Under this arrangement typesetting takes place in a technologically advanced centre, and a kilo or two of film is flown to a country for lithographic printing locally. This arrangement will combine the advantages of easy 'word handling', sophisticated typesetting, and local printing.

We hope that this will be the first step in assisting countries to assemble *all* the appropriate technologies for the clinical aspects of primary care in a systematic form as a series of carefully interfaced microplans.

ADAPT DON'T ADOPT—
Dr Halfdan Mahler

Equipment and supplies

The following supplies are available from Teaching Aids at Low Cost (TALC), c/o The Institute of Child Health, Guildford Street, Great Ormond Street, London, WC1 1EH:

A set of four spoons for preparing glucose–salt solution, as shown in Manual 9–10b. £1 for four sets of spoons, or $2 for five sets, price includes postage and packing by surface mail.

Ten sets of 35 mm transparencies illustrating the contents of the workers' manual, and cross referenced to it. Also a pamphlet listing questions to be asked about the slides and the answers to be expected.

An outfit for the multiple-choice questions containing a perforated plastic overlay (Guide 3–2), three stencils for the answer-sheet, phenolphthalein powder and a powder from which to prepare alkaline ink.

Spare booklets of multiple-choice questions *may* become available in future.

References

We have drawn extensively on too many people and their writings to mention them all. We would however, most particularly like to acknowledge our debt to John Biddulph's *Child care for health extension officers* (Department of Health, Port Moresby, Papua New Guinea), and Jelliffe's *Child health in the tropics* (Arnold). Some of the other works that we have either made particular use of, or refer to, are listed below.

[1] *Primary health care.* A Joint Report by WHO and UNICEF to the International Converence on Primary Health Care at Alma-Ata, September 1978.

[2] KING, M.H. and MARTODIPOERO, S. Health microplanning in the developing world. *Int. J. Hlth Serv.* **8,** no. 4 (1979).

[3] KING, M.H. (ed.). *Nutrition for developing countries,* (ELBS edn.). Oxford University Press (1973).

[4] KING, M.H. *A medical laboratory for developing countries,* (ELBS edn.). Oxford University Press (1971).

[6] KING, M.H. *Medical care in developing countries,* (Section 2.7). Oxford University Press, Nairobi (1956).

[7] CONOVER, W.J. *Practical nonparametric statistics,* (Chapter 6). Wiley, New York (1971).

[8] JONGSMA, E.R. *The Cloze procedure: a survey of the research.* Indiana University, Bloomington. Eric. Ed. 050 893 (1971).

[9] MORLEY, D. *Paediatric priorities in the developing world.* Butterworth, London (1973).

[10] WHO MONOGRAPH SERIES. *Treatment and prevention of dehydration in diarrhoeal diseases—a guide for use at primary level* (1976).

[11] BRADLEY, PATRICIA A. Tetanus and its management in an under-five clinic setting. *J. trop. Pediat.* **20,** 291 (1974).

[12] GUILBERT, J.J. *Educational handbook for health personnel.* WHO Offset Publication No. 35 (1977).

[13] ESSEX, B.J. An approach to rapid problem-solving in clinical medicine. *Brit. med. J.* **3,** 34–6 (1975).

[14] *A growth chart for international use in maternal and child health care.* WHO, Geneva (1978).

Booklet A—Pretests

Booklet A—Pretests

A.1. READING PRETEST

This is a test to see how easily you can understand the manual. If you can understand it easily you can guess the missing words. How many can you guess? Take a piece of paper and write numbers one to 50. Then guess the missing words and write them down (Guide 6.3).

Diarrhoea is common. Many children die (1) ... it and it is especially dangerous (2) ... babies. Fortunately, we can prevent diarrhoea. (3) ... you treat children with diarrhoea carefully, (4) ... of them will die.

The stools (5) ... a normal baby are described in (6) ... 26.29 A healthy older child passes (7) ... once or twice a day, or (8) ... only once in two days. His (9) ... are brown and solid. If he (10) ... many fluid stools he has diarrhoea. (11) ... there is blood and mucus in (12) ... stools, or the stools may be (13) .... Stools become green if they are (14) ... so quickly that the green bile (15) ... not have time to become brown.

(16) ... has many causes, but infection and (17) ... are the most important causes. They (18) ... work together. Organisms inside the gut (19)... most infectious diarrhoea. Often, these organisms (20) ... not dangerous enough to harm adults (21) ... sometimes they are specially dangerous and (22) ... cause diarrhoea at any age. Sometimes, (23) ... is caused by infections outside the (24) ... such as malaria or tonsillitis.

A (25) ... baby is born with no organisms (26) ... him, or in his gut—he (27) ... no flora (2.2) and is sterile (2.2b). During (28) ... first months of his life he (29) ... many organisms for the first time. (30) ... come to him from the skin, (31) ... hands, or the breasts of his (32) .... A few of them are helpful. (33) ... organisms (lacto-bacilli) grow well in (34) ... breast milk and help to keep (35) ... harmful organisms away. As a child (36) ... older other organisms come to live (37) ... his gut. They come to him (38) ... his food and water from the (39) ... of healthy adults. Some of them (40) ... grow in him and cause diarrhoea, (41) ... he has not yet become immune (42) ... them. As he grows older his (43) ... learns to live with the organisms (44) ... meets. This is why older children (45) ... adults get diarrhoea less often.

Gut (46) ... which are not dangerous enough to (47) ... adults, often cause diarrhoea in young (48) .... You will probably see about ten (49)... with this kind of diarrhoea

for (50) ... child with one of the 'special' organisms in the next sections.

Dysentery is the name for any diarrhoea with blood and mucus in the stools. Bacillary and amoebic dysentery are the most common kinds, but some worms can cause it.

A.2. MATHS PRETEST Code 4

1. PITO'S pulse beats 14 times in 15 seconds. In one minute it beats—

A—30 times? B—46 times? C—56 times? D—60 times? E—68 times?

2. A standard teaspoon holds five ml. How many teaspoonfuls of medicine are there in a 100 ml bottle?

A 3   B 5   C 10   D 15   E 20

3. A cup holds about 200 ml. How many cupfuls would make a litre (1000 ml) of water?

A 5   B 6   C 7   D 8   E 9

4. There are 20 drops in one ml. TIBBY needs $1\frac{1}{2}$ ml of tetrachlorethylene. She needs—

A—20 drops? B—30 drops? C—40 drops? D—50 drops? E—60 drops?

5. MIRABEL (15 kg) needs 120 ml/kg of fluid in a day. A cup holds about 200 ml. How many cupfuls of fluid does she need?

A 5   B 6   C 7   D 8   E 9

6. Baby CHRISTMAS (5·5 kg) needs 150 ml of milk each day for each kilo he weighs. He has five feeds a day. At each feed he needs—

A—120 ml? B—165 ml? C—190 ml? D—200 ml? E—285 ml?

7. In which of these are all the measures the same?

A 50 mg, 0·5 g, half a gram.   B 10 mg, 0·1 g, a tenth of a gram.   C 200 mg, 0·02 g, a fifth of a gram.   D 250 mg, 0·25 g, a quarter of a gram.   E 750 mg, 0·75 g, one gram.

8. Which of these would NOT give PITO half a gram of ampicillin?

A 0·5 g of powder   B Half a 1 g tablet   C Half a 1000 mg tablet   D Two 100 mg tablets   E Two 200 mg tablets and a 100 mg capsule

9. THEOBALD'S mother needs a gram of tetracycline. How many 50 mg capsules would you give her?

A 10   B 20   C 30   D 40   E 50

10. Baby TANYA needs 25 mg of isoniazid. You have only got 100 mg tablets. How much would you give her?

A Two tablets **B** 1/3 tablet **C** 0·2 tablet **D** Half a tablet **E** Quarter of a tablet

11. BLAISE (7·5 kg) needs 250 mg/kg/day of aminosalicylate. You only have 500 mg tablets. Which of these would be closest to the dose he needs?

A Four tablets **B** Five tablets **C** Five-and-a-half tablets **D** Six-and-a-half tablets **E** Seven tablets

12. You have dissolved 1 g of streptomycin in 10 ml of water. You want to give baby TRIXIE 150 mg. She needs—
A—0·15 ml? **B**—1 ml? **C**—1 ½ ml? **D**—3 ml? **E**—15 ml?

All these four children in the next figures have had their temperatures taken for three minutes in their rectums.

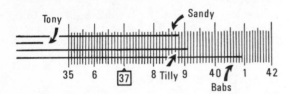

13. SANDY's temperature is—
A—36·9 °C? **B**—37·2 °C? **C**—38·8 °C? **D**—39·0 °C? **E**—29·5 °C?

14. TONY—
A—has a normal temperature? **B**—has hypoglycaemia? **C**—has hypotonia? **D**—may have hypothermia? **E**—has a temperature of 35 °C?

15. TILLY's temperature is—
A—39·0 °C? **B**—39·1 °C? **C**—39·2 °C? **D**—39·4 °C? **E**—29·9 °C?

16. BABS's temperature is—
A—39·8 °C? **B**—40·0°C? **C**—40·7 °C? **D**—40·3 °C **E**—40·9 °C?

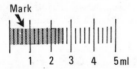

17. This shows a syringe of penicillin ready to give to MARK. How much penicillin is he being given?
A 2·6 ml. **B** 2·8 ml. **C** 3·0 ml. **D** 3·2 ml. **E** 3·5 ml.

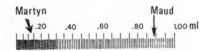

18. MARTYN (30 kg) is being given adrenalin. How much adrenalin is there in the syringe?
A 0·2 ml. **B** 0·3 ml. **C** 3 ml. **D** 3·5 ml. **E** 3·8 ml.

19. If the syringe were filled up to the place marked MAUD, it would contain—
A 0·8 ml? **B** 0·84 ml? **C** 0·89 ml? **D** 0·98 ml? **E** 9·8 ml?

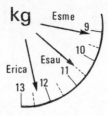

20. ESME weighs about—
A—9·2 kg? **B**—9·5 kg? **C**—9·8 kg? **D**—10 kg? **E**—10·1 kg?

21. ESAU weighs about—
A—9·5 kg? **B**—10·0 kg? **C**—10·1 kg? **D**—10·5 kg? **E**—11·1 kg?

22. ERICA weighs about—
A—10·0 kg? **B**—10·1 kg? **C**—11·5 kg? **D**—12·0 kg? **E**—12·3 kg?

Caspar

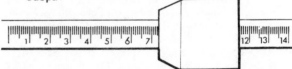

23. CASPAR is being weighed on a beam balance. He weighs about—
A—6·9 kg? **B**—7·0 kg? **C**—7·1 kg? **D**—7·2 kg? **E**—7·4 kg?

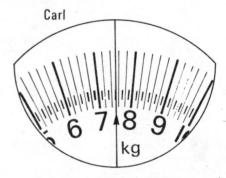

24. CARL is being weighed on bathroom scales. He weighs—
A—6·25 kg? **B**—7·0 kg? **C**—7·1 kg? **D**—7·5 kg? **E**—7·8 kg?

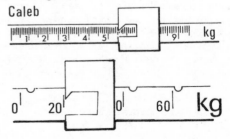

25. CALEB is being weighed on a balance with two beams. He weighs—
A—$5\frac{1}{2}$ kg? **B**—20 kg? **C**—23·8 kg? **D**—25 kg? **E**—25·5 kg?

A.3. MCQs EASY
Questions from all over the microplan Code 1

1. A child should START to eat porridge (any soft food) when he reaches the age of—
A 4 to 5 months? **B** 2 to 3 months? **C** 5 to 7 months? **D** 1 to 2 months? (7.2)

2. A child should breast feed—
A—until he has teeth? **B**—until he is eating mixed food? **C**—until he starts to walk? **D**—until his mother becomes pregnant? **E**— until he is 18 months old or more? (7.2)

3. What is the best time between each child in a poor family?
A One year **B** Two years **C** Three years or more (5.25)

4. Artificial (bottle) feeding should be—
A—prevented as much as possible? **B**—taught to all mothers? **C**—advertised in clinics? (26.14)

5. Which of these would you tell poor village mothers to add to rice to make it a better food for young children?
A Maize **B** Wheat **C** Powdered full-cream milk **D** Beans **E** Meat (6.2)

6. A child CANNOT be immunized against—
A—tetanus? **B**—TB? **C**—polio? **D**—tonsillitis? **E**—whooping cough? (Chapter 4)

7. Which of these is an antibiotic?
A Aspirin **B** Benzyl benzoate **C** Penicillin **D** Crystal (gentian) violet **E** Piperazine (3.11)

8. The most important presenting symptom of TB in children is—
A—cough with blood in the sputum? **B**—loss of weight? **C**—chest pain? **D**—diarrhoea? **E**—wheezing? (13.1)

9. The most important treatment for a child with acute watery diarrhoea is—
A—no solid food until his stools are solid? **B**—antibiotics? **C**—more fluids? **D**—as little fluid as possible? **E**—drugs to make his stools solid? (9.20)

10. Most of the children who come to a clinic with coughs—
A—need an antibiotic? **B**—have lower respiratory infections? **C**—have TB? **D**—are seriously ill? **E**—need cough mixture only? (8.5)

11. Penicillin is useful for treating—
A—thrush? **B**—a large boil with spreading infection round it? **C**—worms? **D**—diarrhoea caused by drinking dirty water? **E**—colds? (11.5)

12. BAMBANG is breast-fed and is given milk from a bottle. The flow of milk in his mother's breasts would become LESS if she—
A—expressed her breast milk? **B**—used a breast-pump? **C**—used a nipple-shield? **D**—let him suck from her breasts less often? **E**—stopped his bottle-feed? (26–9)

13. Which of these makes the LEAST good porridge for a young child?
A Millet **B** Cassava **C** Wheat **D** Rice **E** Maize (7.2)

14. These are the weights of four children. They were 15 months old when they were first weighed. They were 18 months old when they were next weighed. Which of them has had the worst nutrition?
A SAPPHO first weighing 12 kg, second weighing 12·5 kg **B** ZWONKO 10 kg, 10 kg **C** MORO 11 kg, 10 kg **D** HERO 7 kg, 8 kg (7.1)

15. If you do not sterilize needles and syringes before you give injections, you may cause—
A—anaemia? **B**—pneumonia? **C**—TB? **D**—jaundice? (22.11)

16. HUGO (2 years, 39·5°C) has had a cough and fever for 3 days. Which of these would you do FIRST?
A Cool him with water **B** Give him cough mixture **C** Give him penicillin **D** Give him fluids to drink **E** Cover him with warm clothes (10.3)

17. A child who needs an antibiotic needs it for—
B—one day only? **C**—two weeks? **D**—one month? **E**—at least three days? (3.13)

18. The earliest sign of dehydration is—
A—a fast pulse? **B**—a sunken fontanelle? **C**—thirst? **D**—sunken eyes? **E**—loss of skin elasticity? (9.17)

19. About how many glasses (or cups) contain a litre of water?
A 2 **B** 3 **C** 4 **D** 5 **E** 6 (9.22)

20. Which of these children needs penicillin?
A BOSCO with constipation. **B** NIKKO who is breathing fast (70 times a minute). **C** SALKO with malaria. **D** PITO with thirst, a dry mouth, and a sunken fontanelle. **E** LUPO who is bottle-fed and losing weight. (8.21)

21. DELPHINE (3 years) has a large swollen painful red lesion on her knee and some tender lumps in her groin. These lumps are a sign that—
A—she has had her disease a long time? **B**—the swelling on her knee should be opened to let out the pus? **C**—she will soon recover? **D**—viruses are infecting her? **E**—her disease is spreading in her body? (2.4)

22. FRITZ (2 years) has had a fit. The most serious possible cause of his fit is—

A—meningitis? **B**—fever? **C**—tonsillitis? **D**—whooping cough? **E**—measles? (15.6)

23. To make salt-and-sugar water, a mother should measure one litre of water and add—

A—eight level teaspoonfuls of salt and one level teaspoonful of sugar? **B**—one level teaspoonful of salt and eight level teaspoonfuls of sugar? **C**—one heaped teaspoonful of salt and one heaped teaspoonful of sugar? **D**—eight heaped teaspoonfuls of salt and one heaped teaspoonful of sugar? **E**—one heaped teaspoonful of salt and eight level teaspoonfuls of sugar? (9.22)

24. SALVATORE (3 years) has fever and pain in his ear for one day. He probably has an infection of his—

A—middle ear? **B**—outer ear? **C**—inner ear? **D**—mastoid? **E**—skull? (17.9)

25. The most serious cause of abdominal pain and vomiting is—

A—a gut infection? **B**—constipation? **C**—an acute abdomen (peritonitis)? **D**—worms? **E**—pneumonia? (20.2)

A.4 MCQs VARIED
A variety of questions from all over the microplan Code 1

PEDRO (2 years, 7·5 kg) came to the clinic with a mild cough. He has white foamy (bubbly) lesions on both his sclerae at the outer sides of his eyes. The conjunctivae of both his eyes look dry and wrinkled (folded). He is still breast-fed and eats rice and salt twice a day. All your vitamins are finished. He needs more protein and energy food, and—

1. A.—green leaves? **B**—penicillin injections? **C**—cough mixture? **D**—to stop breast feeding? **E**—chlortetracycline eye ointment? (16.14)

NIZAR (3 years, 13 kg) is the son of a rich farmer and has a rising growth curve. He came to the clinic yesterday with a mild sore throat, a temperature of 38 °C, and no other signs. He was given two sulphonamide tablets, three vitamin B tablets, an injection of procaine penicillin, an injection of 'Pyramidon' (amidopyrine), and a small bag of dried skim milk. No health education was given. Today, he has a rash of itchy 1 cm red papules over most of his body. The middle of each papule is paler than its outer part. Which of these things did he need yesterday?

2. A Sulphadimidine. **B** Vitamin B. **C** Procaine penicillin. **D** 'Pyramidon' (amidopyrine injection). **E** None of these things. (3.10, 7.6)

His rash is most likely to have been caused by—

3. A—measles? **B**—vitamin B? **C**—penicillin? **D**—milk? **E**—scabies? (3.15)

4. AMARJEET is two months old. She is breast-fed and her mother has plenty of milk. AMARJEET should be having—

A—breast milk only? **B**—breast milk and fruits? **C**—breast milk and rice porridge? **D**—breast milk and vitamin tablets? **E**—breast milk and fruit juice? (7.2)

RANI (9 years) has just been given an injection of procaine penicillin because she has a cold. A few minutes after the injection she became very ill. She fell down, she had great difficulty breathing, she wheezed and she went blue. She has often had penicillin before but this is the first time this has happened. She is still wheezing and is very ill. She needs—

5. A—ephedrine tablets? **B**—phenobarbitone? **C**—an intramuscular antihistamine injection? **D**—subcutaneous adrenalin? **E**—more penicillin? (3.2)

SUSNIATI (21 years). The doctor is late this morning because he has been to the funeral of Miss Susniati who used to work at the clinic. She fell off her new motor scooter a week ago on a muddy road and cut her foot. She was unconscious for a few minutes but soon woke up. During the last three days she has been unable to open her mouth. She had strong spasms of her muscles. Her head and back bent backwards and the corners of her mouth bent downwards. Treatment could not help her and she died. Her death could have been prevented by—

6. A—early treatment for meningitis? **B**—polio vaccine? **C**—subcutaneous chloroquine? **D**—tetanus toxoid? **E**—BCG vaccine? (18.16)

7. A moderately dehydrated child with diarrhoea who is able to drink should if possible be given a fluid containing—

A—potassium chlorate? **B**—sodium carbonate? **C**—potassium chloride? **D**—potassium bicarbonate? **E**—sodium citrate? (9.21)

8. The simplest way of diagnosing pneumonia in a young child is to—

A—take a history from his mother? **B**—look at the way he breathes? **C**—listen to his lungs with a stethoscope? **D**—tap his chest to see if it sounds solid? **E**—send him for a chest X-ray? (8.9)

9. Which of these drugs do we usually give for the longest time?

A Isoniazid **B** Iron **C** Dapsone **D** Niclosamide **E** Tiabendazole (3.24)

10. RAM'S mother brings him to the clinic every month. Which of these things should we do on every visit?

A Give him dried skim milk **B** Keep a record of his symptoms in the clinic **C** Tell his mother she is doing something wrong **D** Immunize him **E** Weigh him (4.13)

11. Which of these is the most important thing to look for on a child's weight chart?

A Where he is on his weight chart. **B** Whether his growth curve is rising or falling, or staying the same. **C** Whether he is on the 'road to health' or not. **D** How many times he has been weighed. **E** When he first came to the clinic. (7.1)

RAMADAN (4 years). His urine is red and he is passing very little urine. His eyelids are slightly swollen. There are red cells, casts, and protein in his urine. He has no dysuria or frequency. Ten days ago he had fever and a sore throat. He has—

12. **A**—a urinary infection? **B**—schistosomiasis? **C**—the nephrotic syndrome? **D**—acute nephritis? **E**—a stone in his bladder? 23.7)

Which of these would help him?

13. **A** An operation on his bladder **B** Penicillin for ten days **C** Niridazole **D** Trying to pass urine lying on his back **E** Sulphadimidine for two weeks (23.7)

14. Here is a list of symptoms—pallor, sleepiness, sucking weakly or 'not sucking', not gaining weight, abdominal swelling, diarrhoea, vomiting, fits, jaundice and cyanotic attacks. If a one month old baby showed several of these symptoms at the same time his probable diagnosis would be—

A—pneumonia? **B**—bronchitis? **C**—septicaemia? **D**—tetanus? **E**—gastroenteritis? (26.24)

15. Here are five diseases—1. Severe conjunctivitis on the second day of life. 2. Impetigo of the newborn. 3. Urinary infection in a two-year-old boy. 4. Vulvovaginitis in a three-year-old girl. 5. Umbilical sepsis followed by septicaemia.

Which of them are most likely to be caused by gonococci?

A 1 and 2 **B** 2 and 5 **C** 2 and 3 **D** 1 and 4 (26.40, 26.47, 23.4, 23.10, 26—36)

16. Which of these children LEAST needs urgent treatment?

A LEON (12 months, 7 kg) who has giardiasis. **B** GEISHA (3 weeks old) who has a skin rash with large vesicles. **C** SRI with kwashiorkor and diarrhoea. **D** DIO with xerophthalmia and a small corneal ulcer. **E** GOTA (2 months old) who is not sucking and has a swollen fontanelle. (7.10, 16.13, 15.6, 7.9, 9.6, 26.47)

17. A child with kwashiorkor always has—

A—a large liver? **B**—a weight below the road to health? **C**—abnormal hair? **D**—a skin rash? **E**—oedema? (7.10)

18. VYANAKATESH (2 years) has been pulling and scratching his right ear for a week. It is discharging pus. Moving his ear is painful. He looks 'well', eats well, hears well with his right ear, and has had no fever. Unfortunately you have no auriscope. He probably has—

A—acute otitis media? **B**—chronic otitis media? **C**—otitis externa? **D**—a foreign body in his ear? **E**—allergy? (17.9)

19. Fever or vomiting or fits might be the presenting symptom with any of these diseases EXCEPT one. Which one?

A Tonsillitis **B** Otitis media **C** Cerebral malaria **D** Tetanus **E** Meningitis (18.16, 20.15)

20. Which of these is the most dangerous antibiotic for a preterm baby?

A Penicillin **B** Chloramphenicol **C** Streptomycin **D** Ampicillin **E** Tetracycline (3.18)

21. Which of these is NOT true. A nasogastric drip can—

A—be used in children who are vomiting? **B**—be given in a child's home? **C**—be given with glucose–salt solution? **D**—sometimes be used to treat severe dehydration? **E**—be safely given to an unconscious child? (9.24, 9.27)

22. If you were only allowed one of these for treating severe diarrhoea, which would you choose?

A Glucose–salt solution **B** Sulphadimidine **C** Salt, sugar, and water **D** Neomycin **E** Chloramphenicol (9.30)

23. Which of these children is most likely to have lactose intolerance?

A GÖRAN (15 months, 7 kg) who has severe watery diarrhoea. He has stopped breast feeding and is not given any milk. **B** BOGE (1 year, 6 kg) who has watery diarrhoea. He is bottle fed with dried skim milk. **C** GOVEA (4 weeks) who sometimes brings up a few mouthfuls of milk after a feed. Otherwise he is healthy. **D** WARI (4 years, 15 kg, 37·6 °C) who has had soft blood-stained stools for two weeks and who has no signs of dehydration. **E** SISIA (3 years, 12 kg, 38 °C) with soft bubbly stools. She does not drink milk and has not been given any dried skim milk. (9.29)

24. A primary care worker is LEAST able to treat a child who has—

A—an intussusception? **B**—swallowed 20 iron tablets half an hour ago? **C**—a prolapse of his rectum? **D**—a foreign body in his ear? **E**—fractured his upper arm (humerus) during birth? (9.15, 25.7)

25. Which of these children needs a lumbar puncture?

A MARY (8 years, 37·2 °C) who has had fits for several years. **B** MARIA (10 days, 37·4 °C) who has not been sucking well for two days and is having muscle spasms which bend her backwards. **C** MARYLOU (1 year, 38·6 °C) who has not been well for two days and had a fit this morning. **D** MARYAN (1 day, 36 °C) who was born after a difficult labour. She will not suck and has no Moro reflex. (15.9)

A.5 OVERALL PRETEST
Questions from all over the manual Code 5

1. Bacteria which look like very small balls are called—

A—protozoa? **B**—viruses? **C**—bacilli? **D**—spirochaetes? **E**—cocci? (2.2)

2. Which of these ways of treating a child with severe skin sepsis and cellulitis does NOT give him enough antibiotic for long enough?

A Ampicillin four times a day for three days. **B** Two ml of procaine penicillin into each buttock and then sulphadimidine tablets for three days. **C** One ordinary dose of procaine penicillin. **D** One dose of benethamine ('depot') penicillin. **E** Benzyl penicillin four times a day for three days. (3.13)

3. What kind of immunity protects the child of an

immune mother from measles or malaria until he is about six months old?

A Natural active immunity **B** Artifical passive immunity **C** Artificial active immunity **D** Natural passive immunity (4.2)

4. I would use penicillin to treat—

A —malaria? **B** —otitis media? **C** —headache? **D** —a sprained ankle? **E** —infective hepatitis (3.15)

5. Which of these is NOT a sign of marasmus?

A A thin 'old man's face' **B** No fat under the skin **C** Very low weight for age **D** Thin wasted muscles **E** Oedema (7.9)

6. MONTY (3 years) has had a cough for about ten days. He now coughs in spasms. After a spasm of coughing he makes a loud noise as he breathes in and then vomits. Which of these would have prevented his disease?

A Boiling his drinking water **B** Penicillin injections **C** More protein and energy food **D** DPT vaccine **E** BCG vaccine (8.17)

7. Which of these would you examine last?

A A child's skin **B** His nutrition **C** His throat **D** His tonsillar lymph nodes **E** His breathing (5.16)

8. APITON (3 years, 15 kg) has had diarrhoea for a week. He is bottle-fed. His mother gave him salt-and-sugar water. She put eight level teaspoonfuls of salt and one level teaspoonful of sugar in five cups of water. Last night he started to have fits. He is drowsy and irritable, and his mouth is dry, but his skin elasticity feels normal. He will not drink. Lumbar puncture shows clear CSF. Which of these is true?

A He has been given too much salt (hypernatraemic dehydration). **B** He has been given too much sugar. **C** He can easily be rehydrated by mouth. **D** He has meningitis. **E** He is only mildly dehydrated. (9.18, 9.22)

9. The rectal temperature of a healthy child is between—

A—35 and 36 °C? **B**—36·0 and 37·5 °C? **C**—37·5 and 38 °C? **D**—38·5 and 39 °C? **E**—39 and 39·5 °C? (10.1)

10. The best way for a child's mother to treat pyoderma at home is to—

A—wash the lesions in permanganate solution? **B**—wash the lesions in water? **C**—put sulphonamide ointment on the lesions? **D**—wash the lesions in lysol? **E**—put oil on the lesions? (11.6)

11. Which of these children has certainly NOT got leprosy?

A ESPINA with a hot, red, swollen lesion **B** ELINA with an anaesthetic lesion **C** ELENESTO with several large hypopigmented (pale) lesions **D** EVELINA with several large chronic patches **E** ESINETI with tender thickened nerves (12.3)

12. MAURICE (7 years) has TB meningitis. He was probably infected by—

A—another child at school? **B**—an adult with a chronic cough? **C**—an adult with TB meningitis? **D**—eating infected food? **E**—his younger sister who has been coughing for two weeks? (13.3)

13. CONCETTA (5 years) has just been hit by a car. She is weak, cold and pale and her pulse is 140. There are some large bruises on her body. The nearest hospital is many miles away. Which of these things might help her most?

A An injection of adrenaline **B** Oral glucose–salt solution **C** Being nursed sitting up **D** A nasogastric drip **E** Intravenous fluid (14.2)

14. If a child's CSF looks very mildly turbid, and is not blood-stained, you can be sure he has—

A—more than 1000 pus cells in each microlitre of CSF? **B**—virus meningitis? **C**—meningitis? **D**—TB meningitis? **E**—cerebral malaria? (15.6)

15. N'SOUGAN (3 years) has very severe conjunctivitis with much swelling of the eyelids. You should treat him as if it was—

A—impetigo of the newborn? **B**—septicaemia? **C**—a corneal ulcer? **D**—caused by gonococci? **E**—trachoma? (16.8)

16. The healthy ear drum—

A—is pink? **B**—has blood on one side of it and bone on the other side? **C**—has air on one side only? **D**—has the maleus at the bottom of the drum? **E**—has air on both sides of it? (17.2)

17. In young children acute sore throats may present with any of these symptoms EXCEPT—

A—being unable to pass urine? **B**—fits? **C**—abdominal pain? **D**—vomiting? **E**—coughing? (18.1)

18. Where would you MOST expect to find a swelling caused by oedema?

A—over the front of the neck? **B**—at the side of the neck? **C**—over the wrists? **D**—over the ankles? **E**—on the scalp? (19.7)

19. Which of these does NOT cause abdominal swelling?

A Malnutrition **B** Urine infection **C** Heavy infections with *Ascaris* **D** Gut obstruction **E** A very large spleen (20.8)

20. A child most often infects himself with hookworms by—

A—sucking toys which have fallen on infected ground? **B**—eating food which flies have walked on? **C**—walking on ground where an infected person has passed his faeces? **D**—scratching his anus and sucking his fingers? **E**—drinking dirty water? (21.1)

21. Each red cell lives for—

A—about 12 days? **B**—the rest of a child's life? **C**—about 120 days? **D**—about one day? **E**—about 12 months? (22.1)

22. Gums which have become sore because a baby's teeth are coming through can cause—

A—fits? **B**—diarrhoea? **C**—fever? **D**—bronchitis? **E**—none of these things? (25.2c)

23. Contractures are LEAST likely to happen in children who have—

A—severe malnutrition? **B**—polio? **C**—severe burns of their arms and legs? **D**—had a fracture? **E**—tuberculoid leprosy? (7.9, 12.1, 14.3, 24.4)

24. ZACHARY has a cephalhaematoma. What would you do?

A Send him to hospital **B** Inject penicillin **C** Remove the blood from the swelling with a needle **D** Give him vitamin K and leave the swelling to go by itself **E** Put hot compresses on the swelling (26.4)

25. Urinary infections do NOT present as—
A—fever? **B**—coughing? **C**—fever and vomiting? **D**—a child wetting herself (or himself) after she has become dry? **E**—dysuria? (23.4)

A.6 INSTRUMENT—
Breast- and bottle-feeding

What do you think about the way babies should be fed? Take a pencil and paper and write 1 to 20 down the left hand side. Read the sentences and write 'Agree' or 'Disagree' to each of them (Guide 4.7).

(1) **We should advertise bottle feeding in our clinics.**
(2) **We should teach all mothers how to bottle feed their children.**
(3) **When a mother has plenty of breast-milk and is giving her child a bottle we should encourage her to stop breast-feeding and go on bottle feeding.**
(4) **Breast-feeding over the age of one year causes malnutrition.**
(5) **Most children in poor families need extra milk in a bottle.**
(6) **All mothers should breast-feed their children at special times by the clock.**
(7) **Mothers should not breast-feed when they are pregnant.**
(8) **Bottle-feeding is one of the best things that have come with 'modern life'.**
(9) **Poor mothers usually don't have enough breast milk for their babies.**
(10) **Bottle-feeding is useful because it stops a mother's breasts from losing their shape.**
(11) **I am going to breast-feed my children (Or encourage my wife to breast-feed them.)**
(12) **Breast-feeding is the natural way of feeding a child.**
(13) **I think breast-milk alone is usually enough for a child until he is about four months old.**
(14) **Mothers should not be ashamed to breast-feed in public if they have to.**
(15) **Breast-feeding makes a child feel happy and safe.**
(16) **Breast-fed babies get a better start in life.**
(17) **If the child of a poorer village mother is not breast-fed he will probably die.**
(18) **Breast milk can provide about half the protein and energy food a child needs in the second year of his life..**
(19) **Breast-fed children get less diarrhoea than bottle-fed children.**
(20) **If a baby has diarrhoea, his mother should continue breast-feeding him.**

PRETEST MULTIPLE-CHOICE QUESTIONS
OF THE 'CHAPTER SERIES'

DIFFICULT WORDS PRETEST A
Chapter 1: Code 5

1. When we measure how good or how bad something is we—
A—describe it? **B**—record it? **C**—observe it? **D**—notice it? **E**—evaluate it?

2. Which of these is NOT in the thorax?
A Oesophagus **B** Heart **C** Kidneys **D** Lungs **E** The pleural cavities

3. Which of these is a part of the eye?
A Urethra **B** Pharynx **C** Groin **D** Sclera **E** Meninges

4. Which of these is NOT in the abdomen?
A Stomach **B** Pharynx **C** Ureters **D** Bladder **E** Spleen

MATCH these words with the explanation for them—
5. Reduce **6.** Destroy **7.** Increase **8.** Notice **9.** Describe
A See **B** Explain **C** Make larger **D** Break or spoil **E** Make smaller

10. The lips of a cyanosed child are—
A—blue? **B**—yellow? **C**—red? **D**—black? **E**—white?

MATCH each of these with its opposite—
11. Expiration **12.** Relaxation **13.** Negative **14.** General **15.** Painless when touched.
A Inspiration **B** Contraction **C** Local **D** Tender **E** Positive

MATCH each of these with the example of it—
16. Symptom **17.** Complication **18.** Lesion **19.** Sign **20.** Disease
A Hand infection following a cut finger **B** A spleen which can easily be felt **C** Whooping cough **D** An abscess **E** Chest pain

21. Which of these describes the order in which urine flows down the urinary system?
A Kidneys, urethra, bladder, ureter **B** Kidneys, bladder, urethras, ureter **C** Kidneys, ureters, bladder, urethra.

22. A rash which is different on the right and left sides of the body is—

A—general? B—symmetrical? C—gross? D—severe? E—asymmetrical?

23. ANGEL (4 years) was brought by her mother to see you because she has a severe cough. She also has a headache. While she is in the clinic she vomits. When you examine her you find she is anaemic and has some scabies lesions. You diagnose whooping cough and scabies. Her presenting symptom is—
A—cough? B—vomiting? C—whooping cough? D—anaemia? E—scabies?

24. Which of these can only be a symptom and not a sign?
A Anaemia B Scabies C Cough D Headache E Vomiting

25. Which of these words would you use when there is very very much of something, or it is very big?
A Mild B Gross C Moderate D Severe E Doubtful

DISEASE IN THE CHILD A
Chapter 2: Code 2

1. Which of these is the LEAST common cause of disease in children?
A Accidents B Malnutrition C Infection D Tumours E Behaviour diseases (2.1)

2. Which of these is a hereditary disease?
A Iron deficiency anaemia B Whooping cough C TB D Pneumonia E Sickle-cell anaemia (2.1)

3. Which of these is NOT caused by a virus?
A Boils B Polio C Chickenpox D Measles E Herpes simplex (2.2)

4. BABATUNDE has whooping cough. He was infected by—
A—faeces? B—organisms getting into him through his skin? C—droplets? D—by an insect? E—by contact? (2.7)

5. Which of these MUST be completely sterile before they are used?
A Thermometers B Needles used for injection or lumbar puncture C Tongue depressors D Oral glucose saline E An auriscope (2.2b)

6. Septicaemia—
A—does not kill babies? B—is caused by bacteria growing in the blood? C—is usually a chronic disease? D—cannot be treated with penicillin? E—is caused by viruses growing in the blood? (2.4)

7. Which of these is a local symptom of an acute infection?
A Fever B A slow pulse C An 'ill' child D Pain E Not eating (2.4)

8. KUMASO (4 years, 38·5 °C) has a large warm, red tender swelling near his umbilicus. He also has lymphadenitis, lymphangitis, and fever. What kind of organism is causing these lesions?
A Bacteria B Viruses C Protozoa D Fungi E Larvae (2.4, 19–1)

9. KUMASO has signs which show that—
A—he is in no danger from septicaemia? B—he does not need an antibiotic? C—the organisms are spreading beyond his local lesion? D—he is infected by more than one kind of organism? E—he needs local treatment only? (2.4)

10. Which of these drugs could NOT kill the organisms which are causing Kumaso's lesions?
A Sulphadimidine B Penicillin C Tetracycline D Chloramphenicol E Tetrachlorethylene (TCE) (2.4)

11. TB—
A—can cause lesions in many parts of the body? B—is an acute disease? C—causes septicaemia? D—can be treated with penicillin? E—causes acute inflammation? (2.6)

12. Larvae are—
A—a stage in the life-cycle of the malaria parasite? B—bacteria which are going to die? C—old worms? D—young worms? E—a kind of virus? (2.7)

MATCH the following words with the explanation for them—
13. Lymph **14.** Lymphangitis **15.** Lymphadenitis **16.** Cellulitis
A A clear fluid that is formed in the tissue and goes back into the blood. B Inflammation of the lymph nodes. C Spreading inflammation in the tissues. D Inflammation of the lymph vessels. (2.4)

17. Bacteria which look like very small balls are called—
A—protozoa? B—viruses? C—bacilli? D—spirochaetes? E—cocci? (2.2)

MATCH these things with the diseases they prevent—
18. Wearing shoes **19.** Boiling water for ten minutes **20.** Immunization **21.** Plenty of washing with soap and water
A Pneumonia B Skin sepsis C Hookworm anaemia D Syringe abscesses E Whooping cough (2.7)

22. In some hot districts people put many clothes on a child with a fever. This is—
A—a bad custom? B—a good custom? C—a harmless custom? (2.9)

23. KANTUN has secondarily infected ringworm. What kind of organism is causing the primary infection?
A Fungus B Bacteria C Virus D Protozoa E Worms (2.6)

24. What kind of organism is causing KANTUN'S secondary infection?
A Fungus B Bacteria C Virus D Protozoa E Worms (2.6)

25. Which of the organisms that are infecting KANTUN can be killed by drugs?
B The primary organism C The secondary organism D Neither organism E Both organisms (2.6, 11.13)

DRUGS A
Chapter 3: Code 5

1. Which of these drugs or pairs of drugs does NOT work as a broad spectrum antibiotic?

A Penicillin and sulphadimidine **B** Penicillin and streptomycin **C** Tetracycline **D** Chloramphenicol **E** Penicillin (3.13)

2. Which of these is most likely to harm the white cells in a child's blood so seriously that he dies?

A Tetracycline **B** Isoniazid **C** Chloramphenicol **D** Penicillin **E** Streptomycin (3.18)

3. Which of these pairs of drugs can be used for suppressing malaria?

B Paracetamol or chloramphenicol **C** Tetrachlorethylene or tetracycline **D** Pyrimethamine or chloroquine **E** Aminosalicylate or thiacetazone (3.25)

4. Which of these is used to treat poisoning by causing vomiting?

A Benzyl benzoate **B** Ipecacuanha **B** Paraldehyde **D** Thiabendazole **E** Niclosamide (3.47)

MATCH these diseases or symptoms with the drugs that are used to treat them—

5. Fever **6.** Asthma **7.** Tapeworms **8.** TB **9.** Malaria

A Thiacetazone **B** Quinine **C** Niclosamide **D** Adrenalin **E** Aspirin (3.22, 3.25, 3.30, 3.40, 3.41)

10. GWEMBE has thrush. Which of these could you use to treat him?

A Gentian Violet **B** Terramycin **C** Penicillin **D** Chloramphenicol **E** Tetracycline (3.48, 18.15)

MATCH these diseases or symptoms with the drugs you would use to treat them.

11. Acute septic infections **12.** TB **13.** Pain **14.** Leprosy **15.** Hookworm infection

A Penicillin **B** Isoniazid **C** Dapsone **D** TCE (tetrachlorethylene) **E** Paracetamol (3.14, 3.24, 3.20, 3.27, 3.42)

MATCH these diseases or symptoms with the drugs you would use to treat them.

16. Severe dehydration **17.** Scabies **18.** Ringworm **19.** Fever **20.** *Trichuris* infection (3.29, 3.32, 3.42, 3.48)

A Benzyl benzoate **B** Paracetamol **C** Tiabendazole **D** Benzoic acid ointment **E** Darrow's solution (3.9)

21. Which of these would you give to a child as tablets?

A TCE (tetrachlorethylene) **B** Paraldehyde **C** Dapsone **D** Benzyl benzoate **E** Ipecacuanha (3.24)

22. About how much does an ordinary cup contain?

A 100 ml **B** 500 ml **C** 300 ml **D** 400 ml **E** 200 ml (3–2)

23. Which of these should be used in a children's clinic?

A Placebo cough mixture **B** Anabolic steroids **C** 'Pyramidon' (antipyrine) **D** Kaolin **E** Vitamin B_{12} (3.9)

24. CLAUDE (20 kg) needs ethambutol. The dose is 25 mg/kg/day and it has to be given four times a day. How much will he need at each dose?

A 500 mg **B** 100 mg **C** 50 mg **D** 125 mg **E** 250 mg

25. Which of these should be given to a child by mouth?

A Benzyl penicillin **B** Tetrachlorethylene **C** Potassium permanganate **D** Benzyl benzoate **E** Gamma benzene hexachloride (3.27)

HEALTHY CHILD A
Chapter 4: Code 6

1. Which of these is NOT true?

A Put newly arrived vaccine at the back of the refrigerator behind the vaccine you already have. **B** If an ampoule of vaccine is not used at the end of the day, you must throw it away. **C** You can store vaccines in the door of a refrigerator. **D** Keep polio and measles vaccine frozen solid. **E** DPT vaccine is harmed if it is frozen solid. (4.10)

2. Which of these vaccines is killed most quickly if it becomes warm?

A Measles **B** Polio **C** DPT **D** BCG (4.3)

3. Which of these children LEAST need to be put on the special care register? The child—

A—who is one of twins? **B**—whose father has TB? **C**—whose brothers and sisters have died? **D**—whose mother has difficulty with bottle-feeding? **E**—who is breast-fed? (4.14, 6.3)

4. A mother who brings a healthy child to the clinic may need all these things EXCEPT one. Which one?

A Praise for something which is good **B** Blame for anything that is wrong **C** Advice about family planning **D** Explanation about her child's weight **E** Being seen by the same worker each time she comes to the clinic? (4.13, 4.14)

5. Which of these vaccines is given by intradermal injection?

B Measles **C** BCG **D** Polio **E** DPT (4.6)

6. Vaccines must be—

A—given with syringes which have been sterilized in spirit? **B**—reconstituted with water for injection? **C**—kept in the sun as much as possible? **D**—only be given to well nourished children? **E**—given while they are still effective? (4.10)

7. Which of these contains antibodies?

A BCG vaccine **B** DPT vaccine **C** Measles vaccine **D** Tetanus antitoxin **E** Polio vaccine (4.2)

8. Which of these gives a child an artificial passive immunity? An injection of—

A—BCG vaccine? **B**—DPT vaccine? **C**—measles vaccine? **D**—tetanus antitoxin? **E**—none of these? (4.2)

9. Which of these vaccines can if necessary be given at birth?

B Measles **C** Polio **D** DPT **E** BCG (4.6)

10. Which of these has the right ages in the right order for the milestones of smiling, sitting without help, and walking?

A 6 weeks, 9 months, 18 months **B** 1 week, 9 months, 12 months **C** 6 months, 1 year, 2 years **D** 8 months, 13 months, 16 months **E** 6 months, 9 months, 18 months (4.12, 24.16)

MATCH these things with the disease they prevent—

11. Passing faeces in latrines **12.** A capsule of vitamin A every 6 months **13.** Supression with pyrimethamine **14.** Monitoring a child's growth **15.** Immunization

A Xerophthalmia **B** Hookworm anaemia **C** Malnutrition **D** Diphtheria **E** Malaria (4.1, 4.9, 4.11, 22.5)

16. Which of these vaccines causes a scar at the place where it is given?

A DPT **B** BCG **C** Measles **D** Polio (4.6)

17. Which of these kinds of immunity lasts the longest?

A Artificial passive **B** Natural active **C** Natural passive (4.2)

18. What kind of immunity does a child get from his mother when he is born?

A Natural active **B** Artificial active **C** Natural passive **D** Artificial passive (4.2)

19. JARBAS has a dirty cut on his foot and is to have tetanus antitoxin. He will become immune—

B—in a few days? **C**—in a few weeks? **D**—immediately? (4.2)

20. The immunity JARBAS gets will last—

A—a few weeks? **B**—a few months? **C**—a few years? **D**—all his life? (4.2)

MATCH these vaccines with the sentence which describes them—

21. BCG **22.** Measles **23.** DPT **24.** Polio

B A mixture of toxoids and dead bacteria **C** Given with a 1 ml tuberculin ('Microstat') syringe **D** A mixture of three live viruses **E** The most expensive vaccine (4.6, 4.8, 4.8b, 4.9)

25. Which of these children needs special care most?

A DIDI whose weight curve has been below the road to health but is rising. **B** BUDI who is on the road to health but only comes about every three months. **C** KADI who is on the road to health but had mild diarrhoea last week. **D** TITI whose weight fell last month after she had measles. **E** JADI who has *Ascaris* worms.

SICK CHILD A

Chapter 5: Code 2

1. Which of these is NOT necessary every time a child comes to a clinic on a monthly visit?

A He should be weighed. **B** His mother should be told when to bring him back again. **C** His mother should be congratulated about something. **D** His temperature should be taken. **E** A dot for his weight should be put on his weight chart. (4.13, 5.3, 5.28)

2. Which of these has the steps in caring for a sick child in the WRONG order?

A Diagnosis, management. **B** Special tests, diagnosis, management. **C** Weighing, history, examination.

D Explanation, family planning. **E** Management, explanation, weighing. (5.1)

3. When a mother gets integrated MCH care she—

A—can if necessary get antenatal care, family planning, and well- and sick-child care in the same place on the same day? **B**—gets these kinds of care from the same worker but on different days? **C**—is always cared for by the same worker? **D**—gets all the 'ten steps' the manual describes? **E**—gets hospital and health centre care? (5.2)

4. Which of these is NOT part of taking a child's history?

A Letting his mother tell you what is wrong with him in her own way. **B** Asking how much of each symptom there has been. **C** Looking at the way he breathes. **D** Asking what treatment he has had. **E** Giving her a chance to think of any other symptoms he has had. (5.6)

5. Which of these can be used as a milestone?

A Breathing **B** Walking **C** Eating **D** Sleeping **E** Lying down (5.10, 24.10)

6. Which of these is part of a child's family history?

A 'Has he been given any medicine?' **B** 'Has his uncle got a cough?' **C** 'Has he been immunized?' **D** 'Where do you get your water?' **E** 'Was his birth normal?' (5.12)

7. Which of these is NOT true? Poor children are—

A—often malnourished? **B**—more often infected? **C**—in greater need of our help? **D**—more likely to come to our clinic? **E**—more likely to die? **F**—more likely to have brothers and sisters who have died? (5.13)

8. A child is probably not ill if he is—

A—laughing? **B**—restless? **C**—irritable? **C**—sleepy? **E**—quiet? (5.15)

MATCH these diseases with the signs they cause—

9. Severe watery diarrhoea **10.** Obstructive laryngitis **11.** Jaundice **12.** Protein energy malnutrition

A Yellow eyes **B** Bitot's spots **C** Loss of skin elasticity **D** An arm circumference less than 14 cm **E** Stridor (5.17)

MATCH these specimens with the things that a health centre laboratory can find in them—

13. Urine **14.** Blood **15.** A skin scraping **16.** A stool smear

A Protein **B** AAFB **C** *Ascaris* ova **D** Sickle cells **E** Threadworms (5.19)

17. I would use penicillin to treat—

A—headache? **B**—a sprained ankle? **C**—malaria? **D**—infective hepatitis? **E**—otitis media? (17.9)

18. A child is probably well if he—

A—is irritable? **B**—cries and cannot be comforted? **C**—is hungry? **D**—is delirious? **E**—is 'floppy' (hypotonic)? (5–5)

19. Which of these is usually the FIRST sign that a child is ill?

A 'He feels cold.' **B** 'His lips look blue.' **C** 'I cannot wake him up.' **D** 'He has stopped running about and playing.' **E** 'He makes a loud noise when he breathes.' (5.15, 8.9)

20. Fast breathing is the most important sign in diagnosing—

A—obstructive laryngitis? **B**—upper respiratory infection? **C**—TB? **D**—asthma? **E**—lower respiratory infections, especially pneumonia? (5.17)

21. There are many children in your clinic and you cannot spend much time on each of them. Which of these would be the LEAST useful on every child?

A Looking to see if he is 'well' or ill **B** Feeling for his spleen **C** Asking how long he has had symptoms **D** Telling his mother how she can help him **E** Looking at his weight chart (5.27)

22. Which of these is part of a child's treatment?

A Giving him chloroquine **B** Letting him spend the night in the health centre **C** Sending him to hospital **D** Asking him to come back tomorrow **E** Sending him for a special test (5.21, 5.23)

23. Which of these things is LEAST necessary when you are examining a sick child?

A Equipment to measure his height? **B** A torch? **C** A spatula? **D** An auriscope? **E** Batteries for the torch? (5.2)

24. When you make a child's records you should—

A—only record the positive finding? **B**—record how long he has his symptoms? **C**—make two copies, one for the clinic and one for his mother? **D**—use your own special shorthand? **E**—make no records for well children? (5–20, 5.26)

25. If the birth interval is too short, breast-feeding—

A—goes on too long? **B**—is painful? **C**—starts too late? **D**—harms a child? **E**—stops too early? (5.25)

RECORDING AND REPORTING A

Chapter 6: with revision: Code 2

MATCH these signs with the kind of children who show them—

1 Eats hungrily and runs about actively **2** Looks as if he is asleep but cannot be woken up **3** Delirious **4** Irritable and restless all day

A The severely ill child **B** The tired child **C** The moderately ill child **D** The well child **E** The very severely ill child (5:2 (Revision))

5. Which of these is true?

A Everything a health worker does should be recorded and reported. **B** A clinic should only make the records and reports that are helpful in deciding something. **C** A clinic should keep as many records as possible. **D** No patient should be allowed to take his records home. **E** A health worker should wash his hands at the beginning of the clinic only. (6.1)

6. Which of these things should NOT happen to a child's weight chart? His weight chart should be—

A—used to record if he is sensitive to penicillin? **B**—kept in the clinic? **C**—kept in a plastic bag? **D**—explained to his mother? **E**—used to record his more important diseases? (6.2)

7. Which of these things is NOT true? Home-based records are useful because—

A—they can be taken to hospital if necessary? **B**—record files don't need to be searched in clinic? **C**—they help to teach patients about their own health? **D**—they are a copy of the clinic's records? **E**—a patient can take them with him when he moves to another district? (6.2)

8. A special-care register should contain—

A—the children who are at special risk? **B**—all the children in the clinic? **C**—the acutely ill children? **D**—the children from the richest families? **E**—the children who are going to recover quickly? (6.3)

9. Which of these children would you NOT put in your special-care register?

A FRANCINE (1 month) whose mother has died **B** DURGA (6 months) all of whose brothers and sisters have died C VJAY (3 years) with acute otitis media which has now healed **D** IJAKAIT whose mother has TB **E** OMONDI (3 months) whose mother has difficulty breast feeding (6.3)

10. Which of these things are NOT recorded on a child's weight chart?

A The birth dates of his brothers and sisters **B** The date of his BCG immunization **C** His address **D** Notes on family planning **E** The signs and symptoms of each illness he has (6.2, 7.1)

11. A children's tally sheet records—

A—immunizations and some diseases only? **B**—children's names? **C**—where children live? **D**—in blocks of ten 'O's which are crossed off? **E**—all the illnesses children have? (6.4)

PLEASE DON'T WRITE ON THESE QUESTIONS OTHER PEOPLE MAY NEED THEM

---

12. Which of these syringes is sterile? The syringe which has been—

A—washed through with sterile distilled water? **B**—boiled and then used for 20 children? **C**—boiled and then kept in a bowl of water since this morning? **D**—heated in steam at 120 °C for 15 minutes? **E**—washed through with spirit? (6.13)

13. Each health worker should—

A—use the same medical shorthand? **B**—use shorthand for all medical words? **C**—keep changing his shorthand? **D**—use shorthand that mothers can understand? **E**—write only in shorthand (6:1)

14. The medical shorthand for six months is—

C—6/52? **D**—6/12? **E**—6/7? (6:1)

15. Which of these show that something is normal?

A TCA **B** NAD **C** FP **D** NH **E** PN (6:1)

16. Which of these is a way of giving injections?
A PS B HW C SC D AAFB E PN (6:1)

17. A 'high patients per worker per day' score probably shows that—

A—the clinic is giving high quality care? B—most children in the district are getting the care they need? C—the output of the health workers is low? D—the clinic is a large one? E—the staff are working hard? (6.9)

18. Which of these kinds of penicillin last for the longest time in a child's body?

A Procaine penicillin B Benzyl penicillin C Benethamine or benzathine (depot) penicillin D Procaine penicillin forte (PPF) (3.15 (Revision))

19. If an infected syringe is rinsed with sterile distilled water before being used again it—

A—cannot cause jaundice? B—does not infect the distilled water? C—becomes sterile? D—may cause an injection abscess? E—can safely be used? (6.13)

20. Which of these is NOT part of integrated MCH care?

A Antenatal care B Postnatal care C Care for healthy children D Family planning E Care for school children (6.8)

21. Sterilizing in a pressure cooker is better than sterilizing by boiling because—

A—the syringes stay sterile longer? B—it uses less fuel? C—it kills fewer organisms? D—it does not harm any kind of plastic? E—uses more water? (6.13)

22. Which of these kills organisms fastest?

A Steam at 1 kg/cm^2 in a pressure cooker B Lysol solution C Boiling water D Hot water E Ice (6.13)

23. When water is boiled in an open pan the highest temperature it can reach is about—

A—100 °C? B—120 °C? C—200 °C? D—1000 °C? E—1080 °C? (6.13)

24. Five minutes in steam at 120 °C kills—

A—all organisms? B—most harmful organisms? C—bacteria only? D—viruses only? (6.13)

25. A pressure cooker should be opened—

B—while it is still on the stove? C—while the weight is still keeping the steam in? D—while it is still hot? E—after it has cooled? (6.13)

MALNUTRITION A
Chapter 7: Code 5

1. A healthy one-year-old child should weigh about—
A—5 kg? B—12 kg C—7 kg? D—14 kg? E—10 kg? (N 1.1)

2. The best way of monitoring a child's growth is to take monthly measurements of his—
A—arm circumference? B—length? C—weight? D—height? (4.1, 7.1)

3. A child's arm circumference should be measured—
A—with his arm bent? B—with the tape so tight that his skin is wrinkled? C—on his right arm? D—in the middle of his left arm half way between his elbow and his shoulder? E—as high up his arm as possible? (7.1 N 1.6b)

4. Which of these is NOT true?

A A sick child is not completely recovered until he has regained the weight he lost while he was ill. B Until a sick child's symptoms have gone he should be given fluids only. C Severe measles makes a child's mouth sore. D Sick children usually don't eat normally. E When a child has a fever the protein in his body is broken down faster than normal. (7.2)

5. GLORIA (36 months, 9 kg) is very thin. There is very little fat under her skin. Her legs are swollen with oedema and her skin is peeling. Which of these is the best diagnosis for her?

A Keratomalacia B 'Underweight child' C Kwashiorkor D Marasmus E Marasmic kwashiorkor (7.10)

6. Kwashiorkor—

A—is usually more common than marasmus? B—usually makes children very hungry? C—comes on more slowly than marasmus? D—should be treated with high-protein high-energy feeds? E—only happens in children who are below the road-to-health? (7.10)

7. Lack of vitamins causes—
A—kwashiorkor? B—marasmus? C—pellagra? D—goitre? E—caries? (N 4.4)

8. Which of these children is in the GREATEST danger from kwashiorkor? The child whose growth curve—

A—was above the upper line, but lost 3 kg after an attack of measles? B—is above the lower line and is rising slowly? C—is between the lines and has been flat for two months? D—has always been below the lower line and is rising slowly? (7.1)

9. Breast-feeding—

A—causes diarrhoea more often than bottle-feeding? B—gives a 2-month-old baby all the protein and energy food he needs? C—does not contain enough vitamin C so he should have fruit juice? D—must be done at special times by the clock each day? E—should stop before a child is a year old? (7.2 N Chapter 7)

10. Which of these is the best (most complete) meal?

A Maize, dried beans, and spinach? B Sago and mangoes? C Rice, green beans, and onions? D Sweet potatoes, coconut, and banana? E Cassava, pumpkin leaves, and pawpaw? (N Chapter 6)

11. Which of these contains the most protein and thus makes the best porridge for a young child?

A Maize B Cassava C Sago D Plantains (bananas) E Sweet potatoes (7.4)

12. An artificially fed child—

A—gets fewer infections than a breast-fed child? B—must have his bottle sterilized after each feed? C—should be fed with sweetened condensed milk? D—passes softer stools than a breast-fed child? E—costs less to feed than a breast-fed child? (N Chapter 8)

13. All these things EXCEPT one help to cause kwashiorkor in a child. Which one?

A Being sent away from his mother to live with a relative **B** Starting porridge too late **C** Measles **D** Several attacks of diarrhoea **E** Going on breast feeding too long (7.10)

14. Which of these is best for sterilizing a feeding bottle?

A Iodine **B** Permanganate **C** Hypochlorite **D** Lysol **E** Soap and water (N 8–7)

15. Young children usually fall off the road-to-health because—

A—they are breast fed for too long? **B**—they do not get enough vitamins? **C**—their mothers are malnourished? **D**—they are not given porridge often enough or early enough? (7.4)

16. To prevent malnutrition we must teach poor mothers to give their children—

A—powdered milk every day? **B**—eggs three times a week? **C**—more meat and fish? **D**—rice instead of maize? **E**—legumes (beans and groundnuts) and a good staple food? (7.2)

MATCH these diseases with the things that prevent them?

17. Diarrhoea **18.** Caries **19.** Goitre **20.** Anaemia

A Breast-feeding **B** Iodine **C** Iron **D** Fluoride **E** Vitamin A (N 4.4)

21. Which of these would you teach village mothers about?

A Vitamins **B** Amino acids **C** Salt-and-sugar water **D** Reference protein **E** Aflatoxin (N 10:11)

22. Which of these is NOT true? Tube feeding—

A—is useful for treating severely malnourished children? **B**—is useful for children who won't eat? **C**—can be done by mothers? **D**—can be done at home? **E**—must be done with sterile feed? (7.12)

23. Dried skim milk—

A—is useful for treating severely malnourished children? **B**—does not cause diarrhoea? **C**—makes a good artificial feed? **D**—should be given to a child to drink, not added to his porridge? **E**—should be given to children with rising growth curves who are on the road-to-health? (7.6)

24. When should most children start to eat porridge?

A 2 weeks **B** 1 month **C** 2 months **D** 4 months **E** 6 months (7.2)

25. If you want to find out if a child's muscles are wasted, you should feel—

A—his cheeks? **B**—the back of his arms below his axillae? **C**—his abdomen? **D**—his lower arms? **E**—his lower legs? (7.13)

COUGH A
Chapter 8: Code 4

1. Which of these are more common?

C Upper respiratory infections **D** Lower respiratory infections (8.1)

2. Respiratory infections are more dangerous in—
D—older children? **E**—babies? (8.1)

3. All these children are coughing. Which of them needs an antibiotic?

A FEBY who has a respiratory rate of 70 per minute. **B** FILEMON who is six months old with a cough for two days and no other signs. **C** FILIP who has been coughing for two weeks and is 'well'. **D** FRANCIS (3 years) who has been whooping for a week and now vomits after coughing. **E** FILIS (37·2 °C) who has a nasal discharge. (8.5)

4. Postural drainage—

A—kills the organisms causing lower respiratory infections? **B**—helps children to cough up sputum? **C**—must be done with a child standing up? **D**—is only useful with upper respiratory infections? **E**—can only be done by a health worker? (8.5)

5. SAMIR (3 years) has pneumonia. Which of these would you give him?

A One injection of procaine penicillin **B** Benzyl penicillin for one day **C** Streptomycin for 3 days **D** Chloramphenicol for one week **E** An injection of benzathine or benethamine penicillin (depot penicillin) (8.15)

6. Antibiotics do NOT help—

A—pneumonia? **B**—colds? **C**—the early stage of whooping cough in babies? **D**—the secondary infection in measles? **E**—chronic upper respiratory infections with purulent discharge? (8.7)

7. HELOISE (18 months) has obstructive laryngitis with severe insuction. When she breathes in, the lower part of her chest moves—

D—in? **E**—out? (8.9)

8. MULEME (3 years, 37·8 °C) has had a noisy wet cough for two days. She is not eating normally, and does not want to play, but otherwise she is well. Her respirations are 48 per minute, and she has mild insuction. She is not cyanosed. What is her diagnosis?

A Obstructive laryngitis **B** Asthma **C** Bronchiolitis **D** Bronchitis **E** Pneumonia (8.12)

9. Which of these diseases makes a child breathe much more deeply than normal?

A Pneumonia **B** Severe dehydration with acidosis **C** TB **D** Bronchitis **E** Whooping cough (8.15, 9.18)

10. MARYAMU (2 years, 38·3 °C) had a cold a few days ago and started coughing. Her cough is now worse and her mother is worried because she is breathing fast. She sits quietly and will not run about and play. Her nose moves as she breathes, and her respirations are 76 per minute. She is slightly cyanosed and there is mild insuction. What is her diagnosis?

A Bronchiolitis **B** Obstructive laryngitis **C** Asthma **D** Bronchitis **E** Pneumonia (8.15)

11. Which of these diseases causes difficulty breathing, which is worst when a child breathes out?

A Asthma **B** Obstructive laryngitis **C** Severe anaemia **D** Severe dehydration **E** High fever (8.13)

12. Severe anaemia makes lower respiratory infections more difficult to diagnose because it—
A—makes cyanosis worse? **B**—causes insuction? **C**—hides cyanosis? **D**—makes a child breathe more than 60 times a minute? **E**—prevents children breathing fast? (8.9)

13. When would you give an antibiotic to a child with an upper respiratory infection? When he has—
A—a red throat? **B**—a nasal discharge? **C**—acute tonsillar lymphadenitis? **D**—a temperature of 37.5 °C? **E**—a sore throat? (8.6, 18.11)

14. A child is most likely to need a tracheotomy if he has—
A—tonsillitis? **B**—asthma? **C**—bronchiolitis? **D**—obstructive laryngitis? **E**—bronchitis? (8.11)

15. KULISTINA (6 months, 37·5 °C, haemoglobin 13 g/dl) is wheezing and cyanosed. She is breathing with difficulty 50 times a minute. What is her probable diagnosis?
A Bronchitis or tonsillitis **B** Bronchiolitis or pneumonia **C** Whooping cough or diphtheria **D** Anaemia or hyperpyrexia **E** Asthma or a foreign body in her bronchi (8.14)

16. Besides antibiotics which of these doses KULISTINA need?
B Antihistamines **C** Adrenaline **D** Ephedrine **E** Oxygen (8.14)

17. How many times a minute should a child be breathing before you should diagnose pneumonia?
A 60 **B** 40 **C** 50 **D** 70 **E** 20 (8.9)

18. Which of these diseases is LEAST often complicated by TB, malnutrition, or pneumonia?
B Tonsillitis **C** Whooping cough **D** Measles (8.17, 10.6, 18.11)

19. Which of these is most useful in helping you to diagnose pneumonia from bronchitis?
A Insuction **B** Fever **C** How fast a child breathes **D** Stridor **E** The movement of his nose (8.15)

20. A moving nose is a sign of —
A—lower respiratory infection? **B**—upper respiratory infection? **C**—fever? **D**—anaemia? **E**—cyanosis? (8.9)

21. Which of these diseases is most likely to make a child vomit?
A TB **B** Chronic upper respiratory infections **C** Bronchitis **D** Whooping cough **E** Asthma (8.17)

22. Which of these diseases does NOT present as a cough?
A Bronchitis **B** Upper respiratory infections **C** Laryngitis **D** Measles **E** Mumps (19.4)

23. Which of these drugs is LEAST useful in treating asthma?
A Plenty of fluids by mouth **B** Aminophylline **C** Adrenalin injections **D** Ephedreine tablets **E** Antihistamines (8.13)

24. A foreign body in the bronchi—

A—is soon dissolved and is therefore harmless? **B**—may help to cause TB? **C**—can always be removed by turning the child upside down and hitting him on the back? **D**—helps to cause secondary infection in the lung? **E**—can easily be treated in a health centre? (8.18)

25. A child with asthma—
A—has obstruction to his larynx? **B**—should be given penicillin? **C**—has pus in his alveoli? **D**—usually vomits when he has an asthmatic attack? **E**—wheezes loudest when he breathes out? (8.13)

DIARRHOEA A
Chapter 9: Code 6

1. Green stools are caused by—
A—the liver making too much bile? **B**—too little bile in the gut? **C**—stools passing through the gut too quickly? **D**—stools passing through the gut too slowly? **E**—eating too much? (9.1)

2. Which of these does NOT cause diarrhoea sometimes?
A Threadworms **B** Strongyloides **C** Septicaemia **D** Lactose **E** *Giardia lamblia* (9.5, 21.5)

3. Amoebic dysentery can be treated with—
A—isoniazid or streptomycin? **B**—penicillin or sulphadimidine? **C**—tetrachlorethylene or bephenium? **D** —niridazole or niclosamide? **E**—metronidazole or tetracycline? (9.4)

4. Which of these usually causes the most severe dehydration?
A Amoebic dysentery **B** Bacilliary dysentery (9.4)

5. One of these things does NOT help to prevent diarrhoea. Which one?
A Breast-feeding **B** Making sure that a child's growth curve is rising **C** Making sure that a child eats plenty of green leafy vegetables **D** Making sure that a child's food is clean **E** Boiling his drinking water (9.8 to 9.14)

6. Which of these children is MOST likely to need rehydration?
A ROBINSON with fever and about four soft blood-stained stools each day for a week. **B** WINSTON (5 years) with two watery stools yesterday, none in the night, and one today. **C** NELSON (1 month) with liquid stools each time he feeds since birth. **D** LIESON with mild diarrhoea most days for several months. **E** GOODSON (2 years) with watery stools yesterday and last night. He has too many stools to count (9.18)

7. Which of the children in Question 6 is most likely to be malnourished?
A ROBINSON **B** WINSTON **C** NELSON **D** LIESON **E** GOODSON (9.11)

8. Which one of these signs can be caused by marasmus and by dehydration?
A Dry mouth **B** A swollen fontanelle **C** Fast breathing **D** Loss of skin elasticity **E** Swelling of the ankles (9.18)

9. Which of these is the most serious sign in a dehydrated child?

A Thirst B Sunken eyes C Loss of skin elasticity D Fast, weak pulse E Coma (9.18)

10. Children with acute diarrhoea and dehydration lack all these things EXCEPT one. Which one?

A Iron B Sodium C Chloride D Potassium E Water (9.17)

11. KALUSA (21 months, 37·5 °C) has had severe watery diarrhoea for five days and has been treated at home. He is drowsy and is breathing deeply 50 times a minute. He is not coughing and there is no insuction.

A He is only mildly dehydrated? B He probably has acidotic breathing? C He probably has pneumonia? D He should be rehydrated by mouth? E He has been given the right rehydration fluids? (9.18)

12. Which of these is NOT caused by dehydration?

A Swelling of the eyes B Passing little urine C A fast, weak pulse D Thirst E Shock (9.18)

13. Which of these is the best at helping the gut to absorb salt and water?

A Milk B Sodium bicarbonate C Potassium chloride D Ordinary sugar E Glucose (9.21)

14. Which of these is NOT true? Oral rehydration fluids—

A—must have the right amount of salt and sugar? B—can save the lives of many children? C—contain drugs to kill the organisms causing diarrhoea? D—can be made by mothers at home? E—can sometimes be used to treat children who are vomiting? (9.22)

15. SONGEA is moderately dehydrated. Which of these would be most useful in deciding how to manage him?

A Seeing how sunken his eyes are B Asking how much urine is he passing C Seeing how dry his mouth is D Giving him fluid to see if he drinks well E Feeling how elastic his skin is (9.31)

16. AGNESI is being given a scalp vein drip. Which of these would you watch for as a sign that she is being given too much fluid?

A Swelling of her ankles B Swelling of her eyelids C Coughing D Passing dark urine E Vomiting clear fluid (9.28)

17. GODFREE is mildly dehydrated but he will not drink glucose–salt solution, water, or milk. Which of these things would you do FIRST?

A Give him an intravenous drip. B Give him fluid through a nasogastric tube. C Give him an intraperitoneal drip. D Send him home and tell his mother that he will probably be able to drink later. E See if he will eat food. (9.22)

18. Which of these diseases is LEAST likely to cause diarrhoea?

A Tonsillitis B Malaria C Ringworm D Septicaemia in babies E Measles (9.10)

19. MAGALITA (20 months, 8 kg, 39·8 °C) has had mild diarrhoea for several months. During the last few days her diarrhoea has got worse and there is now blood in her stools. She is drowsy, her mouth is dry and her eyes are sunken. Her diarrhoea is—

B—acute? C—chronic? D—acute on chronic? (9.12)

20. MAGALITA'S bloody diarrhoea is most likely to be caused by—

A—bacilliary dysentery? B—amoebiasis? C—giardiasis? D—cholera? E—malnutrition? (9.4)

21. A health centre laboratory is LEAST likely to have special tests for—

A—lactose intolerance? B—the bloody diarrhoea caused by heavy infections with some worms? C—the diarrhoea caused by malnutrition? D—*Giardia?* E—amoebae? (9.5, 9.29)

22. NAKIKU (1 year, 8·5 kg, 37·8 °C) has severe watery diarrhoea with blood and mucus in her stools. She has vomited once. She is breast-fed but is also given porridge and a feeding bottle. Her eyes are moderately sunken, her mouth is dry, and her skin elasticity is moderately reduced. She sucks thirstily. Her feeding-bottle is dirty and contains milky tea. How would you rehydrate her?

B Intravenously C Intraperitoneally D Intragastrically E Orally (9.20)

23. Which of these would a health centre laboratory be most likely to find in NAKIKU's stools?

A Amoebae B Red cells and pus cells only C Giardia D Vibrio cholerae E The bacteria causing her diarrhoea (9.3)

24. What would you say to NAKIKU's mother?

A 'It is time you stopped breast feeding.' B 'Here is some medicine for her (kaolin and streptomycin).' C 'Don't give her anything except salt-and-sugar water until her diarrhoea has stopped and her temperature is normal.' D 'Give her porridge as soon as she can eat.' E 'Give her dried skim milk from a cup and spoon.' (9.31)

25. Whenever NAIKIKU starts passing liquid stools again her mother should—

A—give her an antibiotic? B—take her to the clinic quickly? C—stop giving her fluids? D—give her glucose–salt solution or salt-and-sugar water? E—stop giving her food? (9.22)

FEVER A

Chapter 10: Code 5

1. Which of these diseases most often causes fever which lasts several days or weeks without any other symptoms?

A Pneumonia B Pharyngitis C Ostoemyelitis D Otitis media E Urinary infection (10.10)

2. When a child has a rigor his temperature is—

C—going up? D—staying high? E—going down? (10.1)

3. Hypothermia is the opposite of—

A—hypertonia? B—hypoglycaemia? C—hypopyrexia? D—hyperpyrexia? E—hypernatraemia? (10.1)

4. Fits can be caused by—

A—hypothermia? **B**—hyperpyrexia? **C**—anaemia? **D**—hypotonia? (10.1)

5. The rectum is about half a degree Celsius hotter than the—

D—axilla? **E**—mouth? (10.1)

6. If a child's mouth temperature is 38 °C, his axilliary temperature is—

A—38·5 °C? **B**—36·5 °C? **C**—37·0 °C? **D**—37·5 °C? **E**—39 °C? (10.1)

7. An oral thermometer has a—

C—long, thin bulb? **D**—short, round bulb? (10–1)

8. Which of these is NOT true?

A Malaria causes pus to form. **B** Hyperpyrexia must be treated quickly. **C** Fever is usually caused by infection. **D** Too many clothes can turn an ordinary fever into hyperpyrexia. **E** Any disease which can cause fever may cause hyperpyrexia. (10.7)

9. JACINTA (2 years) has fever caused by pneumonia. She is being given penicillin and aspirin. Penicillin is—

A—symptomatic treatment for her fever? **B**—causal treatment for her pneumonia? **C**—both of these? **D**—neither of them? (10.3)

10. Which of these pairs of drugs helps to lower a child's temperature but does not cure his disease?

A Aspirin or paracetamol **B** Paraldehyde or phenobarbitone **C** Penicillin or sulphadimidine **D** Chloroquine or pyrimethamine **E** Piperazine or tetrachlorethylene (10.2)

11. Which of these diseases is more likely to present as a cough than as fever?

A Bronchitis **B** Malaria **C** Typhoid **D** Otitis media **E** Urinary infection (10.7, 10.8)

12. Otitis media, laryngitis, and kwashiorkor are important complications of one of these diseases. Which one?

A Urinary infection **B** Measles **C** Malaria **D** Chickenpox **E** Polio (106, 10.7)

13. When a child has measles, antibiotics are helpful in treating—

D—the primary infection? **E**—the secondary infection? (10.6)

14. Which of these diseases is most often complicated by conjunctivitis and stomatitis?

A Pneumonia **B** Otitis media **C** Measles **D** Typhoid **E** Malaria (10.6 to 10.8)

15. Which of these diseases is most easily diagnosed by examining a child's blood?

A Polio **B** Bronchitis **C** Measles **D** Malaria **E** Urinary infection (10.6 to 10.8)

16. SAID (4 years) lives in a district where falciparum malaria is common. Your immersion oil is finished, so you cannot examine his blood. He has pneumonia. You should—

A—only treat him for malaria? **B**—only treat him for pneumonia because he will be immune to malaria?

C—only treat him for malaria if you can feel his spleen? **D**—not treat him for malaria because you cannot examine a blood slide? **E**—treat him for malaria and pneumonia? (10.7)

17. RABSON has severe falciparum malaria. He has had several attacks before. Which of these symptoms or signs would you NOT expect him to have?

A Nasal discharge **B** Anaemia **C** Jaundice **D** A large spleen **E** Fits (10.7)

18. LAMEK is ill with fever. You should diagnose measles if he gets—

A—a rash on the second day and spots in his mouth on the fifth day of his illness? **B**—a rash on the third day with normal eyes and mouth? **C**—a mild rash on the first day of the fever? **D**—spots in his mouth on the third day and a rash and mild conjunctivitis on the fourth day? **E**—a cough and mouth ulcers on the first day with an itchy rash round his neck? (10.6)

19. Which of these helps to make measles more severe?

A Treating a child before the rash has come **B** Malnutrition **C** Bathing a child while he has fever **D** Constipation **E** Feeding a child too much while he has fever (10.6)

20. A large spleen is usually a sign of—

A—measles? **B**—TB? **C**—chronic malaria? **D**—acute malaria? **E**—worms? (10.6)

21. Pyrimethamine can suppress—

A—vomiting? **B**—pneumonia? **C**—malaria? **D**—measles? **E**—typhoid? (10.6 to 10.8)

22. HEINRICH has had fever for a week. You have examined him carefully. He has no other signs and diagnosis is difficult. Which of these diseases might he have?

A Tonsillitis **B** Pneumonia **C** Measles **D** Meningitis **E** Typhoid (10.8)

23. Which of these signs would make you think that a child's fever might be caused by infective hepatitis?

A Jaundice **B** Cough **C** Diarrhoea **D** A stiff neck **E** Septic spots on his skin (10.10)

24. Which of these signs would make you think that a child's fever was caused by pneumonia?

A A large spleen **B** A swollen red ear drum **C** Large tonsils **D** Respirations of 80 per minute **E** Wheezing (8.15)

25. The most common cause of fever in a child is—

A—typhoid? **B**—upper respiratory infection? **C**—urinary infection? **D**—lower respiratory infection? **E**—otitis media? (8.6)

SKINS A
Chapter 11: Code 4

MATCH these diseases with the kind of organism which causes them—

1. Herpes zoster 2. Creeping eruption 3. Scabies 4. Pellagra

A An insect B Lack of a vitamin called nicotinic acid C A virus D Bacteria E Worms (11.17, 11.21, 11.10, 11.23)

5. Which of these diseases harms a child's skin and other parts of his body?

A Ringworm B Molluscum contagiosum C Tinea versicolor D Scabies E Measles (10.6)

6. The best way for a mother to treat pyoderma at home is to—

A—wash the lesions in water? B—wash the lesions in permanganate solution? C—put sulphonamide ointment on the lesions? D—put oil on the lesions? E—wash the lesions with lysol solution? (11.6)

7. Lesions which are the same on each side of a child's body are—

A—macular? B—hypopigmented? C—urticarial? D—symmetrical? E—asymmetrical? (11.2)

8. Which of these children is most likely to have leprosy?

A HORACE with itching lesions between his fingers B HYACINTH (2 years, 38 °C) with a nasal discharge, red eyes, and many small red papules C HIRAM with itchy scaly lesions which are worse on the front of his elbows D HERO who has had a pale 3 cm anaesthetic macule on the upper part of his leg for 3 months E HECTOR with several round bald lesions on his scalp (12.3)

9. Impetigo is—

A—a disease with dry scaly lesions? B—very dangerous in newborn babies? C—rare D—not infectious? E—caused by fungi? (11.4)

10. PRITHWI has chronic round scaly lesions on his body. They started as papules which became slowly bigger and began to heal in the middle. They are not hypopigmented and he has no thickened nerves. They—

A—can be treated with benzyl benzoate? B—may make him seriously ill? C—are rare in most communities? D—are probably anaesthetic? E—are probably caused by fungi? (11.13)

11. GANESHBAHADUR (3 years, 38 °C) has a hot, red, swollen, painful lesion on his leg. Red lines on his skin go from it towards some tender swellings in his left groin. He has a fast pulse and is 'ill'. He has all these things, EXCEPT—

A—urticaria? B—lymphadenitis? C—lymphangitis? D—the local signs of septic infection? E—the general signs of a septic infection? (11.3)

12. Which of these diseases would you most expect to see in several people in the same family at the same time?

A Urticaria B Creeping eruption C Impetigo D Kwashiorkor E Cellulitis (11.4)

13. LACHIMADEVI (3 years) is apathetic. The skin on the outer parts of her arms and legs has become dark and is peeling off. Her ankles are swollen. When you press them your finger makes a hole. Her lesions—

A—can be cured with vitamin B? B—will leave her immune when she recovers? C—are caused by lack of protein and energy food? D—are not serious and will soon cure themselves? E—are on her skin only and the rest of her body is normal? (11.22)

14. ANNA has a chronic, symmetrical, dry, red, scaly rash. It is worse on the front of her elbows and behind her knees. She is always scratching.

A Her rash is infected? B It is infectious? C It is easily cured with antihistamines? D When she is older she is more likely to get asthma than other children? E She has scabies? (11.27)

15. SIXPENCE (8 months) has pustules on the palms of his hands and a few between his fingers. Several of his older brothers and sisters have itchy skin lesions. He probably has—

A—ringworm? B—infected scabies? C—pyoderma? D—impetigo? E—chickenpox? (11.10)

16. Tinea versicolor—

A—causes papules? B—causes lesions that are all the same size, shape, and colour? C—causes anaesthetic lesions? D—causes lesions which itch? E—is harmless? (11.14)

17. ADOPA (8 kg, 3 months) is a fat little girl. She has wet red lesions in the folds of her neck and in her axillae. This is probably caused by—

A—the skin in the lesions getting hot and wet? B—malnutrition? C—scabies? D—impetigo? E—eczema? (11.26b)

18. Which of these diseases is most likely to kill a child?

A Scabies B Severe skin sepsis in a malnourished child C Ringworm D Creeping eruption E Tuberculoid leprosy (11.6)

19. Chronic hypopigmented lesions are NOT caused by—

A—tinea versicolor? B—chronic ulcers? C—urticaria? D—leprosy? E—burns? (11.7)

20. Which of these would you NOT be able to feel if you touched it with your finger?

A A macule B A papule C A pustule D A crust E A vesicle (11.2)

21. Which of these diseases does NOT cause macules, papules, vesicles, and pustules?

A Chickenpox B Herpes zoster C Herpes simplex D Leprosy (12.3)

22. Secondary infection may complicate all of these EXCEPT one. Which one?

A Heat rash B Chickenpox C Scabies D Ringworm E Tinea versicolor (11.14)

23. Penicillin is NOT helpful for treating—

A—impetigo of the newborn? B—secondarily infected ringworm? C—cellulitis? D—pyoderma? E—lepromatous leprosy? (11.23)

24. Which of these is NOT true?

A Scabies is a disease of the whole family. B In herpes zoster the pain comes before the skin lesions can be seen. C Permanganate and hypochlorite solutions can be used to treat the same kind of lesions. **D** Eczema is caused by lack of vitamins. **E** Warts are caused by viruses. (11.27)

25. BHIMPRASAD (5 years) has scabies. Where would you LEAST expect to find lesions?

A Along the folds of his axillae **B** On his buttocks **C** On his ankles **D** Between his toes **E** On his face (11.10)

LEPROSY A
Chapter 12: Code 7

1. Which kind of leprosy needs treat... ent for the longest time?

B Indeterminate **C** Borderline **D** Lepromatous **E** Tuberculoid (12.4)

2. Most children with indeterminate leprosy—

A—become severely disabled? **B**—recover without treatment? (12.2)

3. LUKE (10 years) has been treated for lepromatous leprosy for two years. He seems quite well. His treatment—

B—can now stop? **C**—must go on for many more years? (12.4)

4. Which of these children needs two leprosy drugs at the beginning of treatment?

A JOJO with lepromatous leprosy **B** JOAN with tuberculoid leprosy **C** JOSEPH with indeterminate leprosy **D** JORGE with borderline leprosy and few bacilli in his skin scraping (3.24b)

5. Leprosy is serious because it causes severe deformity in—

D—young children? **E**—older children and adults? (12.1)

6. Leprosy causes severe disability in—
C—older children? **D**—young children? (12.1)

7. Leprosy disables a child because his arms or legs are pulled into an abnormal shape by—

B—his normal muscles? **C**—muscles whose nerves have been injured? (12.1)

8. If a child lives with a leprosy patient for several years, what is more likely?

A He will remain well. **B** He too will get leprosy. (12.1)

9. A part of the body in which there is no feeling is—
B—analgesic? **C**—hypotonic? **D**—anaesthetic? **E**—hypopigmented? (12.1)

10. Most children have—
D—little immunity to leprosy? **E**—much immunity to leprosy? (12.2)

11. The most severe anaesthesia is caused by—
B—indeterminate leprosy? **C**—borderline leprosy? **D**—lepromatous leprosy? **E**—tuberculoid leprosy? (12.2)

12. Leprosy treatment should start with—
D—full doses of the drug? **E**—small doses of the drug? (12.4)

13. SASHA'S lesions are completely white (depigmented). He has—

A—has not got leprosy? **B**—might have leprosy? (12.3)

14. AVRAM'S lesions have vesicles. They—
A—might be leprosy? **B**—are not leprosy? (12.3)

15. KAMALA'S lesions are painful. They—
B—might be leprosy? **C**—are not leprosy? (12.3)

16. BIELKE (7 years) has severe tuberculoid leprosy and is being treated. For the last week she has had fever and a rash. The rash does not look like measles or any of the rashes you know. It is probably a drug rash. Her mother will not take her for help. What are you going to do?

A Stop her leprosy drug for two weeks and then start slowly with small doses **B** Stop her leprosy drug completely **C** Go on with her leprosy drug and give her penicillin for her fever (3.24, 12.4)

17. A patient with leprosy usually has—
B—AAFB in his skin *and* anaesthesia? **C**—AAFB in his skin *or* anaesthesia? (12.3)

18. Tuberculoid leprosy makes nerves—
A—thin? **B**—thick? **C**—tender? **D**—thick and tender? **E**—thin and tender? (12.3)

19. Treatment can—
A—make injured nerves grow again? **B**—only stop a child's leprosy lesions getting worse? (12.1)

20. Borderline leprosy is half way between—
C—indeterminate and lepromatous leprosy? **D**—tuberculoid and indeterminate leprosy? **E**—tuberculoid and lepromatous leprosy? (12.2)

21. Which of these drugs would you give to a child with leprosy?

A Isoniazid **B** Dapsone (DDS) **C** Pyrimethamine **D** Niridazole **E** Streptomycin (12.4)

22. A child should take his leprosy tablets—
B—once a month? **C**—three times a day? **D**—once a week? **E**—once a day? (3.24, 12.4)

23. Which of these is NOT the way to examine a child's skin for anaesthesia.

A His eyes should be open all the time. **B** He should be asked to point to the place where he is touched. **C** He should be touched with a piece of cotton wool. **D** He should be examined in a quiet place (12.3)

24. SHOLOM (6 years) is being treated for leprosy. His mother needs to be told these things, EXCEPT one. Which one?

B 'He must take these tablets for several years.' **C** 'These are harmless tablets, you can keep them anywhere.' **D** 'I am going to put him on our special-care register.' **E** 'Bring him to see me every month.' (12.5)

25. TB and leprosy are like one another for all these reasons EXCEPT one. Which one? Both—

A—cause disability? **B**—can be treated with tablets? **C**—are caused by AAFB? **D**—are chronic? **E**—cause death? (12.1, 13.2)

Chapter 13: Code 2

1. MERCY (18 months) is losing weight and is not eating. She has an immunization scar on her right shoulder. This means that—

A—she has been immunized in the wrong way? B—she has not got TB? C—TB cannot kill her? D—she has been immunized with BCG but she might still have TB? E—she will recover quickly? (13.4)

2. TB is caused by—

A—fungi? B—worms? C—viruses? D—protozoa? E—bacteria? (13.1)

3. FRANCISCO has a cough, fever, loss of weight, and is not eating. The midwife who is treating him is not sure if he has TB or not so she gave him chloramphenicol for two weeks. It has not helped him. This—

A—makes it more likely that he has TB? B—makes it less likely that he has TB? C—makes no difference? (13.7)

4. When a child with TB is given TB drugs his symptoms—

A—go in a few days? B—don't go until he has been treated for a year? C—usually get much less in a few weeks, but he needs treatment for a year? D—go when all the TB organisms in his body have been killed? (13.6)

5. A child's lungs are often harmed by TB. Which parts of his body are harmed next most often? His—

A—ureters? B—lymph nodes? C—palate? D—tongue? E—trachea? (13.2)

6. TB is spread by—

A—drinking water that has not been boiled? B—droplet infection? C—contact? D—faeces to mouth infection? E—insects? (13.2)

7. Primary TB infections—

A—usually kill children? B—cause cavities in adults? C—usually cause miliary tuberculosis? D—are so common that most people have them at some time in their lives? E—are so dangerous that fortunately only a few people have them? (13.2)

8. KUO-PIN has TB. He might have presented in any of these ways EXCEPT as—

A—hyperpyrexia? B—painless lumps in his neck? C—pain and swelling in his back? D—failure to get well after measles? E—loss of weight? (13:1)

9. TB is—

C—one of the more difficult diseases to diagnose? D—one of the easiest diseases to diagnose? (13.1)

10. Which kind of TB patient is most infectious? The patient who—

A—has primary TB? B—has TB lymph nodes in his neck? C—has TB of the spine? D—has just started to become ill? E—is an adult and is about to die from TB? (13.2)

11. GUILLERMO has miliary TB. He has lesions—

A—all over his body? B—only in his meninges? C—only in his lymph nodes? D—only in his lungs? (13.2)

12. The course of streptomycin for TB is three times a week for—

A—two years? B—two weeks? C—one year? D—three months? E—six months? (13.6)

13. TB in children commonly presents as—

A—malnutrition? B—cyanosis? C—fits? D—a discharging ear? E—coughing up blood? (13:1)

14. The most useful sign that TB treatment is curing a child is that he—

A—stops coughing? B—has less fever? C—breathes more slowly? D—starts to gain weight? E—coughs up less sputum? (13.6)

15. TB organisms growing in the lungs of an adult most often cause—

A—a high fever? B—a cavity? C—an abscess? D—wheezing? E—bronchitis? (13.3)

16. A newborn child—

A—has a natural passive immunity to TB? B—should be separated from his mother if his mother has active TB? C—can be given BCG vaccine? D—gets a very chronic kind of TB if he is infected by TB bacilli? E—has a stronger immunity to TB than an older child? (13.1, 26.66)

17. When a health centre laboratory reports a patient's sputum as having AAFB + + this means that he—

A—has had TB but it has now healed? B—has been given BCG vaccine? C—has leprosy of his lungs? D—might have TB? E—has TB? (13.3)

18. ANDREAS (3 years, 11 kg) has had a mild fever and a cough for some weeks. His growth curve is falling. He has no BCG scar. He should be treated—

A—with chloramphenicol or another broad spectrum antibiotic? B—for malnutrition? C—for TB? D—with streptomycin to see if he starts gaining weight? E—with cough mixture? (13.2)

19. Which of these is LEAST likely to make a TB infection cause serious symptoms?

A Infection during the first few weeks of life B Severe measles C Whooping cough D Scabies E Malnutrition (13:1)

PLEASE DON'T WRITE ON THESE QUESTIONS OTHER PEOPLE MAY NEED THEM

---

20. Which of these drugs is NOT used to treat TB?

A Thiacetazone B Streptomycin C Isoniazid D Aminosalicylate (PAS) E Penicillin (13.6)

21. The best way of preventing TB from spreading in a community is to make sure that—

A—mothers with TB don't breast feed? B—all adults with TB are diagnosed and properly treated? C—all children finish their treatment? D—adults do not spit on the floor? E—all infectious children are diagnosed early? (13.4)

22. Which of these drugs is NOT used to treat children with TB?

A Metronidazole B Streptomycin C Thiacetazone D Ethambutol E Ethionamide (13.6)

23. A child who is sick with TB should if possible have—

A—two or three TB drugs at the same time? B—penicillin and streptomycin? C—one TB drug only? (13.6)

24. Examining a child's sputum for AAFB is—

A—only possible in small babies? B—seldom possible? C—only possible during the primary infection? D—helpful for diagnosing leprosy? E—the easiest way to diagnose TB in children? (13.3)

25. Which of these diseases is usually most common in children coming to a clinic?

A TB B Typhoid C Lower respiratory infections D Leprosy E Upper respiratory infections (8.1, 13.1)

ACCIDENTS A

Chapter 14: Code 1

1. Which of these would you try to sew up in a health centre?

A Cut skin B Cut tendons C Cut nerves D Broken bones E All of them (14.4)

2. Accidents—

D—happen in the same way in every community? E—differ from one community to another? (14.1)

3. Which kind of burn completely destroys the epidermis and the sweat glands and hair follicles?

A Superficial B Superficial partial thickness C Full thickness D Deep partial thickness (14.3)

4. Which of these is NOT an accident?

A TB B Shock caused by falling out of a tree C Dapsone poisoning because a child ate his father's tablets D Drowning E A broken leg caused by being run over by a car (14.1)

5. NOEL climbed onto a lorry while it was running. He fell out and was hit by a passing car. He is cold and white, pale and sweating. He—

A—is cyanosed? B—has fainted? C—is anaemic? D—is shocked? (14.2)

6. CONCETTA (5 years) has just been hit by a car. She is cold and pale and her pulse is 140. The nearest hospital is many miles away. Which of these things might help her most?

A An injection of adrenalin B Oral glucose–salt solution C Being nursed sitting up D Intravenous fluid E A nasogastric drip (14.2)

7. What kind of burn does boiling hot oil usually cause?

A Superficial B Superficial partial thickness C Full thickness (14.3)

8. A burnt child is NOT in danger from—

A—shock? B—fits? C—loss of protein? D—loss of fluid? E—infection? (14.3)

9. ONOFRIO has come to have a 6 cm superficial partial thickness burn dressed in your clinic. If you don't treat

him properly, his greatest danger is—

A—hepatitis? B—loss of protein and fluid from his burn? C—secondary infection? D—anaemia? E—an injection abscess? (14.3)

10. In which kind of burn does the epidermis have to grow over the burn from the edges?

B Superficial C Superficial partial thickness D Deep partial thickness E Full thickness (14.3)

11. ALPHONSO has burnt himself with a lamp and has a 3 cm burn on his right arm. He should be dressed with—

A—gauze only? B—vaseline gauze? C—vaseline only? D—lint? E—a bandage only? (14.3)

12. Immediately a child is burnt his burn should be—

A—put into hot water? B—painted with gentian violet? C—covered with sauce (a local treatment)? D—put into cold water? E—covered with butter or fat? (14.3)

13. Vesicles (blisters) on a burn show that—

A—all the epidermis is destroyed? B some of the epidermis is still alive? C—it is secondarily infected? D—it is not going to heal? E—it needs a skin graft? (14.3)

14. GUGLIEMO cut himself three days ago. The edges of the skin are wide apart and it is starting to become septic. He needs an antibiotic. His cut should be—

A—sewn up in two or three days' time? B—sewn up now? C—cleaned and dressed and left to heal by itself? (14.4)

15. When a child bleeds into his tissues he has—

A—oedema? B—lymphangitis? C—a fracture? D—a bruise? E—a sprain? (14.5)

16. GULACHAKA has swallowed poison. How long must you probably wait before you are sure there will be no serious symptoms?

A 36 hours B 12 hours C 4 hours D One week E One hour (14.6)

17. RADNIWATI has just swallowed some dapsone tablets. She should be made to vomit—

A—if she has any symptoms of poisoning? B—after she has been given something to drink? C—after she has been given something to eat? D—after the tablets have had time to dissolve in her stomach? E—immediately? (14.6)

18. AMMON (2 years) has swallowed some of his brother's epilepsy tablets half an hour ago. What would you do FIRST?

A Wait and see if he has symptoms. B Give him a purge to remove the tablets. C Rub the back of this throat with a spatula. D Send him for help. E Pass a stomach tube. (14.6)

19. ARUNEE (4 years) is unconscious. He should be put—

B—with his feet lower than his head? C—sitting up? D—on his side with his head lower than his feet? E—on his back? (14.8)

20. Coma is NOT caused by—

A—dehydration? B—upper respiratory infections? C—poisoning? D—cerebral malaria? E—head injuries? (14.8)

21. Which of these would be the most useful treatment for a child in coma for many hours?

A Promethazine **B** Ipecacuanha **C** A nasogastric drip **D** Aspirin **E** Intravenous fluid (14.8)

22. A deeply unconscious child—

A—cannot cough? **B**—coughs normally? **D**—vomits if he coughs? **D**—coughs more easily than normal? (14.8)

23. Which of these is never caused by poisoning?

A Vomiting **B** Meningitis **C** Coma **D** Fits **E** Pneumonia (14.6)

24. Which of these is the LEAST likely complication of a cut foot?

A TB **B** Tetanus **C** Cellulitis **D** Septicaemia (14.4)

25. Which of these is NOT a good way of cleaning a very dirty wound?

A Putting it under a tap **B** Scrubbing it with a sterile brush **C** Putting antibiotic ointment on it **D** Taking out pieces of dirt with forceps **E** Soaking it in saline (14.4)

FITS A
Chapter 15: Code 4

1. A child who has had febrile convulsions—

A—will have epileptic fits all his life? **B**—will have more fits as he grows older? **C**—is more likely to get convulsions again than other children? **D**—will never have a convulsion again? **E**—will certainly not develop normally? (15.5)

2. All these children are three years old. Which of them is most likely to have a damaged brain?

A OLA who has had two febrile convulsions lasting less than five minutes. **B** ALAIDA (38·5 °C) who had a fit lasting three minutes. **C** ANESI who had tonsillitis with febrile convulsions lasting ten minutes. **D** ABISA who did not have a lumbar puncture when he had a febrile convulsion. **E** SNAKE who has just had a fit which lasted 30 minutes. (15.9)

3. ORANGE (2 years) has been ill for several days. His head and back are bent backwards. Which of these signs would make you think that he has tetanus and not meningitis?

A Muscle spasms during which he stays conscious **B** Coma **C** Fits **D** A cloudy CSF **E** A record of being immunized with DPT (15.1)

4. Healthy CSF is—

A—milky white? **B**—clear, like water? **C**—slightly cloudy? **D**—pale yellow? **E**—slightly red with blood? (15.2)

5. All of these children have had a fit, and should have a lumbar puncture. Who needs a lumbar puncture most urgently?

A JULIUS (18 months) who has had diarrhoea for a week and is bottle-fed. He has a sunken fontanelle. **B** JENNY (13 months, 37·5 °C) whose left ear-drum is red and swollen.

C STONE (3 years, 39·2 °C) who has large tonsils with pus on them and tender tonsilar lymph nodes. **D** WEDSON (2 years, 38·7 °C) who had febrile convulsions twice last year. He now has a cough and a nasal discharge. **E** ZAWINYA (5 months, 38·2 °C) who has been vomiting for two days. Her fontanelle is swollen. (15.9)

6. A lumbar-puncture needle should be sterilized in—

A—iodine? **B**—boiling water or steam? **C**—hypochlorite? **D**—sterile distilled water? **E**—lysol? (15.3)

7. On a lumbar-puncture needle there should be—

D—no live organisms of any kind? **E**—very few live organisms? (15.3)

8. Which of these is NOT a symptom of meningitis?

A Vomiting **B** Drowsiness **C** Not sucking **D** Abdominal pain **E** Fever (15.6)

9. When a child has a lumbar puncture—

A—he should be sitting on his mother's knees? **B**—his arms and legs should be tightly held so that his back is bent? **C**—the needle should be put in above his first lumbar spine? **D**—the health worker should not get iodine on his fingers? **E**—a 0·45 × 10 mm needle should be used? (15.3)

10. TARZAN (3 years) has had a fit. Which of these would be LEAST helpful in making the diagnosis?

A Taking his temperature **B** Examining his throat **C** Examining his ears **D** Making him put his head between his legs **E** Feeling his fontanelle (15.6)

11. GINGER has a *very* mildly positive Pandy's test.

A His CSF may be normal? **B** He certainly has meningitis? **C** He has febrile convulsions? **D** He has mild pyogenic meningitis? **E** He has mild TB meningitis? (15.3b)

12. Which of these is the most common but least serious cause of fits?

A Cerebral malaria **B** Dehydration **C** Febrile convulsions **D** Meningitis **E** Epilepsy (15.5)

13. Febrile convulsions are more common in—

A—malnourished children? **B**—children under six months? **C**—children between 6 months and 4 years old? **D**—children over four years? **E**—bottle-fed babies? (15.5)

14. Which of these children are MOST likely to recover by themselves without treatment?

B JAIME with cerebral malaria **C** JAMES with pyogenic meningitis **D** JOHN with virus meningitis **E** JACK with TB meningitis (15.6)

15. ARTOO (3 years) is having a fit. *P. falciparum* is common in his district. Which of these does he need NOW?

A Subcutaneous quinine **B** Subcutaneous chloroquine **C** Oral chloroquine **D** Intravenous chloroquine **E** Intramuscular chloroquine (15.7)

16. A child who is having a fit should be made to—

C—sit up? **D**—lie on his back? **E**—lie on his front or his side? (15.9)

17. DAMINA (6 years, 39 °C) has fits about every two or three months and quickly recovers after them. For the last few days she has not been well. She had a fit this morning and vomited. Does she need a lumbar puncture?

A Yes B No (15.9)

18. POSTUMUS (2 years) has had two fits during last night. He has no signs of dehydration or infection. Does he need a lumbar puncture?

B Yes C No (15.9)

19. MARCEL. During the last three days he has had several attacks in which he had sudden jerky movements of his right arm and the right side of his mouth. Does he need a lumbar puncture?

C Yes D No (15.9)

20. MERLE (5 months) has had a fit. Her fontanelle is swollen. Does she need a lumbar puncture?

A Yes B No (15.9)

21. MAUREEN (4 years, 38·2 °C) has not been well for three days. This morning she vomited three times and had a fit. Her neck is stiff and she cannot put her head between her legs. Unfortunately you have not been taught how to do a lumbar puncture. What would you say to her mother?

A 'I must try to do a lumbar puncture.' B 'I will give her paraldehyde and send her for help.' C 'I am sorry, I cannot help her.' D 'We must treat her for meningitis and send her for help.' E 'Daily penicillin will cure her.' (15.6)

22. All these children have meningitis. Which of them is most likely to have a positive Kernig's sign and a stiff neck?

B AZIZ (1 day) C AZIZUL (1 week) D ABDUL (1 year) E ABDULLA (5 years) (15.6)

23. INDRA (4 years, 38·2 °C) has had a cough for four days. Her nose is moving, her respirations are 66 per minute, and there is insuction. Kernig's sign is positive and her neck is mildly stiff. Does she need a lumbar puncture?

E Yes D No (8.15, 15.6)

24. DOLIKA (3 years, 39·5 °C) has just had a fit. The FIRST thing you should do is to—

A—give her phenobarbitone? B—give her chloroquine? C—examine her throat and ears? D—cool her with water? E—do a lumbar puncture? (15.9)

25. Meningitis causes all of these symptoms EXCEPT—

A—not eating? B—headache? C—coma? D—fits? E—cough? (15.6)

EYES A

Chapter 16: Code 8

1. Blindness can be prevented by—

B—clean drinking water? C—using latrines? D—the right early treatment of eye disease? E—eating plenty of vitamin D? (16.1)

2. The conjunctival sac is a pocket between—

A—the eyelids and the eyeball? B—the cornea and the iris? C—the pupil and the lens? D—the retina and the cornea? (16.2)

3. The cornea is—

A—the soft pink tissue under the eyelids? B—part of the back of the eye? C—the white part of the eye? D—a circle of blue or brown tissue? E—the window at the front of the eye? (16.2)

4. A healthy cornea contains—

B—blood vessels? C—no blood vessels? (16.2)

5. Many small pink swellings in the conjunctiva of the upper eyelid can be caused by—

A—vitamin A deficiency? B—trachoma? C—corneal ulcers? D—phlyctenular conjunctivitis? E—measles? (16.3, 6.9)

6. A stye is—

A—a white spot on the cornea? B—a small abscess round one of the eyelashes? C—a swelling under the eyelids? D—a swelling at the outer edge of the cornea? (16.3)

7. Red watery eyes are caused by—

A—measles? B—chickenpox? C—typhoid? D—malaria? E—meningitis? (16.4)

8. PATRICK (12 years) has been hitting a piece of iron with a hammer. A small piece of iron has broken off and gone into his eye. If it has gone into the inside of his eye—

A—he will be able to see it? B—his eyes will bleed? C—you may not be able to see the hole where it went in? D—it will cause no harm? E—it will not cause sepsis? (16.5)

9. When a health worker examines a child's eyes for foreign bodies he should turn over the child's—

D—lower eyelids? E—upper eyelids? (16.5)

10. Fluorescein is useful for diagnosing—

B—foreign bodies? C—acute conjunctivitis? D—corneal ulcers? E—phlyctens? (16.5)

11. If a foreign body has been removed from a child's eye but he still feels it—

C—he must have some other disease? D—there must be another foreign body on his eye? E—he may only be feeling the soreness the foreign body has caused? (16.5)

12. A corneal ulcer looks like a piece of the cornea which—

A—is not as smooth and shining as it should be? B—is round with sharp edges? C—is a dirty white? D—is red and inflamed? E—is swollen? (16.7)

13. Conjunctivitis—

A—often spreads to other parts of the body? B—makes the sclera red near the cornea only? C—is not infectious? D—makes the sclera red all over? E—is usually in one of a child's eyes only? (16.7)

14. Children with kwashiorkor or marasmus—

A—are usually growing normally? B—often have vitamin A deficiency? C—are usually too young to have keratomalacia? D—should be given plenty of pale coloured vegetables? E—should be treated with protein and energy food alone and don't need extra vitamins? (7.11)

15. Many children have mild conjunctivitis for a few days only. It is usually caused by—
A—vitamin A deficiency? B—trachoma? C—bacteria and viruses that seldom cause serious harm? D—gonorrhoea? E—measles? (16.8)

16. Acute purulent conjunctivitis can be caused by—
A—gonorrhoea? B—malaria? C—whooping cough? D—TB? E—trachoma? (16.8)

17. LUIGI (3 years) has acute conjunctivitis with grossly swollen eyes that discharge pus. The health centre laboratory has found Gram negative intracellular diplococci in the pus. He was probably infected by—
A—organisms in water? B—droplets? C—contact from his friends? D—flies? E—contact from his parents? (16.8)

18. Which of these children are most likely to have trachoma?
A BIDDY (18 months) with dry corneae and Bitot's spots. B BILLY (12 years) with pannus, and follicles under his upper lids. C BOBBY (14 years) with follicles only and no pannus. D BARRY (5 years) with a small yellow–grey swelling beside his corneae. E BARNY (4 years) with swollen eyelids and pus coming from them. (16.9)

19. FERNANDO (5 years) has mildly red watery eyes. If these are caused by trachoma, what stage is it?
B Fourth C First D Second E Third (16.9)

20. BLODWYN (3 years) has a painful yellow–grey 1 mm swelling at the outer side of her cornea. She has—
B—vitamin A deficiency? C—a corneal ulcer? D—phlyctenular conjunctivitis? E—allergic conjunctivitis? (16.11)

21. Vitamin A deficiency is usually diagnosed in children who present with symptoms of—
A—vitamin A deficiency? B—malnutrition or infection? (16.5)

22. Xerophthalmia means that a child's eyes are—
A—ulcerated? B—blind? C—red? D—dry? E—watery? (16.13)

23. Vitamin A—
A—is harmful if much more than the right dose is given? B—can be made by the body from proteins? C—cannot be given by injection? D—is not stored by the body? E—is found in rice? (16.13)

24. Bitot's spots are—
A—a sign of vitamin B deficiency? B—a sign of TB? C—found on the sclera? D—usually found in one eye only? E—dark red? (16.13)

25 OTFRIED has corneal lesions in one eye caused by vitamin A deficiency. Which of these does he MOST need now?
A Vitamin A by mouth B Oily vitamin A by injection C Chlortetracycline eye ointment D Water miscible (soluble) vitamin A by injection E Procaine penicillin by injection (16.15)

EARS A

Chapter 17: Code 8

1. A discharging ear can cause—
A—deafness? B—meningitis? C—mastoiditis? D—any of these things? E—none of these things? (17.1)

2. The healthy ear-drum—
A—has air on both sides of it? B—has air on one side only? C—has blood on one side of it and bone on the other side? D—is completely flat? E—has the handle of the maleus at the bottom of the drum. (17.2)

3. The ear-drum is between—
A—the middle ear and the mastoid? B—the outer ear and the mastoid? C—the outer and the inner ear? D—the middle and inner ear? E—the outer and middle ear? (17.2)

4. Which of these is most often diseased in children?
A The outer ear B The inner ear C The middle ear D The mastoid (17.2)

5. The Eustachian tube joins—
A—the outer and the middle ear? B—the pharynx and the middle ear? C—the pharynx and the outer ear? D—the back of the nose and the inner ear? E—the pharynx and the mastoid? (17.2)

6. You should examine a child's ears—
A—at the beginning of the examination before he starts to cry? B—at the end of the examination? C—at the same time as you examine the other parts of his head? D—while he lies on a couch? E—while his mother is out of the room? (17.3)

7. When you examine a child's ear you should use—
A—the largest speculum that will go into his ear without hurting him? B—the smallest speculum you have? (17.3)

8. The handle of the maleus goes from—
C—the top of the ear-drum towards its middle? D—the middle of the ear-drum towards its side? E—the side of the ear drum towards its bottom? (17.3)

9. Which of these immunizations is specially important for a child with a discharging ear?
A Measles B Polio C Diphtheria D BCG E Tetanus (17.5)

10. When you syringe an ear the syringe should—
A—block the meatus? B—go as far into the meatus as possible? C—point downwards and forwards? D—be filled with warm water? E—point straight at the drum? (17.6)

11. Which of these is NOT a cause of ear discharge?
A Acute otitis media with a perforation B Chronic otitis media with a perforation C Otitis externa D Foreign body E Mumps (17.8)

12. A perforation is a hole in—
A—the drum? B—the middle ear? C—the inner ear? D—the outer ear? E—the mastoid? (17.7)

13. You have got all of these drugs. Which of them would you give to a child with acute otitis media?

A Penicillin B Sulphadimidine C Streptomycin D Penicillin and sulphadimidine E Chloramphenicol

14. 'All painful swellings behind the ear are caused by mastoiditis'

A True? B False? (17.12)

15. QUINTUS (4 years) has had discharge from his left ear for one year. For the last five days he has had fever and pain in his ear. Antibiotics will probably—

C—help him? D—not help him? E—cause serious side effects? (17.10)

16. Moving a child's ear hurts him if—

A—he has otitis externa? B—he has otitis media? C—he has otitis interna? D—he has a perforated ear drum? E—his ear drum is about to perforate? (17.9, 17.12)

17. The complications of otitis externa are—

A—deafness? B—meningitis? C—mastoiditis? D—all of these diseases? E—none of these diseases? (17.12)

18. GUS (4 years, 38·6 °C) is ill with pain and discharge from his ear. There is a swelling behind his ear which has pushed it forwards. He has—

A—mumps? B—mastoiditis? C—otitis externa? D—otitis media? E—meningitis? (17.11)

19. When there is pus in the air spaces behind a child's ear he has—

A—lymphadenitis? B—meningitis? C—mastoiditis? D—severe otitis media? E—otitis externa? (17.11)

20. When a child has otitis media a discharge from his ear means that—

A—he has mastoiditis? B—he has otitis externa also? C—his Eustachian tube has opened? D—his ear-drum has perforated? E—the infection has spread to his outer ear and pus is coming from it? (17.9)

21. The best way way to prevent chronic otitis media is to—

A—treat all upper respiratory infections with chloramphenicol? B—diagnose and treat acute otitis media before the drum perforates? C—immunize children? D—keep children on the road to health? E—weigh children? (17.9)

22. If you cannot send a child with mastoiditis to hospital you should treat him as if he had—

A—lymphadenitis? B—acute otitis media? C—otitis externa? D—osteomyelitis? (17.11)

23. CHAMBO (1 year) keeps pulling at his left ear. He is LEAST likely to have—

A—tonsillitis? B—acute otitis media? C—'itchy ears'? D—a foreign body in his ear? E—otitis externa? (17.9)

24. Which of these does NOT cause deafness?

A Chronic otitis media B Obstruction of the meatus by wax C Otitis externa without obstruction of the meatus D Obstruction of the meatus by a foreign body E Acute otitis media (17.10, 17.12)

25. RENATO (5 years) has a tender bean-shaped swelling behind his right ear, and some septic lesions in his scalp. Moving his ear does not hurt him. There is wax in his

meatus and you cannot see his drum. He has probably got—

A—otitis externa? B—acute otitis media? C—chronic otitis media? D—pyoderma and acute lymphadenitis? E—mastoiditis? (17.12)

MOUTH AND THROAT A
Chapter 18: Code 5

1. In young children acute sore throats may present with any of these symptoms EXCEPT—

A—fever? B—fits? C—vomiting? D—cough? E—constipation? (18.1)

2. ROSE has tonsillitis. In two or three weeks' time this may cause disease in her—

A—lungs? B—stomach? C—kidneys? D—bladder? E—spleen? (18.11)

3. The best way to sterilize throat spatulae before using them again is to wash them in—

A—permanganate solution? B—sterile water? C—hot soapy water? D—water and boil them? E—an antiseptic solution? (18.2)

4. Tender tonsillar lymph nodes are a sign of—

A—thrush? B—an acute throat infection? C—chronic lymphadenitis? D—any kind of upper respiratory infection? E—TB? (18.2)

5. Which of these things would you examine before you examine a child's throat?

A His weight B His temperature C His tonsillar lymph nodes D His respirations E All of these things (18.2)

6. Which of these diseases cause lesions in a child's mouth and on his skin?

A Tinea versicolor B Ringworm C Scabies D Measles E Impetigo (18.4)

7. Which of these diseases does NOT cause lesions in a child's mouth or lips?

A Thrush B Herpes stomatitis C Scabies D Vitamin B deficiency E Cancrum oris (18.3)

8. FUNLADE (3 years) has had fever for a week. His mouth is sore and his lips are crusted. His mother should wash out his mouth with—

A—saline? B—hypochlorite? C—permanganate? D—lysol? E—any local medicine? (18.4)

9. Which of these children would you LEAST expect to have thrush?

A OSMAN who has been given tetracycline for three weeks. B TAREK who has polio. C SHERIF who is newborn. D ISMAIL who has severe TB. E HAZIZ who is malnourished. (18.5)

10. The same organism that causes sores on a mother's lips may infect her baby and cause—

A—herpes stomatitis? B—thrush? C—Vincent's stomatitis? D—cancrum oris? E—chickenpox? (18.6)

11. Which of these diseases causes the worst smell in a child's mouth?

A Vincent's stomatitis **B** Thrush **C** Mumps **D** Tonsillitis **E** Herpes stomatitis (18.7)

12. A child with cancrum oris needs all these treatments EXCEPT—

A—hydrogen peroxide mouth washes? **B**—as little food as possible until his lesion has healed? **C**—plenty of fluids? **D**—the removal of dead tissue? **E**—an antibiotic? (18.1)

13. You can treat thrush with—

A—penicillin? **B**—tetracycline? **C**—sulphadimidine? **D**—any of these drugs? **E**—none of these drugs? (18.5)

14. FUAD ($4\frac{1}{2}$ years, 11 kg) has a deep ulcer on his gum and on the inside of his left cheek. He is probably an early case of—

A—measles? **B**—diphtheria? **C**—cancrum oris? **D**—herpes stomatitis? **E**—thrush? (18.9)

15. Angular stomatitis is caused by lack of—

A—vitamin E? **B**—vitamin D? **C**—vitamin C? **D**—one of the B vitamins? **E**—vitamin A? (18.10)

16. Which of these diseases is LEAST likely to cause fever?

A Tonsillitis **B** Diphtheria **C** Pneumonia **D** Bronchitis **E** Thrush (18.5)

17. A child who has had tetanus and recovered from it—

A—should be given DPT or tetanus toxoid? **B**—is now immune to tetanus? **C**—must NOT be given tetanus toxoid? (18.16)

18. Many sore red throats are caused by viruses, and are not helped by antibiotics.

D True? **E** False? (18.11)

19. Diphtheria organisms can make a toxin which harms the—

B—heart? **C**—brain? **D**—skin? **E**—lungs? (18.12)

20. Which of these is white and easiest to remove from a child's mouth or throat?

A A diphtheritic membrane **B** The lesions caused by thrush **C** Milk curds **D** The lesions caused by herpes **E** The lesions of Vincent's stomatitis (18.5)

21. A child is most likely to need a tracheotomy (a hole made in his trachea) if he has—

A—tonsillitis? **B**—pneumonia? **C**—diphtheria? **D**—bronchitis? (18.12)

22. Which of these is NOT part of the treatment of a child with tetanus?

A Penicillin **B** Antitoxin **C** Paraldehyde to make the spasms less **D** Enough food and fluids **E** Cooling with water to lower his temperature (18.16)

23. Tetanus organisms are LEAST likely to get into a child through—

A—his lungs? **B**—a discharging ear? **C**—a wound? **D**—his umbilicus if he is newborn? **E**—carious teeth? (18.16)

24. BRAVO (4 years) had a very small cut on his leg last week. It is healing well. He has not been immunized.

B He cannot possibly get tetanus from such a small cut? **C** His cut is healing well, so he cannot get tetanus? **D** He might get tetanus in the next week or two? **E** He has now passed the danger time for tetanus? (18.16)

25. Tetanus bacteria—

A—cause pus to be formed? **B**—stay in the local lesion? **C**—go to other parts of the body and harm them? **D**—cause cellulitis? **E**—grow in the blood (18.16)

SWELLINGS A

Chapter 19: with revision: Code 8

1. Swellings almost anywhere in the body can be caused by—

A—hernias? **B**—lymphadenitis? **C**—mastoiditis? **D**—cellulitis? **E**—goitre? (19.1)

2. Oedema most often causes swelling—

A—over the ankles? **B**—in the middle of the neck? **C**—in the groin? **D**—at the umbilicus? **E**—on the back? (19.9)

3. Osteomyelitis usually causes a painful tender swelling—

A—over a lymph node? **B**—in the groin? **C**—in the middle of the abdomen? **D**—in front of the ear? **E**—over a bone? (19.9, 24.5)

4. Which of these children have a swelling that is most likely to be helped by penicillin?

A JIM has a swelling at his umbilicus which gets larger when he coughs. **B** JANE (14 years) has a swelling in the middle of her neck which moves when she swallows. **C** JACK (5 years) has had a hot tender painful swelling in the muscles of his right leg for three days. **D** JULES has swollen ankles. **E** JUSTIN has had a large spleen for several months. (24.5b)

PLEASE DON'T WRITE ON THESE QUESTIONS OTHER PEOPLE MAY NEED THEM

---

5. SARINA has some painless, 1 cm, bean-shaped swellings under both the angles of her jaw. She is eating well and has no symptoms. She has—

A—a goitre? **B**—chronic septic lymphadenitis? **C**—acute septic lymphadenitis? **D**—TB lymphadenitis? (19.2)

6. Whenever a health worker finds a large, tender lymph-node the first thing he should do is to look for signs of—

A—septicaemia? **B**—a septic local lesion? **C**—TB? **D**—malnutrition? **E**—anaemia? (19.2)

7. A child with acute septic lymphadenitis usually needs—

A—an antibiotic? **B**—no treatment? **C**—isoniazid? **D**—to be sent for help? (19.2)

8. The lymph nodes which are most often seen and felt to be enlarged because of TB are the nodes—

A—in the axilla? **B**—under the chin? **C**—at the sides of the neck? **D**—in the groin? **E**—at the back of the neck? (19.2)

9. When lymph nodes at the sides of the neck open and discharge through the skin the disease is probably caused by—

A—protozoa? **B**—leprosy? **C**—chronic sepsis? **D**—acute sepsis? **E**—TB? (19.3)

10. Which of these swellings would not be helped by penicillin?

A Pyomyositis **B** Cellulitis **C** Mastoiditis **D** TB lymphadenitis **E** Acute septic lymphadenitis (19.3)

11. RAWYA has mumps. What are you going to say to her mother?

A 'She needs hospital treatment.' **B** 'She is not infectious.' **C** 'She may get a second attack of mumps.' **D** 'Penicillin will help her.' **E** 'Her swellings will go by themselves in about two weeks.' (19.4)

12. Lack of one of these things in a child's food causes swelling of the feet. Which one?

A Protein **B** Iodine **C** Vitamin C **D** Vitamin A **E** Potassium (7.10, 19.7)

13. NADIA has a swelling in the lower front part of her neck which moves up and down when she swallows. It is a swelling of her—

A—larynx? **B**—lymph nodes? **C**—parotid gland? **D**—thyroid gland? **E**—uvula? (19.6)

14. Iodine-lack in a community is most serious because it can cause—

A—neck swellings? **B**—backward children? **C**—keratomalacia? **D**—oedema? **E**—anaemia? (19.6, 24.14b)

15. The most useful sign or special test for diagnosing the nephrotic syndrome from other kinds of swelling is—

A—oedema of a child's eyelids? **B**—severe anaemia? **C**—protein + + + + in his urine? **D**—oedema of his ankles? **E**—to measure the protein in his blood? (19.7)

16. There are no lymph nodes—

A—round the eyes? **B**—under the jaws? **C**—in the axilla? **D**—in the groins? **E**—behind the ear? (19–1, 19–16)

MATCH these families with the disease you would expect them to get.

17. The family where an uncle has a cavity in his lung. **18.** The poor family who eat maize and little other food. **19.** The family who eat no green leafy vegetables. **20.** The family where someone has a sore on his lip.

A Thrush **B** A dark, scaly symmetrical rash on the parts of a child's body on which the light shines **C** The child who cannot find his toys as it gets dark in the evening **D** A baby with herpes stomatitis **E** A child with TB meningitis (11.23, 13.11, 16.13, 18.16 (Revision))

MATCH these children with the drugs you would give them.

21. The child with leprosy **22.** The child who is having fits **23.** The child who has swallowed 30 iron tablets **24.** The child with scabies. (3.47, 11.10, 12.4, 15.9 (Revision))

A Ipecacuanha **B** Dapsone **C** Benzyl benzoate **D** Paraldehyde

25. Which of these diseases does NOT make lymphnodes swell?

A Acute lymphadenitis? **B** Chronic septic lymphadenitis? **C** TB lymphadenitis? **D** Malaria? (19.2)

ABDOMEN A
Chapter 20: with revision: Code 1

1. Hernias—

A—may become bigger or smaller quickly? **B**—are found in any part of the body? **C**—get smaller when a child coughs or cries? **D**—are caused by bacterial infection? **E**—always need a surgical operation? (20.4)

2. In a child with an acute abdomen I should NOT expect to find—

A—abdominal tenderness? **B**—abdominal swelling? **C**—abdominal pain? **D**—vomiting? **E**—a swollen fontanelle? (20.2)

3. When we examine a child's abdomen we can find out—

A—if he has a urine infection? **B**—what he has eaten? **C**—how large his spleen is? **D**—how long his gut is? **E**—if he has worms? (20.3)

4. Which of these children has an acute abdomen?

A TOKS with peritonitis **B** JIM with hepatitis **C** JACK with gastroenteritis **D** JILL with nephritis **E** SUKIE with tonsillitis (20.2)

5. Which of these children has NOT got an acute abdomen?

A HUGH with a tender hernia, vomiting, and a swollen abdomen. **B** HENRY with a heavy *Ascaris* infection, a swollen abdomen, vomiting, and constipation. **C** HARRY with vomiting, abdominal pain, and constipation. **D** HERBERT with abdominal pain, fever, and pus on his tonsils. **E** HUMPHRY with a swollen abdomen and a painful hernia that cannot be reduced (20.11, 20.14)

6. JAKE (4 years). You have examined his abdomen and cannot feel his spleen.

A He has chronic malaria? **B** He cannot have malaria? **C** He has hookworm anaemia? **D** His spleen is normal as far as you are able to find out? (20.3)

7. A child's liver is on his—

C—right? **D**—left? (20.3)

8. ANDREW has a tender place at the right side of his abdomen. As you try to touch it his muscles contract and prevent you from touching it. He has—

A—rebound tenderness? **B**—guarding? **C**—rigidity? **D**—spasticity? **E**—hypotonia? (20.3)

9. Which of these swellings can be reduced when a child lies down?

A The swellings caused by mumps **B** The swelling caused by an acute septic infection **C** A hernia **D** An enlarged spleen **E** Large lymph nodes (20.4)

10. NUBUO (3 years, 38·2 °C) has a severe septic lesion on his right buttock. This would cause lymphadenitis—

A—near his anus? **B**—at his umbilicus? **C**—in his right axilla? **D**—in his left groin? **E**—in his right groin? (19:1, 20.5)

11. A strangulated hernia is dangerous because it may cause—

A—lymphadenitis? **B**—peritonitis? **C**—malnutrition? **D**—cellulitis? (20.5)

12. RARUA (3 years) has two hernias. Which of them will probably cure itself as he grows older?

C His inguinal hernia **D** His umbilical hernia (20.5, 20.7)

13. Which of these does NOT cause abdominal swelling?

A Malnutrition **B** A urine infection **C** Heavy infection with *Ascaris* **D** Gut obstruction **E** A very large spleen (20.8)

14. Which of these is most serious? Abdominal swelling for—

A—3 months with mild diarrhoea? **B**—1 year with fever sometimes? **C**—2 days with vomiting and constipation? **D**—6 months with passing worms sometimes? **E**—2 months with normal stools? (20.8)

15. Most children with an acute abdomen—

C—keep moving about? **D**—lie still? (20.3)

16. SHILLING (3 years, 38·5 °C) has had vomiting and abdominal pain for one day. He has no diarrhoea and no abnormal signs in his abdomen or anywhere else. He should be—

A—given glucose–salt solution and observed carefully? **B**—given an antibiotic? **C**—sent to hospital quickly? **D**—given intravenous fluids? **E**—given a drug to stop him vomiting (20.14)

17. If a child with an acute abdomen is not treated, he will probably—

A—get more attacks like this? **B**—become severely malnourished? **C**—become severely anaemic? **D**—recover by himself? **E**—die soon? (20.13)

18. Which of these is a sign that a child with abdominal pain has NOT got an acute abdomen?

A Constipation **B** Vomiting **C** Large inflamed tonsils and fever **D** Looking 'ill' **E** Abdominal rigidity (20.13)

19. The commonest cause of vomiting in a young child is—

A—acute abdomen? **B**—worms? **C**—constipation? **D**—an acute mild infection somewhere in his body? **E**—meningitis? (20.14)

20. Which of these worms obstructs the gut?

A *Trichuris* **B** *Ascaris* **C** Tapeworms **D** Hookworms **E** Threadworms (20.15)

21. All these children have abdominal pain and have vomited once. Which of them is most likely to have an acute abdomen?

A JURG with a temperature of 39 °C. **B** BO with respirations of 84 per minute. **C** SUNE with pus cell + + + in his urine. **D** STIG with an abnormally red throat and tender tonsilar lymph nodes. **E** HANS with abdominal tenderness and guarding. (20.15)

22. Which of these diseases does NOT sometimes cause abdominal pain? **A** Malnutrition **B** Tonsillitis **C** Pneumonia **D** Bacillary dysentery **E** Malaria (20.13)

23. Which of these diseases LEAST often causes diarrhoea?

A Food poisoning **B** Gut obstruction **C** Measles **D** Giardiasis **E** Lactose intolerance (20.13)

24. Which of these is the MOST serious sign in a dehydrated child?

A Shock **B** Loss of skin elasticity **C** Sunken eyes **D** A pulse of 120 per minute **E** A dry mouth (9.18 (Revision))

25. Which of these kinds of cough would you expect to last longest? The cough caused by—

A—acute bronchitis? **B**—pneumonia? **C**—whooping cough? **D**—measles without any complications? **E**—tonsillitis? (8.17 (Revision))

WORMS A
Chapter 21: with revision: Code 5

MATCH these organisms with the diseases they cause—

1. Acid-fast bacilli. **2.** Plasmodia. **3.** Fungi **4.** Insects

A Amoebic dysentery **B** Scabies **C** Malaria **D** Tinea versicolor **E** Leprosy (12.3, 10.7, 11.13, 11.10 (Revision))

MATCH these chemicals with the number of grams of them needed to make a litre of glucose–salt solution.

5. Potassium chloride **6.** Sodium bicarbonate **7.** Ordinary salt **8.** Glucose

A 20 g **B** 4·5 g **C** 3·5 g **D** 2·5 g **E** 1·5 g (9.21 (Revision))

9. PEDA'S vulva itches so that she scratches it. Which of these might be causing her symptoms?

A Tapeworms **B** Threadworms *(Enterobius)* **C** *Ascaris* **D** Hookworms **E** Ringworm (21.5)

10. With which of these worms can a child make his load heavier by infecting himself with his own faeces on his own hands?

A *H. nana* **B** *Strongyloides* **C** *T. solium* **D** *T. saginata* **E** Hookworms (21.4)

11. Which kind of worm would you look for by using pieces of 'Sellotape' ('Scotch tape')?

A Threadworms **B** Tapeworms **C** *Trichuris* **D** Hookworms **E** Ascaris (21.5)

12. Which of these worms would you NOT treat with niclosamide?

A *T. solium* **B** *Ascaris* **C** *T. saginata* **D** *H. nana* (3:1b)

13. ANUP has threadworms. He needs—

D—one dose of piperazine? **E**—piperazine for several days? (21.3)

14. Which of these worms obstructs the gut?

A Hookworms **B** *Taenia* **C** *Ascaris* **D** *Trichuris* **E** *Strongyloides* (21.3)

15. Which of these worms does NOT hold on to the wall of the gut?

A Hookworms **B** *Taenia* **C** *H. nana* **D** *Ascaris* (21.3)

16. CORA (8 months) cannot walk yet, but she is often left to play on soil where there is faeces. Sometimes she eats earth.

A She is too young to be infected by hookworms but *Ascaris* might infect her? **B** Hookworms might infect her but not *Ascaris?* **C** Only *Trichuris* can infect her? **D** Only *Strongyloides* can infect her? **E** Any of these worms might infect her? (21.1, 21.3, 21.6, 21.7)

17. Which of these is the best way of preventing worm infections?

A Making sure that everyone uses latrines **B** Boiling water **C** Immunization **D** Early treatment **E** Keeping all children on the road-to-health (21.7)

18. Which of these is one of the 'danger signs' in diarrhoea?

A Pale lips and conjunctiva **B** A swollen fontanelle **C** Oedema **D** Sunken eyes **E** Noisy breathing (9.31 (Revision))

19. A child's worm-load usually depends on—

B—how many worms get into him? **C**—how they multiply when they are in him? **D**—both these things? (21.1)

20. OLA's anus itches. What worm might be causing this?

A *Trichuris* **B** Tapeworms **C** Threadworms **D** *Strongyloides* **E** *Ascaris* (21.1)

21. Which of these drugs kill the most kinds of worms?

A Tetrachlorethylene **B** Bephenium **C** Pyrantel pamoate **D** Piperazine **E** Penicillin (3:1b)

22. SITA is vomiting and is dehydrated. Her mother says she has vomited a worm. It is probably—

A—*Strongyloides?* **B**—*H. nana?* **C**—a threadworm? **D**—a tapeworm? **E**—*Ascaris?* (21.3)

23. Which would you treat first?

A SITA'S dehydration **B** Or her worms **C** Both at once (9.20)

24. Which of these is the smallest?

B *T. solium* **C** *T. saginata* **D** *H. nana* (21.4)

25. Which of these worms can go from one child straight to another child, or from a rat to a child?

A *Strongyloides* **B** *H. nana* **C** *T. solium* **D** *T. saginata* **E** *Ascaris* (21.4)

ANAEMIA AND JAUNDICE A
Chapter 22: Code 5

1. In a healthy child haemoglobin is—

C—dissolved in the plasma? **D**—in the white cells? **E**—in the red cells? (22.1)

2. You can most easily diagnose anaemia by looking at the conjunctiva of a child's—

C—lower eyelids? **D**—upper eyelids? **E**—sclerae? (22.1)

3. ROSA is mildly anaemic. PEPA is moderately anaemic. PABLO is severely anaemic. They all became anaemic slowly. Which of them would you expect to have symptoms?

B All of them **C** PEPA and PABLO **D** PABLO probably (22.1)

4. Which of these healthy people do you expect to have the highest haemoglobin?

A A woman **B** A full-term newborn baby **C** A two-month-old child **D** A one-year-old child **E** A man (22.2)

5. All these children have infective hepatitis. Which of them has NOT got one of the danger signs you would be worried about in a child with infective hepatitis?

A BLODWYN with severe jaundice **B** GWYNNETH with severe vomiting **C** GLYNNIS who is very drowsy **D** ELUNED who is bleeding from her nose **E** GWEN who has pale urine and dark stools

6. Dactylitis is a sign of—

A—malaria? **B**—hookworm anaemia? **C**—iron deficiency anaemia. **D**—sickle-cell anaemia? **E**—hepatitis?(22.8)

7. LISELOTTE has a haemoglobin of 2 g/dl. She is—

B—normal? **C**—severely anaemic? **D**—mildly anaemic? **E**—moderately anaemic? (22.2)

8. Sickle-cell anaemia—

A—is inherited by a child from his parents? **B**—is infectious? **C**—should be treated with iron? **D**—is difficult to diagnose in a health-centre laboratory? **E**—is not made worse by infections? (22.8)

9. All these children have a haemoglobin of 9 g/dl. Which of them most needs iron?

A ARCHIMEDE with malaria **B** ARISTIDE with chronic dysentery **C** ADOLPHE with sickle-cell anaemia (22.4)

10. Which of these does NOT cause anaemia? Lack of—

A—vitamin A? **B**—protein? **C**—folic acid? **D**—iron? (22.3)

11. Iron medicine makes a child's stools—

A—black? **B**—white? **C**—yellow? **D**—green? **E**—red? (22.4)

12. Which of these most often causes anaemia?

A *Trichuris* **B** Hookworms **C** *Ascaris* **D** Tapeworms **E** Threadworms (22.5)

13. SIRAYUL has yellow eyes, mild fever, dark urine, and pale stools. He will not eat. He probably has—

A—malaria? **B**—sickle-cell anaemia? **C**—infectious hepatitis? **D**—syringe jaundice? **E**—either infectious hepatitis or syringe jaundice? (22.11)

14. Which of these children needs iron?

C YUMMY who is bleeding into his gut. **D** YUCKY whose red cells are being destroyed while they are in her blood vessels. (22.3)

15. Which of these children most needs iron?

A The small-for-dates baby **B** The jaundiced baby **C** The breast-fed baby **D** The preterm baby **E** The bottle-fed baby (22.4)

16. Which of these can be used again by the body many times to make blood?

A Vitamin C **B** Glucose **C** Vitamin A **D** Folic acid **E** Iron (22.3)

17. FAUSTUS is anaemic and has a large spleen. Which of these would probably help him most?

A Folic acid and chloroquine **B** Iron **C** Penicillin **D** Vitamin A and calcium **E** Ampicillin (22.3)

18. Which of these foods contains the LEAST iron?

A Dark green leafy vegetables **B** Liver **C** Meat **D** Rice **E** Legumes (22.4)

19. A child is most likely to suffer from anaemia caused by lack of iron in his food during his—

B—first year? **C**—second year? **D**—third year? **E**—fourth year? (22.4)

20. A double dose of iron medicine will—

B—cure a child's anaemia quicker? **C**—make no difference? (3.33, 22.5)

21. Which of these treatments is the cheapest?

A *Ascaris* treated with piperazine **B** Threadworms treated with piperazine **C** Hookworms treated with TCE (tetrachlorethylene) **D** Hookworms treated with bephenium (22.5)

22. Which of these diseases causes a haemolytic anaemia?

A Chronic bleeding **B** Hookworms **C** Malnutrition **D** Lack of iron **E** Malaria (22.7)

23. Which of these diseases may cause mild jaundice and anaemia?

A Sickle-cell anaemia **B** Iron deficiency anaemia **C** Hookworm anaemia **D** Hepatitis **E** PEM (22.7)

24. A child with 63 hookworms in a standard faecal smear would probably—

A—have bloody diarrhoea? **B**—have a haemoglobin of 12 g/dl? **C**—be dead? **D**—be severely anaemic? **E**—have a large spleen? (21.1, 22.5)

25. Which of these should NOT be given by intramuscular injection?

A Iron **B** Darrow's solution **C** Iodized oil **D** Quinine **E** Vitamin A (22.5)

URINARY SYMPTOMS A
Chapter 23: Code 6

1. Dysuria is—

A—pain in the bladder? **B**—blood in the urine? **C**—pain while passing urine? **D**—not being able to pass urine? (23.1)

2. WILLY wants to pass urine but he cannot. He has—

A—retention? **B**—frequency? **C**—polyuria? **D**—urgency? **E**—dysuria? (23.1)

3. Which of these diseases are most likely to make a child's urine dark?

B Urinary infection **C** Nephrotic syndrome **D** Anaemia **E** Dehydration (23.1)

4. Which of these diseases makes the urine red?

B Acute nephritis **C** Fever **D** Dehydration **E** Meningitis (23.1)

5. Examining a child's urine for pus cells is helpful in diagnosing—

A—dehydration? **B**—malaria? **C**—urinary infection? **D**—meningitis? **E**—backwardness? (23.2)

6. Which of these children MOST needs to have his urine examined? The child with—

A—fits? **B**—chest pain? **C**—a discharging ear? **D**—a chronic cough? **E**—fever which has lasted 10 days? (10.10)

7. Which of these things is a health-centre laboratory LEAST likely to be able to do with a specimen of urine?

A Examine it for protein **B** Examine it for pus cells **C** Look for the ova of *Schistosoma haematobium* **D** Culture (grow) bacteria (23.2)

8. Which of these does NOT cause dysuria?

C Threadworms **D** Nephritis **E** Urinary infection (23.7)

9. A urinary infection can cause any of these EXCEPT—

A—fever? **B**—dysuria? **C**—pus in the urine? **D**—bacteria in the urine? **E**—bile in the urine? (23.4)

10. Schistosomiasis can be treated with—

A—niridazole? **B**—tiabendazole? **C**—penicillin? **D**—piperazine? **E**—mepacrine? (23.8)

11. Urinary infections do NOT present as—

A—fever? **B**—cough? **C**—dysuria? **D**—fever and vomiting? **E**—a child 'wetting herself' after she has become dry? (23.4)

12. AMIE (5 years) has rigors, pain when she passes urine, and frequency. Unfortunately, your health centre has not got a laboratory in which to examine her urine. Which of these would you give her?

A Sulphadimidine **B** Penicillin **C** Amidopyrine **D** Sulphaguanidine (23.4)

13. Chronic urinary infections are dangerous because they—

A—cause haematuria? **B**—cause a child to lose protein from his kidneys? **C**—cause dehydration? **D**—cause septicaemia? **E**—destroy his kidneys? (23.4)

14. FARIDA has had several urinary infections. She—

A—will probably not get any more attacks? **B**—is now immune? **C**—may have a congenital abnormality of her kidneys? **D**—can get the special tests she needs at a health centre? **E**—may get acute nephritis? (23.4)

15. BHOOMI has had a urinary infection. What would you tell his mother?

A 'He is cured and we need not worry.' **B** 'His brothers and sisters may become infected.' C 'He will never get attacks like this again.' D 'I am going to write URINARY INFECTION on his weight chart.' (23.4)

16. A child who is having sulphadimidine needs to drink plenty of water so that—

A—if he gets haematuria the blood will be washed away? B—the sulphadimidine will not block the small tubes in his kidneys? C—his body has plenty of fluid to sweat with? D—his urine becomes pale? E—the sulphadimidine is absorbed better? (23.4)

17. Which of these worms are most likely to make a child's urine red?

A Hookworms B *Schistosoma haemotobium* C *Ascaris* D Threadworms E Tapeworms (23.8)

18. Which of these children has the nephrotic syndrome?

B PRAKASH with swollen eyelids, protein +, red cells, and casts in his urine. C SATISH with swollen eyelids, swollen ankles, and protein + + + + in his urine. D IMRANA with swollen ankles, a 'flaking paint rash', apathy, and a normal urine. (19.8, 23.1)

19. Which of these diseases does NOT cause swelling of the eyes or feet?

B Nephrotic syndrome C Acute nephritis D Acute urinary infection E Kwashiorkor (23:1)

20. *Schistosoma haematobium* is most common in—

A Schoolchildren B Babies C Children before they go to school D Adults E Mothers (23.8)

21. Which of these diseases is often caused by gonococci?

A Pneumonia B Diarrhoea C Vulvovaginitis in a young girl D Acute nephritis (23.10)

22. Which of these would you LEAST expect to cause a sore red vulva in a young girl?

B Gonococci C Foreign body D Threadworms E *Ascaris* (23.10)

23. ARA is a week old. His mother is worried because she cannot pull back his foreskin. What are you going to tell her?

A 'He should be circumcised.' B 'This is normal.' C 'He needs a small operation.' D 'Try pulling down his foreskin a little bit more each day.' (23.11)

24. A boy's foreskin should be able to be pulled back—

C—at birth? D—when he is about four? E—when he is about 12 years old? (23.11)

25. Which of these children are most likely to have a urinary infection?

B MIRA with fever for 2 days. C ABHAYA with fever and cough. D LALIT who has had fever for two weeks but no other signs. E KAMALA with fever and severe meningeal signs. (23.4)

NOT WALKING A
Chapter 24: Code 3

1. KIEM is late speaking but is normal with his other milestones. We should examine his—

A—stools? B—haemoglobin? C—urine? D—abdomen? E—hearing? (24.16)

2. MULOBEZI (4 years, 38·2 °C) cannot walk. He has had a large, firm, warm, tender swelling in his left thigh for four days. He has had rigors and is ill. The swelling seems to be in the muscles of his thigh, not the bone. He probably has—

A—Osteomyelitis? B—Septic arthritis? C—Pyomyositis? D—Polio? E TB? (24.5b)

3. BAN is eighteen-months old. He used to walk normally, but for the last three days he has stopped walking. This might be caused by—

A—poliomyelitis? B—cerebral palsy? C—Down's syndrome? D—cretinism? E—some other disease which has made him backward? (24.1)

4. Cerebral palsy is caused by—

A—cerebral malaria only? B—birth injury only? C—meningitis only? D—severe jaundice only? E—all of these diseases? (24.12, 24.15)

5. Which of these helps to prevent cerebral palsy?

A Immunizing pregnant mothers against tetanus B Treating hookworm anaemia early C Diagnosing hepatitis early D Giving mothers good care in childbirth E Polio vaccine (24.12, 24.15)

6. Penicillin is useful for treating—

A—polio? B—leprosy? C—acute osteomyelitis? D—a TB hip? E—Down's syndrome? (24.5)

7. Which of these children need treatment most urgently?

A IVOR whose legs have been weak because of polio for a month. B IGOR with osteomyelitis for two days. C IOLO with a TB hip. D ION who is late walking and talking. E IVAN (2 years) who limps because he has a club foot (24.5)

8. Acute osteomyelitis is caused by—

A—viruses? B—pyogenic bacteria? C—TB bacilli? D—worms? E—fungi? (24.5)

9. The organisms which cause polio first harm a child's—

A—muscles? B—nerves? C—bones? D—joints? E—tendons? (24.4)

10. The organism which causes polio infects—

C—a few unfortunate children? D—most children unless they have been immunized? (24.2)

11. Most children who are infected with the polio virus have—

A—no symptoms? B—mild fever only? C—meningeal signs? D—paralysis of their legs? E—mild diarrhoea? (24.2)

12. HO (3 years). His legs became severely paralysed by polio ten days ago. What would you say to his mother?

A 'Operations don't help his disease.' **B** 'He will not be able to walk again.' **C** 'Put his legs through all their movements several times a day.' **D** 'Penicillin will help him.' (24.4)

13. MACHMOED (4 years, 39 °C) has a severe pain in his right leg. The middle of his right thigh is tender. Bending his hip and knee does not hurt him. He is 'ill' and he will not eat. His left leg and his arms are normal. What is his probable diagnosis?

A Injury **B** TB **C** Polio **D** Septic arthritis **E** Osteomyelitis (24.5)

14. SUKHDEY ($3\frac{1}{2}$ years, 38 °C) has had an acutely painful lesion in one of the bones in his lower arm for four days. There is no weakness or wasting, but moving his wrist hurts him. He needs antibiotics for at least—

A—3 days? **B**—4–6 weeks? **C**—6 months? (24.5)

15. Which of these does NOT show muscle wasting?

A Chronic polio **B** Leprosy where the nerves have been harmed **C** Acute polio **D** Marasmus **E** Chronic joint disease (24.4)

16. Which of these diseases causes anaesthesia and muscle wasting?

A Chronic joint disease **B** Malnutrition **C** Polio **D** Leprosy (24.8)

17. Which of these diseases does NOT cause contractures?

A Leprosy **B** Chronic joint disease **C** Polio **D** Malnutrition (24.8)

18. Severely backward children—

A—are seldom hidden by their families? **B**—cannot be made normal again? **C**—are about one in ten thousand of all children? **D**—cannot be helped? **E**—are found in some communities only? (24.9)

19. HIN is backward. What are you going to tell his mother?

A 'You will have to do everything for him yourself, you cannot teach him.' **B** 'There are some expensive drugs which will cure him.' **C** 'Don't be ashamed of him.' **D** 'He needs hospital treatment.' (24.11)

20. Which of these causes of backwardness is more common in the children of mothers over 40?

A Down's syndrome **B** PEM **C** Cretinism **D** Cerebral palsy **E** Severe jaundice (24.13)

21. HAP (3 years) is backward, deaf, and cannot speak. He walks abnormally and has thick, dry skin and a big tongue. There are several children like HAP in the village. HAP'S backwardness could have been prevented by—

A—better care during childbirth? **B**—immunizing his mother during pregnancy? **C**—giving him vitamins? **D**—immunizing him? **E**—injecting his mother with iodized oil early in pregnancy? (24.14b)

22. In communities where many adults have goitres there will be more children than usual who are backward because of—

A—meningitis? **B**—lack of vitamins? **C**—Down's syndrome? **D**—iodine embryopathy? (24.14b)

23. Which of these diseases is MOST likely to cause cerebral palsy?

A Polio **B** Tonsillitis **C** Smallpox **D** Typhoid **E** Meningitis (24.12)

24. The muscles of a spastic child are—

A—hypertonic? **B**—hypotonic? **C**—normal? (24.15)

25. During their lives children with cerebral palsy usually—

A—get steadily worse and die? **B**—stay about the same? **C**—slowly recover so they are normal by the time they are adults? (24.15)

OTHER SYMPTOMS A
Chapter 25: with revision: Code 4

MATCH these signs with the diseases that cause them

1. Not speaking by the time a child is aged 23 months **2.** A large spleen **3.** Itching anus **4.** A contracture of the knee

A Threadworms **B** Chronic polio **C** Iodine embryopathy **D** Measles **E** Sickle-cell anaemia (23.10, 24.4, 24.14, 22.8, 20.3 (Revision))

5. Which of these is LEAST likely to be a symptom of a behaviour disease?

A A child of five wetting his bed **B** Not going to school **C** Not eating **D** Stealing **E** Not walking by the time a child is aged 3 years (25.2)

6. YETUNDE passes hard stools. They are painful to pass and there is some bright red blood with them. She probably has—

A—faecal incontinence? **B**—a fissure? **C**—amoebic dysentery? **D**—bacilliary dysentery? **E**—rectal prolapse? (25.6)

7. ASHVIN has a foreign body in his ear. What would you use FIRST to try to remove it?

D An ear syringe **E** A bent wire (25.11)

8. Which of these is best given intravenously, but can if necessary be given by intramuscular injection?

A Chloroquine **B** Pyrimethamine **C** Glucose–salt solution **D** Quinine **E** Mepacrine (3.25)

MATCH these children with the examination or special test they need—

9. HO (5 years) has swollen feet. **10.** LO (6 months) has fits, fever, and vomiting. **11.** KO (7 years) was hit in his right eye and it is now painful, red, and watering. **12.** GO (2 years) has not started to talk.

A Staining with fluorescein. **B** Urine for protein. **C** Examining his hearing. **D** A skin scraping for AAFB. **E** Lumbar puncture. (15.6, 24.10, 19.8, 16.7)

MATCH these children with the kind of immunity they have got—

13. MATTHEW was given measles vaccine. **14.** MARK was given tetanus antitoxin. **15.** LUKE got polio. **16.** JOHN (3 days) whose mother had measles when she was a child?

A Synthetic active **B** Natural active **C** Artificial active **D** Artificial passive **E** Natural passive (4.2) (Revision)

17. Constipation is a serious symptom when—

A—there is also abdominal pain, distension, and vomiting? **B**—it has lasted for over a year? **C**—the child has not gained weight for two months? **D**—a bottle-fed baby passes small, dry stools? **E**—a breast-fed baby only passes stools every 3 days? (25.6)

18. Which of these is LEAST likely to cause a behaviour disease?

A. A child being sent away to live with his aunt **B** An uncle staying in the house who has a chronic cough and blood-stained sputum **C** An angry, drunken father **D** Parents who fight **E** A newborn baby sister (25.2)

19. Which of these is most likely to help cause rectal prolapse?

A Hookworms **B** *Ascaris* **C** Malnutrition **D** Constipation (25.7)

20. In which part of the body does a foreign body most commonly present as a blood-stained discharge?

A Nose **B** Ear **C** Bronchi **D** Gut **E** Larynx (25.11)

21. KWANG (2 months). His mother has brought him to see you because she thinks that his breathing is not normal. You examine him and find no abnormal signs. What will you tell her?

A 'He needs penicillin.' **B** 'He needs an X-ray.' **C** 'You have wasted my time. There is no need for you to have come.' **D** 'I am glad we have been able to help you, this is nothing to worry about.' **E** 'Don't bring KWANG again unless you are sure he is ill.' (25.1)

22. JANE (2 years) had rings put in both her ears about three weeks ago. The holes of her ears are swollen and inflamed. Injections and ointment have not helped. What would you tell her mother?

C 'The gold in her ears is too pure.' **D** 'If you leave the rings in long enough the swelling will slowly go.' **E** 'We must take out the rings.' (25.9)

23. HWAN has been sucking a sweet and it has stuck in his throat. He is choking and cyanosed. What would you do FIRST?

B Look for the sweet in his throat **C** Get out the sweet with your finger **D** Send him for help **E** Turn him upside down immediately and hit him on his back (25–1)

24. A foreign body is most serious if it gets into a child's—

A—vagina? **B**—nose? **C**—gut? **D**—bronchi? **E**—ear? (8.18 (Revision))

25. JOEY (3 years, 11 kg) has been brought to the clinic with a wet, red swelling coming out of his anus. It does not cause much pain and he has had it once before. This is most likely to be—

A—an abscess? **B**—a lump of worms? **C**—an intussusception from higher up the gut? **D**—a rectal tumour? **E**—a rectal prolapse? (25.7)

NEWBORN BABY A
Chapter 26: First part: Code 6

1. Which of these things may be NORMAL for a baby during the first few minutes of his life?

A Not moving when he is pinched **B** Not coughing when his mouth is sucked out **C** Irregular breathing **D** Hypotonia (26.1)

2. A newborn baby breathes—

A—most easily through his nose? **B**—most easily through his mouth? **C**—through his mouth and nose equally easily? (26.4)

3. When a baby has just been born his pulse is about—

A—50? **B**—60? **C**—80? **D**—90? **E**—180? (26.1)

4. A baby's cord should usually be tied—

B—after it has stopped beating? **C**—before it has stopped beating? (26.2)

5. If a mother is infected with gonoccocci she is most likely to infect her newborn child's—

A—skin? **B**—mouth? **C**—eyes? **D**—vagina? **E**—urethra? (26.2)

6. How much milk does an artificially fed baby usually need each day for each kilo of his weight?

A 25 ml **B** 50 ml **C** 100 ml **D** 125 ml **E** 150 ml (26.16)

7. When a newborn baby is resuscitated, he should be placed with—

B—his body flat (horizontal)? **C**—his head higher than his legs? **D**—his head lower than his legs? (26.3)

8. The most dangerous complication of mouth-to-mouth resuscitation is—

A—blowing up the baby's stomach? **B**—becoming infected yourself from the baby? **C**—infecting the baby? **D**—bursting the baby's lungs? **E**—bruising the baby's head? (26.3)

9. You are examining a newborn baby and find that the edge of one of his skull bones is on top of one of the others. This—

A—will last all the baby's life but will not be dangerous? **B**—is a sign of skull fracture? **C**—is a sign of brain injury? **D**—is a sign of dehydration? **E**—is caused by moulding and will go by itself in a few days? (26.4)

10. Which of these babies needs the most milk?

A JAMES who is small-for-dates **B** JOSE who is preterm (26.22)

11. Which of these is NORMAL in a newborn baby six hours old?

A A pulse which is less than 100 **B** A Moro reflex **C** Insuction **D** A rooting reflex on one side but not on the other (26.6)

12. A sick newborn baby who cannot suck needs—

A—tube feeding? **B**—vitamin A? **C**—bottle feeding? **D**—as much handling as possible? **E**—glucose–salt solution? (26.6)

13. Early breast-feeding—

A—causes sore nipples? **B**—makes jaundice worse in newborn babies? **C**—causes diarrhoea? **D**—makes less milk come in the breasts? **E**—helps to prevent breast abscesses? (26.7)

14. The quantity of milk made by a mother's breasts—
A—is always the same? **B**—decreases if a baby sucks too often? **C**—increases if a baby sucks more often? **D**—decreases if a baby sucks in the night? **E**—increases if a baby sucks from one breast only at each feed? (26.7)

15. A baby can suck milk through—
C—a breast pump? **D**—a nipple shield? **E**—a nipple shell? (26–15)

16. KEVAU'S mother has engorged breasts. She should—
A—leave the milk in her breasts? **B**—express the milk from her breasts with a breast pump or by hand? **C**—stop her baby sucking from her breasts? **D**—bottle feed her baby? **E**—drink less fluids? (26.10)

17. JIM was born this morning. His mother is worried because very little milk has come into her breasts yet. What are you going to tell her?
A 'You must not let him lose any weight.' **B** 'Don't worry, your breasts may not be full of milk for four or five days.'**C** 'Let me show you how to make a clean, safe bottle feed.' **D** 'We must see that he gets plenty of fluids on his first day.' **E** 'Don't let him suck until your breasts feel full.' (26.13)

18. MABATA (4 months). His mother says she has not got enough milk. What is the FIRST thing you should do?
A Tell her to give MABATA porridge **B** Examine her breasts **C** Look at MABATA'S growth curve **D** Explain how to make a clean, safe artificial feed **E** Tell her to eat and drink more herself (26.14)

19. Artificial feeds—
A—are safest when they are given from a plastic feeding bottle? **B**—are made with seven heaped spoonfuls of milk powder to a cup of boiled water? **C**—can safely be made as strong as a mother wishes? **D**—should be made with equipment that has been sterilized for each feed? **E**—can safely be stored in a vacuum flask? (26.14)

20. HELMUT (2 months). His growth curve is falling off the road to health. His mother says 'I have very little milk in my breasts and no money to buy milk powder.' What would you say to a mother who said this?
A 'Give him porridge after he has fed from the breasts.' **B** 'Stop breast feeding.' **C** 'Give him porridge before he has fed from the breasts.' **D** 'Cassava will make the best porridge for him.' **E** 'Give him this dried skim milk from a bottle.' (26.15)

21. Which of these babies have breast nodules which are easy to feel, cartilage in their ears, and creases on their heels?
C Small-for-dates babies **D** Preterm babies (26.22)

22. Which of these diseases is most likely to cause serious vomiting and weight loss in a baby three to five weeks old?
A Posseting **B** Intussusception **C** Inguinal hernia **D** Amoebic dysentery **E** Pyloric stenosis (26.27)

23. A preterm baby—

A—is not easily infected? **B**—cannot cough, so milk easily gets into his lungs? **C**—has a good store of iron? **D**—is hypertonic? **E**—is good at keeping his body at a normal temperature? (26.22)

24. A preterm baby is in special danger from—
A—hyperglycaemia? **B**—malaria? **C**—rigors? **D**—haemorrhagic disease? **E**—harmful organisms in his mother's milk? (26.22)

25. A healthy breast-fed baby should have got back to his birth weight by the time he is—
A—two days old? **B**—three weeks old? **C**—two months old? **D**—ten days old? (26.21)

NEWBORN BABY A
Chapter 26: Second part: Code 3

1. When a newborn baby becomes jaundiced after the fifth day of life you should look for signs of—
A—hypothermia? **B**—dehydration? **C**—malnutrition? **D**—tetanus? **E**—infection? (26.23)

2. Jaundice is most serious if you can see it in a newborn baby's—
A—face? **B**—sclerae? **C**—feet? **D**—abdomen? **E**—chest? (26.23)

3. If jaundice starts between the second and fifth days of life the most likely cause is—
A—physiological jaundice? **B**—septicaemia? **C**—a serious anaemia? **D**—hepatitis? **E**—none of these things? (26.23)

4. An older baby's gums which have become sore because his teeth are coming through can cause—
A—fits? **B**—fever? **C**—bronchitis? **D**—diarrhoea? **E**—none of these things? (26.65, 25.2c)

5. When you diagnose septicaemia you need to look for—
C—one sign only? **D**—several signs? (26.24)

6. ZAHRA is a hypothermic baby. You are warming him. Which of these would you give him?
A Tetracycline **B** Penicillin **C** Penicillin and streptomycin **D** Chloramphenicol (26.25)

7. MUTEMEKWA (3 hours old). His left foot is turned inwards. His mother can bend it backwards so that its outer side touches the outer side of his leg. He has—
A—true talipes? **B**—false talipes? (26.52)

8. Penicillin is useful treatment for—
A—diarrhoea caused by dirty bottle feeding? **B**—a sticky umbilicus with red skin round it? **C**—thrush? **D**—most urinary infections? **E**—a nappy rash? (26.43)

9. ·LAYI (1 month) has a swelling in his scrotum. It becomes larger when he cries. It is a—
A—hydrocele? **B**—hernia? **C**—swollen lymph gland? (26.59)

10. Which of these babies is likely to have the hardest faeces?

C DAVID who is breast-fed **D** DAMON who is bottle-fed (26.29)

11. What is the commonest cause of diarrhoea in a baby at any age?

A Gut infection **B** Septicaemia **C** Umbilical sepsis **D** Skin sepsis (26.32)

12. MUSTAFA (2 months) has severe watery diarrhoea. His skin elasticity is reduced, his mouth is dry, and his eyes are sunken. He is breast-fed and is too weak to suck. You have no intravenous fluid and you cannot send him for help. What would you say to his mother?

A 'These capsules (chloramphenicol) will cure him.' **B** 'Your milk is not right for him.' **C** 'We will give him glucose–salt solution down a tube.' (26.32)

13. Haemorrhagic disease of the newborn may cause bleeding—

B—from the umbilicus? **C**—into the stomach? **D**—into the lower gut? **E**—from any of these places? (26.33)

14. FRANK (one week). The skin round his umbilicus is red and is starting to swell. A little pus is coming from round his cord. He is in the greatest danger from—

A—umbilical hernia? **B**—septicaemia? **C**—haemorrhage? **D**—tetanus? (16.36)

15. Which of these things is NOT true? Gonococcal conjunctivitis—

A—easily causes blindness? **B**—is very infectious? **C**—can be prevented by giving mothers vitamin A during pregnancy, **D**—is caused by bacteria? **E**—is caught by a baby from his mother? (26.40)

16. Which of these is most likely to cure itself without treatment during the first six months of a child's life?

A Erb's paralysis **B** A cleft palate **C** An inguinal hernia **D** A hydrocele **E** Talipes (26.59)

17. SHIGEO (7 days) makes sudden movements. His jaw closes, the ends of his lips are pulled back, and his neck and body bend backwards. These movements are made worse by noise or by moving him. He has—

C—fits? **D**—the spasms of tetanus? (26.42)

18. A child with talipes should start treatment—

A—during the first month? **B**—in the first two days of life? **C**—during the second year? **D**—during the first year? **E**—when he tries to walk? (26.52)

19. The size of a newborn baby's fontanelle—

A—is very important because big fontanelles don't close? **B**—shows us how clever a baby is going to be? **C**—is seldom of any importance? (26.50)

PLEASE DON'T WRITE ON THESE QUESTIONS OTHER PEOPLE MAY NEED THEM

---

20. KUNLE'S mother was given three doses of tetanus toxoid during her last pregnancy. She is pregnant again. How many doses of toxoid does she need during this pregnancy?

A One **B** Two **C** Three **D** None (26.42)

21. NARIMAN'S mother is worried because her tongue seems to be tied to the floor of her mouth by a fold of mucosa. What would you tell her?

C 'NARIMAN needs an operation later.' **D** 'She needs an operation now.' **E** 'Don't worry, she will be able to speak as well as any other child.' (26.53)

22. DOREEN (2 days) has passed a few drops of blood from her vagina. What would you say to her mother?

A 'This injection (vitamin K) will help her.' **B** 'She has haemorrhagic disease.' **C** 'She needs iron medicine.' **D** 'Don't worry, this will soon stop.' (26.56)

23. Which of these diseases needs to be treated with penicillin injections and with a freshly made penicillin solution?

A Dacrocystitis **B** Impetigo of the newborn **C** Paronychia **D** Umbilical sepsis **E** Gonococcal conjunctivitis (26.40)

24. HANNE has just been born after a forceps delivery. One side of her face does not move. She—

A—will probably recover by herself? **B**—needs treatment? **C**—will have a facial palsy all her life? **D**—has polio? (26.60)

25. A child should be given his weight chart—

A—at the antenatal clinic? **B**—at birth? **C**—when he is a month old? **D**—when he first comes to the clinic? (26.67)

Booklet B——For the Student or Worker to Teach and Evaluate Himself

Booklet B—For the Student or Worker to Teach and Evaluate Himself

B.1. For workers implementing the microplan

You will be given this booklet at the beginning of a programme to improve child care in your district. Read the manual and look at what happens in your clinic now. *In what ways is the care you now give less than the care described in the manual?* What things could you do to improve it? The things that you don't do and could do now are your targets. Targets are things we try to reach. For example, one target is *'We must give every child a weight chart'*. Another target is *'We must be able to make salt-and-sugar water'*. If we don't do these things now, perhaps we should do them.

Some targets only workers can reach. For example, *'We show that we know about diarrhoea by passing instrument (test) DIARRHOEA A, B, or C'* depends on you, not on your manager. Some targets only the manager can reach, for example *'All the important 20 items of equipment are available'*. Only he and the service you both work for can supply the equipment. But many targets can be reached by managers and workers together. These are the joint (together) targets. For example, workers and managers together can reach the target *'We keep a special-care register'*. These joint targets are listed here so that you and your managers can both choose from them.

Decide what targets you could reach, and make a list of them. Talk about them with other workers and with your manager. Then agree on the targets you are going to reach—and try to reach them. Some of these targets will be skills targets, some knowledge targets, and some joint targets. Choose the important targets and the targets you can most easily reach. We have put stars beside the targets as being specially important—the 'star targets.'

B.2. For the students learning the microplan

You will be given this booklet at the beginning of a course in child health. If you are going to be able to care for children, you must know the knowledge in the manual, and be able to do the tasks (skills) it describes. These are your educational targets (objectives). There are three multiple-choice instruments (tests) to measure your knowledge of each chapter in the manual. There is one instrument for each chapter in this booklet. Your teacher has two more booklets. One (Booklet A) contains pretests to measure how much you know before you begin to learn. The other (Booklet C) contains postests to measure how much you know after you have tried to learn. Fill in your scores on the special page at the back of the manual. We are not going to list the knowledge targets for every chapter, because they are all the same. Here are two examples.

WORKERS' KNOWLEDGE TARGETS
'We show that—
— we understand skin disease by passing instrument SKINS C etc.'
— we understand the whole manual by passing instrument OVERALL POSTEST.'
The knowledge targets for DRUGS, COUGH, and DIARRHOEA are 'star targets'.

B.3. Joint targets for workers and managers

These are targets for managers and workers to try to reach together. It is the longest list. There are many targets for some chapters and few for others.

JOINT TARGETS
INTRODUCTION (1)
★ 'We teach other health workers, such as traditional midwives.' ....
....
'We show that we are able to —
— understand and use the manual by passing any of the SICK CHILDREN instruments with our manuals open.' ....
....

★ — use the manual by passing the MANUAL POSTEST.'...

DISEASE IN THE CHILD (2)

'We have —

— studied, discussed, evaluated, and recorded the beliefs and customs in our community concerning child care.'...

— made the community diagnosis of disease in children and listed the most common causes of illness and death.'...

— made and recorded a health-education plan complete with visual aids and methods of evaluation.'..

★ — decided on and recorded the five most important health education messages.'...................

★ — encouraged the community to take health action in (a) nutrition, (b) water supply, and (c) sanitation.'..

'We can list the resources for child care in our community.'...

★ 'We are helping a community group and being helped by one.' The community group could be a women's club, a party organization, or a scout group..
....

DRUGS (3)

'We show that we are able to use the dose tables in the manual by passing the DOSES POSTEST, Booklet C.'...

'We know which local medicines are probably harmful, and which are probably harmless.'...........

★ 'We do not give injections when we could give tablets, or other medicines.'....................................

'We do not give more drugs than necessary to each child.'...

★ 'We treat pyogenic infections with an adequate dose of antibiotics lasting not less than three days.'...

'We have stuck the dose tablets on the wall of our clinic, or put them under a glass table-top, or a transparent plastic sheet on our work table.'..........

'We keep adrenalin and a sterile syringe immediately available to treat an allergic reaction.'...........

'We have taught mothers to bring empty bottles for medicine to the clinic.'...

★ 'We do not use such medicines as vitamin B12, liver injections, amidopyrine injections, antihistamine injections, any mixtures of antibiotics, steroids —especially anabolic steroids—papaveretum, diphenoxylate ("Lomotil"), kaolin, pectin, bismuth, tannalbumin, chalk, enterovioform, charcoal, or coramine, etc.'...

'We prescribe all drugs by their generic titles.'....

'We have taken down the drug- and milk-advertisements in our clinic.'...

'We do not use vitamins, such as C and D, to treat deficiencies we never see.'.....................................

'We have prepacked the more commonly used drugs.'...

'We measure mixtures in 5 ml teaspoons.'..........

★ 'We give a child his first dose of mixture or tablets before he goes home.'.................................

'We teach mothers that a child does not have to have an injection each time he comes to the clinic.'....

'We always keep a small store of life-saving drugs for the very seriously ill children whose lives we might save.'...

HEALTHY CHILD (4)

'We are able to find out what immunizations a child has had.'...

'We know what our immunization targets are, and what percentage of children in the community we are immunizing completely or partly.'.........................

★ 'We follow *all* the rules for immunization in Section 4.10 of the manual.'.................................

'We do not do useless examinations, such as feeling a child's fontanelle to see if it is closed, or routinely feeling his spleen or measuring his height.'.

'When mothers come on a follow-up visit we say we are pleased to see them.'.................................

SICK CHILD (5)

★ 'We give mothers integrated care. This means we care for well and sick children, and we give antenatal care, postnatal care, and family planning on the same day.'...

'We give integrated care six days a week.'..........
....

★ 'We spend an average of at least four minutes with each child.' ....
....

★ 'We have arranged our clinic so that, if possible, a mother always sees the same worker whenever she comes to the clinic—continuity of care.' ....

★ 'We have arranged the furniture and equipment so that (a) we are not separated from a mother by a desk, (b) mothers sit on a chair, (c) all the equipment we need is close beside us, and we have (d) water, (e) soap, and (f) a towel to wash with.' ....
....

'We have taught sweepers to watch for sick children waiting in the queue and to bring them to see us quickly.' ....

'We speak to mothers and children by name, if they like it.' ....
....

'There are some toys or playground equipment at our clinic.' ....
....

RECORDING AND REPORTING (6)
★ 'We know, (a) how many children we are caring for in the community, and (b) what percentage of all the children in the community this is.' ....
....

'We have calculated the average number of children we see each day (Manual 6.9).' ....

'We have calculated the average number of visits per child under five for our clinic area.' ....
....

★ 'We keep a special-care register and write a large "S" on the weight charts of all the children who are in it.' ....
....

'We spend less than a quarter of our time recording and reporting.' ....
....

★ 'We give *safe* injections by (a) boiling or sterilizing all syringes in steam, (b) using a separate sterile needle for each child, (c) using one syringe for not more than ten children (ideally one each), (d) picking up sterile needles with sterile forceps, (e) storing needles dry. We do not use "sterile" water to "sterilize" syringes.' ....
....

NUTRITION (7)
★ 'We show that we understand the weight chart by passing the WEIGHT-CHART POSTEST.' ....
....

'We use the weight chart satisfactorily as shown by the children in our clinic averaging more than seven with the WEIGHT-CHART SCORE (Guide 4.10).' ....
....

★ 'We give such good nutrition education that most children stay on the road to health. If they do fall off, they climb back (Guide 4.9).' ....
....

'We give such good care that two or more years after we have started using the weight charts there is an average of six or more attendances per child.' ...

'We or our wives all breast-feed our children.' .....
....

★ 'We do NOT encourage bottle feeding!' ....
....

'We do not have feeding bottles, or free samples of artificial milk in our clinics.' ....
....

'We do not give dried skim milk to healthy breast-fed babies. We only give it to children over six months old with flat or falling weight curves. We give them enough to be useful (Manual 7.6).' ....
....

'We know the fraction of the local basic wage which is needed to feed a child artificially.' ....
....

★ 'We have worked out and recorded the local best buy for (a) a litre of milk (Table 12, N 5.7b), (b) 40g of protein (N 6.10a), 10 megajoules of energy food (N 6.10a).' ....
....

'We know the best weaning-food ('porridge') to give children.' ....
....

★ 'We can give mothers APPROPRIATE nutrition advice for their children.' ....
....

'We have made and recorded the community diagnosis of malnutrition.' ....
....

'We have made a nutrition education plan, complete with written out lessons, a list of visual aids, and questions that will help in evaluation (N 10.4).' ...
....

COUGH (8)
★ 'We treat lower respiratory infections with adequate doses of antibiotics for not less than three days.' ....
....

★ 'We can recognize (a) movement of the nose, (b) fast breathing, (c) cyanosis, (d) insuction.' ....
....

DIARRHOEA (9)
★ 'We have a rehydration tray in our clinic. (Salt, sugar, teaspoon, cup or mug, water).' ....
....

★ 'We can teach mothers how to measure a litre of water with local measures.' ....
....

★ 'There is water and a clean latrine in our clinic. The latrine is safe for children.' ....
....

FEVER (10)

'We give chloroquine to all children with fever.'..
....

SKINS (11)

★ 'When we treat scabies, we give mothers complete instructions as to how to do it.' ....

LEPROSY (12)

'When a child has a chronic patch on his skin, we test him for anaesthesia, and feel for thickened nerves.'..
....

TB (13)

'When a child has a falling growth curve we enquire if there is a relative with TB.' ....

ACCIDENTS (14)

'We can sew up cuts in our clinic.' ....
....

EYES (16)

'If a child might have an ulcer, we stain his eyes with fluorescein before we examine it.' ....

★ 'We look for signs of vitamin A deficiency in malnourished children, and, if necessary, treat it.'..

EARS (17)

★ We swab discharging ears, and teach mothers to swab them.' ....

'We use our auriscopes.' ....
....

THROAT (18)

★ 'We always examine the throats of children with fever.' ....

★ 'If necessary, we give DPT or tetanus toxoid to children with lesions that might be infected by tetanus bacteria.' ....

ABDOMEN (20)

'We examine a child's abdomen when he has abdominal pain or vomiting.' ....

NEWBORN BABY (26)

'We have breast pumps and nipple shields to sell or lend to mothers.'..

OTHER JOINT TARGETS

....
....
....
....

B.4. Measuring your skills

On the next few pages there is a list of the skills you must all learn. They all come from the manual. Beside each skill is a list of the things you must do. For example, when you give a young child tablets, you must read the label on the tin, and crush the tablets, etc. You get one point for doing each of these things. For example, there is a possible total of eight points for giving tablets. Your teacher will explain how you can use these check-lists. You may only need to learn some of them. He will explain which ones.

Practise using these in a clinic, and in school. If possible, practise with someone else. Where necessary use a child or a large doll.

SKILLS CHECK-LISTS

'We are able to —

— give a young child tablets.' **Manual 3.4 (Label on tin read, tablets crushed, given with spoon, mixed with water or sugar; explains how often to give tablets, importance of finishing the course, and safe-keeping of tablets; drugs recorded. (8 Points))**........
....

— give a young child liquid mixtures.' **Manual 3.4 (*Mixture shaken*, cork topside down, mixture poured away from label, 5 ml spoon; explains sizes of spoon, how often to give mixture, and the importance of finishing the course; drug recorded. (8 Points))**.......
....

★ — give a SAFE intramuscular injection to a child under five.' **Manual 3.5 (Procedure explained, outer side of thigh used, sterile syringe, sterile needle, skin cleaned with spirit, skin stretched, syringe held vertically, plunger withdrawn a little before injecting, needle pushed in quickly, *shaft of needle not touched*, swab put on hole. (11 Points))**.................
....

★ — give a SAFE subcutaneous injection.' **Manual 3.5 (Procedure explained, outside of upper arm used, skin cleaned with spirit swab, sterile syringe, sterile needle, skin pinched up, needle put in at 45°, plunger withdrawn, *shaft of needle not touched*, swab put on hole. (10 Points))** ....
....

— give BCG vaccine.' **Manual 4.6 (Procedure explained, sterile tuberculin syringe, sterile, 0.45 × 10 mm needle, bevel faces graduations, needle spits when flamed without getting red hot, right upper arm, skin stretched, first drops of vaccine discarded, *needle flat into skin*, bevel uppermost, small wheal raised. (11 Points))**.......................................

— give measles vaccines.' **Manual 4.8a (Child between 6 months and 2 years, *mother asked if the child has already had measles*, possibility of fever explained, continue as for subcutaneous injection. (12 Points))**...
....

— give polio vaccine.' **Manual 4.8b (Procedure explained, mother told when to come for next polio immunization or that immunization is complete,**

vaccine not given if child is ill or has diarrhoea, child given vaccine as drops or tablet. (4 Points)) ....
....

— give DPT vaccine.' **Manual 4.9** (Possibility of fever explained, mother told when to come for next immunization or that immunization is complete, continue as for subcutaneous injection. (11 Points))..

★ — write a 'hospital letter' when referring children.' **Manual 5.22** (Name and address of the clinic, date, child's name, age, important items of history, important signs, any special tests done, diagnosis made, *any treatment given*, any significant information, worker's name. (11 Points))..............................
....

— weigh a test object.' **Manual 7.1** (*Balance set to zero beforehand*, weight correct to within 100g. (2 Points))..
....

— make a local events calendar and use it to find out a child's age.' **Nutrition manual 1.6e** (One point for each event with a date, 5 points if age is correct to within three months)..

★ — count a child's respirations.' **Manual 8.9** (Respirations counted over half a minute, counted correctly to within plus or minus four breaths. (2 Points))..
....

★ — give oral rehydration with salt and sugar.' **Manual 9.22** (Procedure explained, mother adds salt and sugar, *level spoonfuls*, half spoonful of salt, eight spoonfuls of sugar, child given fluid to drink; *worker explains the dangers of adding too much salt and sugar*, the importance of persuading the child to drink, the need to go on as long as child has liquid stools, and the 'danger signs.' (10 Points))..............

★ — give oral rehydration with glucose–salt solution.' **Manual 9.22** (Solution made by mothers, worker explains the correct volume of water, *the dangers of making the solution too strong*, the importance of persuading the child to drink, the need to go on as long as child has liquid stools, the 'danger signs'. (6 Points))..

★ — give a nasogastric drip.' **Manual 9.24** (Procedure explained, hands washed, glucose–salt solution or salt-and-sugar water, tube measured from mouth to umbilicus, marked with tape, extra 15 cm, end smoothed with match, oiled, pushed down nose, fixed with tape, *throat examined, tube sucked*, stomach listened to while 10 ml of air injected, correct rate of drip set, level of fluid explained to mother. (15 Points))....................................
....

★ — take a child's rectal temperature.' **Manual 10.1** (Procedure explained, *thermometer shaken down*,

vaseline, child on his back, feet up, thermometer 2 cm into anus, one minute, wipe, read, wash, back in lysol. (10 Points))..
....

— take a child's axillary temperature.' **Manual 10.1** (Procedure explained, thermometer shaken down, bulb deep in the axilla, child's arm by his side, bulb covered, thermometer held, *three minutes*, read, back in lysol. (9 Points))..................................

— take a child's oral temperature.' **Manual 10.1** (Procedure explained, *thermometer shaken down*, thermometer at the side of the tongue, lips closed, two minutes, read, wash, back in lysol. (8 Points)) .

For the three preceding skills the worker must be able to read a thermometer correct to within plus or minus 0·1 ˚C.

— wash out a child's mouth.' **Manual 10.1** (Procedure explained, half a teaspoonful of salt in a cup of water, mouth rinsed, lips wiped. (4 Points)) ....
....

★ — treat hyperpyrexia in very hot districts.' **Manual 10.4** (Procedure explained, child lies on a plastic sheet, naked, water poured over him, temperature taken, pouring continued until his temperature is below 38 ˚C. (6 Points)) ....
....

— treat hyperpyrexia in colder districts.' **Manual 10.4** (Procedure explained, child naked, child made wet with cloths, temperature taken, sponging continued until his temperature is below 38 ˚C. (5 Points)) ....
....

— treat hypothermia in a small baby.' **Manual 10.4** (Procedure explained, baby close to his mother, blanket round them both, temperature taken each hour until it reaches 36 ˚C. (4 Points))..................
....

— treat hypothermia in an older child.' **Manual 10.4** (Procedure explained, bottles of hot water, well covered with cloth, *near the child but not touching*, temperature taken each hour until it reaches 36 ˚C. (5 Points))..
....

— test a lesion for anaesthesia.' **Manual 12.3** (Procedure explained, child in quiet place, child seated, cotton wool used, child asked to point to where he is touched, *lesions and normal skin tested*, first eyes open then eyes shut. (7 Points))..............
....

— examine a child for tender thickened nerves.' **Manual 12.3** (Procedure explained, *both sides examined together*, behind the ears, inside the elbows, below and outside the knees, in the skin round each of the lesions. (6 Points))..............................
....

— sew up a cut.' **Manual 14.4** (Procedure explained, worker's hand washed, cut washed if dirty,

instruments sterilized, needle held in toothed forceps, one side of the skin pierced at a time, interrupted sutures, sutures not too tight, dressing applied, ATS or tetanus toxoid given. (10 Points)) ..
....

★ — *examine a child for meningitis.'* **Manual 15.6 (If the child is less than a year old his fontanelle is looked at and felt, hand placed behind the child's head and his neck is bent forwards, attempt made to place the child's head between his legs, one of the child's legs is bent at the hip and an attempt is made to straighten his knee. (4 Points))** ....
....

— *examine the eye of an older child.'* **Manual 16.2 (Procedure explained, hands washed, taken into a good light, sat on his mother's knee, asked to look up and down right and left, lower lid pulled down and cornea examined, upper eyelid turned upwards and outwards over a matchstick, upper eyelid examined with magnifying glass. (8 Points))** ....
....

★ — *examine the ear of a young child.'* **Manual 17.3 (Procedure explained, at the end of the examination, sideways on his mother's knee, one of his arms behind her back, outer ear and skin around the ear examined, ear pulled backwards. (6 Points))** ....

— *swab a child's ear.'* **Manual 17.5 (Procedure explained, hands washed, child on his mother's knee, applicator sterilized, cotton wool pulled out flat, wool wrapped round applicator, swab looks like Picture 4 Fig. 17–4 in the manual, swab flamed, ear swabbed until the swab comes out clean. (9 Points))** ....
....

— *syringe a child's ears for wax.'* **Manual 17.6 (Procedure explained, warm water, child on his mother's knee, towel over child's shoulder, another towel on her knees, mother holds kidney dish under the ear, ear held and pulled gently backward, end of syringe points slightly upwards and forwards, ear syringed until no more wax comes out, ear looked at with auriscope. (10 Points)) This check-list can be modified for syringing pus—gentle syringing.** ....
....

— *test an older child for deafness.'* **Manual 17.7 (Procedure explained, child's head turned away from the worker, *finger moved about over ear not being tested*, asked to repeat words, progressively further away. (5 Points))** ....
....

— *remove a foreign body from a childs ear.'* **Manual 17.13 (Procedure explained, child on his mother's knee, ear syringed——see above, paper-clip straightened out and small hook made in one end of it, hook flat against skin of meatus, hook pushed past foreign body, foreign body removed. (7 Points))** ....
....

★ — *examine a child's throat.'* **Manual 18.2**

(Procedure explained, cervical lymph nodes felt using both hands, child on his mother's knee, one arm behind her back, worker's head low enough to see into child's mouth, lighted torch, boiled spatula, tongue, teeth and gums looked at, cheeks looked at, spatula put on tongue and pressed down, spatula put in a dish. (11 Points))** ....
....

— *examine the abdomen of an older child for tenderness and enlargement of the spleen and liver.'* **Manual 20.2 (Procedure explained, child lies flat, abdomen relaxed, worker's hand placed *flat* on the abdomen *fingers together*, abdomen gently felt all over, worker's left hand now placed under lower left chest while edge of his right hand faces the spleen, child asked to take deep breaths right hand getting nearer the ribs each time, worker's left hand now put under the child's lower right chest, edge of right hand brought closer to the ribs as child takes big breaths. (9 Points))** ....
....

— *examine the legs of an older child.'* **Manual 24.2 (Procedure explained, *both legs looked at together*, abnormal leg felt all over for tenderness, each joint of the abnormal leg is put through its full range of movement, same done with normal leg, both legs moved about to feel for tone, strength of knee and ankle examined, hips examined by bending them and then opening them out, child asked to try to walk. (9 Points)) This check-list can be adapted to a child's arms.** ....
....

— *examine an older child's back.'* **Manual 24.2 (Procedure explained, child's back looked at standing straight, child asked to touch his toes, asked to bend to right and left, back gently hit with fist. (5 Points))** ...
....

— *to deliver a normal newborn baby.'* **Manual 26.2 (*Hands washed*, clock looked at, baby held head downwards, sucked out, held lower than the uterus, cord felt, two clamps applied, cord cut between clamps, cord tied 5 cm from umbilicus, eyes cleaned from nose outwards, ointment or silver nitrate in eyes, wiped, labelled, wrapped, given to his mother. (15 Points))** ....
....

— *resuscitate a newborn baby.'* **Manual 26.3 (*Hands washed*, clock looked at, baby held head downwards, sucked out, 'Your baby does not breathe', cord clamped, and cut quickly, baby's head bent backwards, worker blows gently from his cheeks, 40 times a minute, worker's mouth over baby's nose and mouth, worker does NOT blow from his lungs, oxygen tube in worker's mouth, oxygen tube left in baby's nose. (13 Points))** ....
....

— *examine a newborn baby.'* **Manual 26.4 (Hands washed, baby's cheek rubbed, baby held in both** hands and quickly lowered and palate examined, hands examined, testes felt for, lower end of spine examined, arms looked at, feet looked at, weighed, put to the breast. (10 Points.))...............................

....

★ — *show a mother how to express her breast milk.'* **Manual 26.8** (Procedure explained, mother's hands washed, worker's hands washed, clean bowl or cup, mother holds up left breast with front of left hand, breast pressed from edge towards nipple, part of breast behind nipple squeezed, procedure repeated several times on all segments of breast. (8 Points)).....

....

— *show a mother how to sterilize feeding-bottles by boiling.'* **Manual 26.15a** (Procedure explained, several bottles, bottles and teats washed, pan with lid, boiled, water tipped out, bottles left in empty pan with lid on. (7 Points))...

....

— *show a mother how to sterilize feeding-bottles with hypochlorite.'* **Manual 26.15a** (Procedure explained, domestic hypochlorite bleach, bowl filled with water, 10 ml of bleach to a litre, bottle and teats washed, placed in hypochlorite solution, no air bubbles, left for at least an hour, hands washed again, hypochlorite solution poured out. (10 Points))......................

....

— *show a mother how to make an artificial feed.'* **Manual 26.15a** (Procedure explained, hands washed, sterilized feeding-bottle, *boiled water*, *seven level teaspoonfuls* of full-cream milk powder to a cupful of water, one heaped teaspoonful of sugar to a cupful of water, mix well. (7 Points)) ....

....

★ — *tube-feed a child.'* **Manual 26.18** (Procedure explained, hands washed, polythene tube with 1·5 mm bore, syringe and needle and tube sterilized, tube fitted to needle, needle fitted to syringe, tube pushed through nose into stomach, throat examined, tube sucked, milk poured into syringe barrel, *plunger NOT used.* (11 Points))...

....

— *care for a newborn child weighing less than 2 kg.'* **Manual 26.22** (*Hands washed*, mouth sucked out, vitamin K given, wiped, *NOT bathed*, heels looked at, breasts felt, ears felt, put to lie with his head on one side, covered with blanket, bottles of warm water beside him, *NOT touching* him. (10 Points))...........

....

— *feed a small baby.'* **Manual 26.22** . Tell the worker whether the baby is small for dates or preterm, how much he weighs, and how many days old he is (Procedure explained, hands washed, put to the breast, 'The baby does not suck', baby fed by one of the methods in Manual 26.18, *equipment sterile*, correct volume of feed given, baby given eight feeds a day, baby put with his head up after feed. (8 Points)) ..

....

— *make a penicillin solution for treating gonococcal conjunctivitis.'* **Manual 26.40** (Procedure explained, boils water, sterilizes cup, hands washed, cup half full of cold boiled water, sterile syringe, 600 mg vial of benzyl penicillin, penicillin dissolved in saline and put into cup, pus wiped out of baby's eyes with cotton wool and warm water, solution dropped into baby's eyes, ten minutes each hour for six hours, intramuscular penicillin given, hands washed, parents treated. (14 Points))..

....

— *treat a newborn baby with talipes.'* **Manual 26.52** (Procedure explained, ankle bent to see if the outer side of his foot can touch the outer side of his lower leg, 'His foot will not touch his lower leg', benzoin tincture put on leg, cotton wool over knee, cotton wool over outer malleolus, cotton wool covered with strapping, first long piece of strapping put on correctly, second piece of strapping correct, third piece correct, toes felt and counted. (10 Points))....

....

'SELF EVALUATION MULTIPLE-CHOICE QUESTIONS OF THE 'CHAPTER SERIES'.

DIFFICULT WORDS B
Chapter 1: Code 7

MATCH these words with the explanations for them—
1. Hypo- 2. Turbid 3. Intra- 4. Primary 5. Hyper-
A First B Cloudy C Inside D Too little E Too much
These words describe the things we do for children.

MATCH them with their explanations—
6. Observe 7. Manage 8. Care 9. Treat 10. Cure
A Do everything you can do for a child who comes to a clinic. B Plan what to do for him. C Watch him carefully.

D Give him a drug or put on dressing. E Make him well again.

MATCH these words with their explanations—
11. Meconium 12. Discharge 13. Cyanosed 14. Pus 15. Mucus
A Blue B The yellow liquid inside a boil C A thick transparent fluid D Any abnormal fluid coming from the body E The first stools of a newborn baby

MATCH these words with the description of them—
16. Contracture 17. Scrotum 18. Inguinal region 19. Spasm 20. Stools

A An arm or leg that a child cannot bend straight B Muscles contracting too strongly C The bag containing the testes D The fold between the abdomen and the legs E Faeces

21. Which of these words shows that something is happening most often?

A Usually B Always C Occasionally D Seldom E Rarely

22. Which of these lists the parts of the gut in the WRONG order?

A Mouth, pharynx, oesophagus B Small intestine, large intestine, rectum C Stomach, small intestine, large intestine D Rectum, anus E Oesophagus, stomach, rectum, small intestine

23. Which of these things does NOT happen in the abdomen?

A Expiration B Digestion C Absorbtion D Making urine E Storing urine

24. If you saw a child with a very very large spleen, how would you record it on his card?

C Spleen + + + + D Spleen + + + E Spleen + + + + +

25. Dehydration means that a child has—

A—too much water in his body? B—hypertonic muscles? C—a temperature which is too low? D—frequency? E—too little water in his body?

DISEASE IN THE CHILD B
Chapter 2: Code 1

1. Which of these causes most disease in the children in a clinic?

A Malnutrition B Accidents C Behaviour diseases D Hereditary diseases E Tumours (2.1)

2. Which of these diseases most often make one another worse?

A Accidents and hereditary diseases B Malnutrition and tumours C Infection and accidents D Hereditary diseases and congenital diseases E Malnutrition and infection (2.1)

3. Which of these is usually a behaviour disease?

A Swelling of the lymph nodes B Cleft palate C Bed wetting D Malaria E Cholera (2.1)

4. Which of these CANNOT be used to kill microorganisms?

A Cold B Boiling C Antiseptics D Disinfectants E Drugs (2.2b)

5. Which one of these is NOT a danger sign in acute septic skin infections?

A Severe lymphadenitis B Spreading swelling and redness C Lymphangitis D A slow pulse E An ill child (2.4)

6. Which of these diseases is NOT caused by protozoa?

A Giardiasis B Malaria C Amoebic dysentery D TB (2.2a)

7. Which of these is a health centre laboratory NOT able to find in specimens from a child?

A Fungi B Protozoa C Viruses D The larvae of worms E The ova of worms (2.2a)

8. BEATRICE has a large boil on her right cheek. What kind of organisms are probably causing it?

A Bacilli B Cocci C Protozoa D Viruses E Fungi (2.3)

9. Where would you look for lymphadenitis when you examined BEATRICE?

A In front of her right ear B Below her right jaw C In front of her right ear and below her right jaw D Behind her right ear E In the lower part of her neck (2.3)

10. The pus inside BEATRICE'S boil contains—

A—red blood cells and organisms? B—organisms only? C—white cells only? D—organisms and fat from her cheek? E—white cells and organisms? (2.3)

11. The skin round BEATRICE'S boil is hot and red and her temperature is 38·5 °C. She is 'ill'. She has lymphadenitis, but no lymphangitis. She has got—

A—signs which show that the organisms are staying inside her local lesion? B—the general signs of an acute septic infection? C—signs that organisms are growing in her lymph vessels? (2.3)

12. Which of these drugs would certainly NOT kill the organisms that are infecting BEATRICE?

A Tetracycline B Penicillin C Sulphadimidine D Paracetamol E Chloramphenicol (2.3)

MATCH these words with the descriptions for them—
13. Pyogenic **14.** Immune **15.** Toxin **16.** Carrier

A A healthy person with harmful organisms on him or in him B Pus-making C Able to fight a disease so as not to be made ill by it D Poison E An organism used in vaccines (2.4, 2.6)

17. Which way does lymph flow in the vessels of the arm?

C Down the front of the arm and up the back D Away from the axilliary lymph nodes E Towards them (2–4)

MATCH these diseases with the way they spread
18. Hookworm **19.** *Ascaris* **20.** Malaria **21.** TB **22.** Scabies

A By contact B By mosquitoes C Faeces to skin D Faeces to mouth E By droplets (2.7)

23. ESTER has measles. Secondary infection has now caused pneumonia. Have we got drugs to kill the organisms causing her primary infection?

A Yes B No (2.2, 2.6)

24. Have we got drugs to kill the organisms causing ESTER'S secondary infection?

A Yes B No (2.2, 2.6)

25. Which of these is a behaviour change that the people in your community will certainly NOT need?

A Making homes safe for young children B Eating green and yellow fruits to prevent vitamin A deficiency C Stopping breast feeding before a child is a year old D Starting to give a child porridge when he is four months old E Keeping flies away from a child's food (2.12)

DRUGS B
Chapter 3: Code 8

MATCH these drugs with the length of their course—
1. Iron mixture **2.** Piperazine for threadworms
3. Piperazine for *Ascaris* **4.** Isoniazid **5.** Procaine penicillin

A Daily for a week **B** Not less than three days **C** One year **D** Not less than three months **E** One dose only (3.14, 3.20, 3.28, 3.33)

MATCH these diseases or symptoms with the drugs you would use to treat them—
6. Giardiasis **7.** An abscess with spreading cellulitis round it **8.** Haemorrhagic disease of the newborn **9.** Fits **10.** Haematuria caused by *Schistosoma haematobium.*

A Penicillin **B** Metronidazole **C** Vitamin K **D** Metrifonate **E** Paraldehyde (3.14, 3.26, 3.38, 3.43, 3.48)

11. Which of these ways of treating a child with severe skin sepsis and cellulitis does NOT give him enough antibiotic for long enough?
A Ampicillin four times a day for three days. **B** Two ml of procaine penicillin and then sulphadimidine tablets for three days. **C** One dose of benethamine penicillin ('depot' penicillin). **D** Benzyl penicillin four times a day for three days. **E** One dose of procaine penicillin. (3.15)

PLEASE DO NOT WRITE ON THESE QUESTIONS SOMEONE ELSE MAY NEED THEM

---

12. Penicillin is helpful in treating—
A—boils with spreading cellulitis? **B**—backache? **C**—urticaria? **D**—most urinary infections? **E**—diarrhoea caused by a gut infection? (3.15)

13. CARLOS (10 kg) is to have 100 mg/kg/day of chloramphenicol. This drug has to be given four times a day. How much does he need at each dose?
A 500 mg **B** 1000 mg **C** 100 mg **D** 250 mg **E** 25 mg

14. Sulphadimidine is helpful for treating—
A—diarrhoea? **B**—lower respiratory infections? **C**—worms? **D**—ringworm? **E**—virus diseases? (3.14)

15. Which of these drugs is usually made into a mixed tablet with another drug?
A Metrifonate **B** Tiabendazole **C** Thiacetazone **D** Niclosamide **E** Bephenium (3.22)

MATCH these side effects with the drugs that cause them—
16. Yellow teeth **17.** Blood in the urine or not being able to pass urine **18.** Black stools **19.** A rash, fever, pain **20.** Kills small babies.

A Tetracycline **B** Children's iron mixture **C** Dapsone **D** Chloramphenicol **E** Sulphadimidine (3.14, 3.17, 3.18, 3.24, 3.33)

21. Which of these drugs CANNOT be used to treat bacterial infections?

A Penicillin **B** Piperazine **C** Tetracycline **D** Chloramphenicol **E** sulphadimidine (3.13, 3.28)

22. DIOGO has just had a severe allergic reaction to procaine penicillin. His mother needs to be told all these things EXCEPT one. Which one?
A 'I am going to write SENSITIVE TO PENICILLIN on his weight chart.' **B** 'He must not have any kind of penicillin again.' **C** 'He must not have ampicillin again.' **D** 'We can easily prevent these reactions by injecting penicillin mixed with an antihistamine.' **E** 'Sulphadimidine will not harm him.' (3.2, 3.15)

23. Which of these is an antiseptic?
A Iodine **B** Benzyl benzoate **C** Chloramphenicol **D** Isoniazid **E** Niridazole (3.48)

24. Which kind or worm would you treat with tiabendazole?
A *Schistosoma haematobium* **B** Hookworms **C** *Strongyloides* and *Trichuris* **D** Tapeworms **E** *Ascaris* and *H. nana* (3.29)

25. About how many drops are there in 1 ml?
A 1 **B** 2 **C** 5 **D** 20 **E** 200 (3.3)

HEALTHY CHILD B
Chapter 4: Code 3

1. Antitoxins—
A—are poisons made by bacteria? **B**—help to kill bacteria and viruses? **C**—can be given by mouth? **D**—are used to treat TB? **E**—prevent bacterial toxins causing harm? (4.2)

2. Live vaccines—
A—are not harmed by sunlight? **B**—can be used for up to a week after a vial has been opened? **C**—must be kept in a refrigerator? **D**—should be given with a syringe that has been kept in spirit? **E**—are destroyed if they become too cold? (4.3)

3. Which of these would you certainly NOT examine when a child without symptoms comes to a clinic for his monthly visit?
A His fontanelle to see if it is closed **B** His ears for discharge **C** His skin and scalp for sepsis **D** His eyes for signs of xerophthalmia **E** His lips and conjunctivae for anaemia (4.12)

4. Which of these vaccines is usually given only once?
C DPT **D** Polio **E** Measles (4.8a)

5. Very many children in your district have *Ascaris* worms. You may need to—
A—examine every child's stools every month? **B**—do nothing because they will be quickly reinfected? **C**—give children with pain a double dose of treatment? **D**—treat every older child in the clinic twice a year? **E**—treat every child every month? (4.11)

6. Your kerosine (paraffin) finished last week and your refrigerator has not been working. If you get a new supply of paraffin next month and the refrigerator starts working again, your—

A—vaccine will all be harmful? **B**—live vaccines will be useless but your killed vaccines can still be used? **C**—vaccines will all be useless? **D**—live vaccines will work again when they have been cold for 24 hours? **E**—live vaccines will still be alive, but your killed vaccines will be useless? (4.3)

7. Which of these would you give into the skin of a child's right shoulder?

A DPT **B** BCG **C** Polio **D** Measles (4.6)

8. Vaccines—

A—are less useful than cough mixture? **B**—must be stored in a refrigerator? **C**—can cure most diseases? **D**—can be made to protect children against any disease? **E**—must only be given to children one at a time, one vaccine at each visit? (4.3)

MATCH these ways of protecting a child with the length of the protection they give—

9. A vitamin A capsule **10.** A pyrimethamine tablet **11.** A complete course of polio vaccine **12.** TCE (tetrachlorethylene) **13.** An injection of iodised oil

A For the child's whole life **B** For 6 months **C** No time because this treats a child and does not protect him **D** A week **E** Three years (4.8b, 4.11, 10.7)

14. Which of these vaccines is dead?

A Polio **B** DPT **C** Measles **D** BCG (4.3)

15. One kind of antibody—

A—is made by each kind of organism? **B**—can 'fight' any organism? **C**—can only 'fight' the organisms for one disease? **D**—is made by each child? (4.2)

16. What kind of immunity does a child get after he has been injected with tetanus antitoxin (ATS)?

A Artificial active **B** Natural active **C** Natural passive **D** Artificial passive (4.2)

MATCH these vaccines with the sentences describing them—

17. BCG **18.** Polio vaccine **19.** Measles vaccine **20.** Tetanus toxoid **21.** DPT

A Is made from a toxin **B** A live vaccine which is given three times **C** One dose only should be given at nine months **D** Prevents TB **E** Protects against three diseases (4.6, 4.8a, 4.8b, 4.9)

22. Which of these diseases cannot yet be prevented by immunization?

A Polio **B** Whooping cough **C** TB **D** Malaria **E** Tetanus (10.7)

23. DILIP was immunized a few weeks ago. There is an ulcer at the place where he was immunized and some firm swellings under his arm. Which vaccine has caused this?

A Tetanus toxoid **B** Measles **C** Polio **D** DPT **E** BCG (4.6)

24. How would you treat DILIP's ulcer?

A Put a dressing on the ulcer and let it heal itself **B** Give him penicillin **C** Send him for help **D** Give him

streptomycin injections **E** Give him BCG into his other arm (4.6)

25. JAKE has had a road accident and has never been immunized. Which of these would give him immediate immunity against tetanus?

A Tetanus toxoid **B** Tetanus antitoxin (ATS) **C** DPT vaccine

---

SICK CHILD B
Chapter 5: Code 3

1. When you examine children in a clinic you should—

A—use the same spatula for all of them? **B**—start with their hair and examine them from their heads downwards? **C**—see specially sick children in turn with everyone else? **D**—leave their clothes on them? **E**—have water, soap, and a towel near you? (5.2)

2. Every time a child comes to a clinic you should—

A—take his temperature? **B**—find his weight chart in the clinic files and give it to him? **C**—find something to praise his mother for? **D**—record his history on his weight chart and in a book? **E**—measure his length? (5.2)

3. The easiest way to find out if a child is 'well' or 'ill' is to—

A—watch him carefully from the time you first see him? **B**—examine him carefully from head to toe? **C**—weigh him? **D**—see if he will drink glucose–salt solution? **E**—take a complete history? (5.15)

4. Which of these has the steps in caring for a sick child in the WRONG order?

A Diagnosis, management **B** Special tests, diagnosis **C** Management, treatment **D** Treatment, explanation, family planning **E** Examination, history taking, weighing (5.1)

5. Which of these people should be looking for seriously ill children in a busy clinic?

A Nurses only **B** Everyone in the clinic, except clerks and sweepers **C** Doctors and nurses only **D** Everyone in the clinic **E** Doctors only (5.15)

6. A child is probably only mildly ill if he is—

A—comatose? **B**—drowsy? **C**—sucking strongly from the breast? **D**—hypothermic? **E**—breathing 80 times a minute? (5:2)

7. When a mother is seen by the same person each time she comes to a clinic she gets—

A—integrated care? **B**—continuity of care? **C**—personal care? **D**—concentrated care? **E**—independent care? (5.2)

8. Which of these diseases does NOT cause signs in a child's face?

A Anaemia **B** Tapeworm infection **C** Jaundice **D** Kwashiorkor **E** Dehydration (5.17)

MATCH these diseases with the signs that help you to diagnose them—

9. Marasmus **10.** Kwashiorkor **11.** Leprosy **12.** Meningitis

A Skin anaesthesia **B** 'Old man's face' **C** Stiff neck **D** Apathy **E** Stridor (15.17, 5.18)

13. A child's presenting symptom is—

A—always something a health worker can see? **B**—his most serious symptom? **C**—his oldest symptom? **D**—his newest symptom? **E**—the symptom his mother tells you about first? (1.4, 5.1)

14. Which of these CANNOT be used as a milestone for a child's development?

A Talking short sentences **B** Sucking **C** Sitting **D** Standing **E** Talking single words (24.10, 5.10)

15. Which of these is part of a child's past history?

A 'What food did you give him yesterday?' **B** 'What is his father's job?' **C** 'What diseases has he had before this disease began?' **D** 'What symptoms has he got?' **E** 'Have any of his brothers or sisters died?' (5.9)

16. Which of these diseases is MOST likely to be shared by the whole family in a short time?

A Leprosy **B** Umbilical hernia **C** Tetanus **D** Scabies **E** Marasmus (5.12)

MATCH these specimens with the things that a health-centre laboratory can find in them—

17 Blood **18** Stool **19** Skin scraping **20** Pus

A Pyogenic bacteria (Gram's stain) **B** Lactose **C** Fungi **D** Haemoglobin **E** Protein (5.19)

21. Which of these would you examine LAST?

A A child's skin **B** His nutrition **C** His tonsillar lymph nodes **D** His breathing **E** His throat (5.16)

22. Which of these children need to be followed up for the longest time?

A KABOMPO (15 months, 11 kg) who is recovering well from pneumonia. **B** SOLWEZI (23 months, 13 kg) with tonsillitis. **C** KABWE (30 months, 13 kg) with malaria. **D** KALABO (3 years, 10 kg) who has had many attacks of respiratory infection and diarrhoea. **E** FIWILA (4 years, 16 kg) with scabies. (5.28, 6.3)

23. When a child is seen at a follow-up visit—

A—he should be seen by a different person from the person who saw him the first time? **B**—all the 'ten steps' should be followed? **C**—there is no need for any recording? **D**—he need not bring his weight chart? **E**—his mother should learn something? (5.28)

24. Which of these diseases can harm a child's lungs for a long time afterwards?

A Measles **B** Tonsillitis **C** Jaundice **D** Mumps **E** Typhoid (5.9)

25. A child's history should be taken—

A—after the examination? **B**—while you are looking at him carefully? **C**—by asking several questions at a time? **D**—without leaving time for his mother to ask questions? **E**—while his mother is standing? (5.4)

RECORDING AND REPORTING B
Chapter 6: with revision: Code 7

MATCH these descriptions with the drugs below—

1 Best for treating septicaemia in newborn babies **2** Tablets for treating TB **3** May kill newborn babies **4** May harm a baby's teeth if given late in pregnancy

A Tetracycline **B** Isoniazid **C** Chloramphenicol **D** Penicillin and streptomycin **E** Penicillin (3.16, 3.20, 3.17, 3.18, 3.24 (Revision))

5. Penicillin is useful for treating the diarrhoea caused by—

A—dirty bottle feeds? **B**—giardiasis? **C**—cholera? **D**—chronic malnutrition? **E**—septic infections in babies? (3.15, 26.32 (Revision))

6. Which of these should be kept in a clinic?

A A copy of a child's weight chart? **B** His weight chart? **C** The special-care register? **D** None of these? **E** All of these? (6.1)

7. Home-based records—

A—are lost too often for them to be useful? **B**—are ready for you to see in a child's home when you visit him? **C**—take up too much of the time of the clinic staff? **D**—are used less and less all over the world? **E**—are best on ordinary paper? (6.2)

8. Which of these drugs is NOT useful for treating malaria?

A Promethazine **B** Pyrimethamine **C** Chloroquine **D** Quinine (3.25 (Revision))

9. Which of these children are you LEAST likely to put in your special-care register?

A JAMES who is the last child in a large family. **B** JOSE who has leprosy. **C** JIMENEZ who has no father. **D** JOAQUIN who has scabies. **E** JUSTIN (3 weeks) whose mother has difficulty breast-feeding. (6.3)

10. A special-care register should contain—

A—only the underweight children? **B**—only children with chronic infections? **C**—the children a clinic can help least? **D**—as many sick children as possible? **E**—the children who should be visited at home if they don't come to the clinic? (6.3)

11. Which of these things is NOT true? A child's weight chart should be—

A—kept in a plastic bag? **B**—explained to a child's mother? **C**—used to record whether he has been given vitamin A? **D**—have the dots for each weighing joined up to make a growth curve? **E**—used to record a child's weight and nothing else? (6.2)

12. Which of these children are MOST likely to need our help. The children—

A—of rich families? **B**—whose fathers have good jobs? **C**—in very small families? **D**—in very poor families? **E**—whose families have plenty of land? (6.3)

13. Which of these is the shorthand for a disease?

A URI **B** PS **C** PH **D** EBM **E** NAD (6:1)

14. Medical shorthand—

A—is necessary so that patients do not understand their records? B—saves time? C—makes any other kind of writing unnecessary? D—should be used in a different way by each health worker? E—makes records more difficult to read? (6.6)

15. Which of these would be best for a newborn baby who cannot suck?

A PEM B DSM C EBM D IVF E PPD (6:1)

Antibiotics—

16. A—can harm children if you use them in the wrong way? B—are used to kill organisms on infected dressings and instruments, etc.? C—kill viruses? D—kill all micro-organisms? (3.11 (Revision))

17. Penicillin and the other common antibiotics we use in the clinic can kill—

A—all viruses? B—some fungi? C—some kinds of bacteria? D—protozoa? E—worms? (3.11)

18. Which of these children are you most likely to put in a special-care register?

A KHALED with tonsillitis B FUSAKO with septicaemia C SUHADI with cerebral malaria D SHINGO with TB E ARIFIN with meningitis (6.3)

19. Water must cover the instruments which are being sterilized in—

A—a pressure cooker? B—a pan? C—both of these things? D—neither of them? (6.13)

20. Which of these kills harmful organisms fastest?

A Boiling water B Air and steam at 120 °C C Lysol D Spirit E Steam at 120 °C (6.13)

21. A pressure cooker should—

A—never be cooled under a tap? B—never be allowed to boil dry? C—make a loud hissing noise all the time that it is being used? D—be filled to the top with water? (6.13)

22. When a pressure cooker is used for sterilizing—

A—the flame of the stove should be as high as possible all the time? B—it should be as full as possible? C—air should not be allowed to escape from it? D—any tins or bottles being sterilized should be kept closed? E—plungers should be taken out of syringes? (6.13)

23. Which of these is NOT used for treating TB?

A Dapsone B Isoniazid C Streptomycin D Aminosalicylate E Thiacetazone (3.19 (Revision))

24. Steam at 120 °C kills all harmful organisms—

B—immediately? C—in 15 minutes? D—in 5 minutes? (6.13)

25. When you start to use a pressure cooker the vent should be—

D—closed by the weight? E—open? (6.13)

NUTRITION B
Chapter 7: Code 6

1. A normal child should be three times his birthweight at the age of—

A—2 years? B—6 months? C—one year? D—8 months? (N 1.1)

2. A child's arm circumference is helpful in measuring his nutrition—

A—from his first birthday until his fifth birthday? B—during his second year of life only? C—from his second to his fourth birthday? D—from the age of six months to four years? (7.1 N 1.5)

3. Which of these things does NOT help to cause marasmus in a child?

A Too little milk in an artificial feed B Advertisements for artificial feeding in a poor community C Diarrhoea D Treating diarrhoea by starving a child E Breast feeding a child until he is two years old or more (7.9)

4. In most communities the most common time for a malnourished child to start falling off the road to health is between—

A—birth and six months? B—six months and one year? C—one year and 18 months? D—18 months and two years? (7.2)

5. Which of these is NOT a sign of marasmus?

A A thin 'old man's face' B No fat under the skin C Oedema D Very low weight for age E Thin wasted muscles (7.9)

6. Dehydration can cause all these signs. Marasmus can cause all EXCEPT one. Which one?

B Loss of skin elasticity C Sunken eyes D Sunken fontanelle E Thirst (7.9, 9.18)

7. Which of these will you see most often? The child—

A—with keratomalacia? B—with marasmus? C—with marasmic kwashiorkor? D—who is underweight for his age? (7.8)

8. Which of these is NOT true?

A Most foods are mixtures of nutrients. B The child who gets enough protein and energy food usually gets enough vitamins also. C Maize or rice are better foods for children than cassava or sago. D Vitamin tablets will make an underweight child grow. E A good staple gives a family much of the protein it needs (N 1.2)

9. Which of these is NOT true about breast milk? Breast milk—

A—contains no harmful organisms? B—contains exactly the nutrients a baby needs? C—gives a young baby all the water he needs? D—prevents diarrhoea? E—gives a baby all the food he needs until he is a year old? (N 7.1, N 8.1)

10. Artificial feeds should NOT be made from—

A—sweetened condensed milk? B—full-cream dried milk? C—evaporated milk? D—boiled fresh cows' milk? E—special baby milks in tins? (N 8.4)

11. Lack of minerals can help to cause all these EXCEPT one. Which one?

A Anaemia B Pellagra C Goitre D Caries (19.6, 22.4, 11.23)

12. A baby of six months or more—

A—can eat almost any food if it is made for him in the right way? B—needs only two meals a day? C—should not breast feed if his mother is pregnant? **D**—should not be given fish because of their bones, or beans because of their hard skins?**E**—should stop breast feeding suddenly? (N 7.4)

Which foods fit these descriptions?

13. Contains one nutrient only. 14. Prevents xerophthalmia. 15. Contains about 50 per cent lactose and no fat. 16. Contains about 10 per cent protein.

A Breast milk **B** Rice or maize **C** Green leafy vegetables **D** Dried skim milk **E** Sugar (N 3.5, N 5.3)

17. Artificial feeds—

A—can safely be kept warm in a vacuum flask? **B**—cause diarrhoea more often than breast feeds? **C**—are made by adding seven heaped teaspoonfuls of skim milk powder to a cupful of water? **D**—are best given in plastic feeding bottles? **E**—can safely be made in a bottle which is sterilized once a week? (N Chapter 8)

18. Which of these children are most likely to lack vitamin C?

A A breast-fed baby **B** A very active two year old child **C** An artificially fed baby **D** A school boy who is growing normally (N 8.14)

19. DIAZ lacks iron, folic acid, and vitamin A. Which of these would give him all of them?

A Orange or yellow fruits and vegetables **B** Maize **C** Bananas **D** Any dark green leaves **E** Cooking oil or palm oil (N 4.5, N 4.7, N 4.10)

20. Which of these children would you expect to have the lowest weight for his age?

A PHOBOS with marasmus **B** DEMOS with kwashiorkor (7.9, 7.10)

21. Which of these is NOT one of the signs of kwashiorkor?

A Oedema **B** Thin pale hair **C** Jaundice **D** Anaemia **E** Apathy (7.10)

22. Mothers should be taught about—

A—nutrients? **B**—joules? **C**—nicotinic acid? **D**—minerals? **E**—why a child's growth curve should rise? (N 10.11)

23. Protein energy malnutrition—

A—usually presents by a mother saying that her child is malnourished? **B**—makes infections worse and is made worse by infection? **C**—is best prevented by giving children vitamins? **D**—can only be diagnosed in hospital? **E**—is most easily monitored by measuring a child's height for his age? (7.7)

24. Which of these is usually the cheapest high protein food?

A Eggs **B** Spinach **C** Meat **D** Beans or groundnuts **E** Milk (N 6.4)

25. Which of these is a severely malnourished child LEAST likely to need?

A Chloroquine **B** Glucose saline **C** Tetrachlorethylene (TCE) **D** 'Lomotil' (diphenoxylate) (7.11)

COUGH B
Chapter 8: Code 2

1. Which of these are the most dangerous?

D Lower respiratory infections **E** Upper respiratory infections (8.1)

2. The most common symptom of a respiratory infection is—

A—movement of the nose? **B**—wheezing? **C**—fast breathing? **D**—stridor? **E**—cough? (8.1)

3. The blood of a cyanosed child has—

A—too little oxygen? **B**—too much oxygen? **C**—too little haemoglobin? (8.2)

4. The upper respiratory tract is separated from the lower respiratory tract by—

A—the palate? **B**—the pharynx? **C**—the larynx? **D**—the trachea? (8.2)

5. Which of these has the parts of the respiratory tract in the RIGHT order?

A Trachea, bronchioles, bronchi **B** Nasal cavities, pharynx, larynx, trachea **C** Bronchioles, bronchi, alveoli **D** Nasal cavities, larynx, trachea, pharynx (8.2)

6. Antibiotics can usually cure respiratory infections caused by—

A—viruses? **B**—bacteria? (8.5)

7. Moderate or severe insuction is a sign—

A—of upper respiratory infection? **B**—of TB? **C**—of acidosis caused by dehydration? **D**—of obstruction to the flow of air into the lungs? **E**—that there is not enough oxygen in the blood? (8.9)

8. Which of these is NOT one of the complications of whooping cough?

A Diarrhoea **B** Marasmus **C** Pneumonia **D** Fits **E** TB (8.17)

9. You are not sure if CEMMO (2 years) has bronchitis or pneumonia. Which of these would be most useful in deciding which of these diseases she has?

A Stridor **B** Insuction **C** How fast she is breathing **D** Coughing **E** Her age (8.14)

10. The respiratory tract can become blocked in all these ways EXCEPT one. Which one?

A Too much purulent mucus in the small tubes of the lung **B** Large lymph nodes pressing on the bronchi **C** Thickening of the bronchial mucosa **D** A foreign body in one of the bronchi **E** Twisting of one of the bronchi (8–4)

11. 'Noisy breathing' is—

A—serious only if there are signs of respiratory obstruction also? **B**—always serious? **C**—never serious? (8.9)

12. A child's respirations should be counted—

A—after his upper respiratory tract has been examined? **B**—after he is undressed? **C**—at the end of the examination? **D**—at the beginning of the examination? (8.9)

13. KITALA (4 years) has had severe asthma since last night. Which of these would help him quickest?

A An adrenalin injection **B** Ephedrine tablets **C** An antihistamine injection **D** Procaine penicillin **E** Aspirin (8.13)

14. Wheezing in older children is usually caused by asthma. In younger children it is usually caused by bronchiolitis. At about what age do children stop getting bronchiolitis and start getting asthma?

A 5 years **B** 36 months **C** 6 months **D** 1 year (8.14)

15. Which of these causes the most severe stridor?

A Pneumonia **B** Obstructive laryngitis **C** Bronchitis **D** Bronchiolitis **E** Upper respiratory infection (8.11)

16. For which of these diseases is hospital treatment always necessary?

A Bronchitis **B** Pneumonia **C** Foreign body in the bronchi **D** Asthma **E** TB (8.18)

17. Antihistamines should be used to treat—

A—asthma? **B**—tonsillitis? **C**—bronchitis? **D**—chronic upper respiratory infections? **E**—none of these diseases? (3.45)

18. Which of these signs would make you think that a child with a respiratory infection needed an antibiotic?

A Koplik's spots **B** A nasal discharge **C** Pus on his tonsils **D** Fever **E** Not eating (8.6, 18.11)

19. ALIMA (3 years) has whooping cough. Her 3-month-old brother SEMBAYWE has started to cough. When will SEMBAYWE start whooping?

A In 3 days **B** In three weeks **C** In ten days **D** Probably never **E** Tomorrow (8.17)

20. Which of these is a sign of a chronic upper respiratory infection?

A Cyanosis **B** Membrane on the tonsils **C** Insuction **D** Koplik's spots **E** Pus dripping down the pharynx (8.8)

21. Which of these is the LEAST likely complication of an upper respiratory infection?

A Otitis media **B** Anaemia **C** Bronchitis **D** Pneumonia (8.7)

22. Which of these diseases makes a child breathe abnormally in a way which is sometimes confused with pneumonia?

A Diarrhoea with severe dehydration **B** Jaundice **C** Marasmus **D** Tonsillitis **E** Peritonitis (8.15, 9.18)

23. Which of these diseases causes a noise which is louder as a child breathes in?

A Obstructive laryngitis **B** Asthma **C** TB **D** Tonsillitis **E** Worms in the lungs (8.9)

24. Which of these causes the fastest breathing?

A Asthma **B** Pneumonia **C** Bronchitis **D** Bronchiolitis **E** Whooping cough (8.15)

25. BITRIS has pneumonia. You only have procaine penicillin. How would you give it to her?

A One injection only **B** Three injections each day for 3 days **C** Two injections a day for 3 days **D** Two injections a day for two days **E** One injection each day for at least 3 days (3.13, 8.15)

DIARRHOEA B
Chapter 9: Code 8

1. Which of these forms a 'vicious circle' that helps to cause diarrhoea?

B Dehydration and malnutrition **C** Infection and dehydration **D** Malnutrition and infection (9–7)

2. Which of these does NOT help to break the vicious circle in Question 1?

A Preventing accidents **B** Giving children more protein and energy food **C** Breast-feeding a child until he is two years old as well as giving him other foods **D** Clean drinking water **E** Measles immunization (9.11)

3. Glucose–salt solution—

A—should be made with level tablespoonfuls of salt and sugar? **B**—should only be made up in a clinic and not by mothers? **C**—can be made any strength that is convenient? **D**—should be given to a child as a few spoonfuls only like other 'medicine'? **E**—should be clean but need not be sterile? (9.21)

4. ISIAH (2 years) has severe watery diarrhoea, but his stools are brown and not like rice water. There is cholera in the district. He—

A—has certainly not got cholera? **B**—certainly has cholera? **C**—might have cholera? (9.7)

5. OSAMU (4 years) has diarrhoea, fever, and vomiting. There is much chloroquine-resistant falciparum malaria in the district. His blood slide is positive. He is severely dehydrated. Which of these would you give him?

A A chloroquine injection and glucose saline **B** Intravenous fluid with quinine in his drip **C** Glucose saline **D** Chloroquine tablets **E** Chloroquine tablets and glucose saline (3.25, 9.9)

6. Which of these does NOT cause diarrhoea?

A Dried skim milk **B** Boiled water **C** Infected food **D** *P. falciparum* **E** Water which contains even a little human faeces (9.29)

7. Which of these is the earliest sign or symptom of dehydration?

A Thirst **B** Dry mouth **C** Sunken fontanelle **D** Loss of skin elasticity **E** Fits (9.18)

8. Both these children are breathing abnormally. MAJID is breathing abnormally deeply. He has diarrhoea, his eyes are sunken, and his skin elasticity is reduced. MOHSEN'S breathing is fast and shallow. He has a cough and fever. Who has acidotic breathing?

C MAJID **D** MOHSEN (9.18)

9. REZA (1 year) has diarrhoea. You might find the cause of his diarrhoea by examining any of these, EXCEPT—

A—his throat? **B**—his stools? **C**—his feeding bottle? **D**—his growth curve? **E**—his urine? (9.10)

10. All these children have diarrhoea. Which of them would probably be MOST difficult to rehydrate?

A TEENY who has fever. **B** WEENY who is malnourished. **C** HUMPTY who has diarrhoea only. **D** DUMPTY who is vomiting. (9.23)

11. APITON (3 years, 15 kg) has had diarrhoea for a week. He is bottle-fed. His mother gave him salt-and-sugar water. She put eight level teaspoonfuls of salt and one level teaspoonful of sugar to five cups of water. Last night he started to have fits. He is drowsy and irritable, and his mouth is dry, but his skin elasticity feels normal. He will not drink. Lumbar puncture shows clear CSF. Which of these is most probable?

A He has been given too much sugar. **B** He is only mildly dehydrated. **C** He can easily be rehydrated by mouth. **D** He has meningitis. **E** He has been given too much salt. (9.18)

12. Which of these is true?

A A mother should go on breast feeding when her child has diarrhoea **B** All children with diarrhoea need drugs **C** When a child has diarrhoea his gut should be rested by not giving him anything to eat **D** None of the organisms which cause diarrhoea are resistant to antibiotics **E** Swelling of the eyelids is a sign that children are being given too little fluid (9.30)

13. Which of these is a sign of dehydration?

A Oedema **B** A swollen fontanelle **C** Muscle wasting **D** Loss of skin elasticity **E** Passing much urine (9.18)

14. The powder for making glucose–salt solution—

A—does not change colour or go soft when it gets damp? **B**—must be added to the right volume of water? **C**—should not be sold in village shops? **D**—is always sold in packets to make 100 ml of fluid? **E**—contains potassium bicarbonate? (9.21)

15. Intragastric rehydration—

A—requires sterile fluids? **B**—should only be given in hospitals? **C**—may make a child's eyelids swell if too much fluid is given? **D**—is useless if a child is vomiting? **E**—can only be used for mildly dehydrated children? (9.24)

16. The most important part of treating acute diarrhoea is to—

A—put back the fluid that a child has lost? **B**—give him antibiotics to kill the organisms that are causing his diarrhoea? **C**—rest his gut? **D**—stop breast-feeding for one or two weeks? (9.20)

17. FEBI (2 years, 10 kg) has had diarrhoea for several days. She is drowsy and her skin elasticity is reduced. Her abdomen has swollen during the last few days but is not tender. She has been treated at home with tea and sugar. Her swelling is probably caused by—

A—too much fluid by mouth? **B**—malaria? **C**—malnutrition? **D**—peritonitis? **E**—lack of potassium? (9.29b)

18. Which of these stools are most likely to be caused by *Giardia*?

A Stools with blood and mucus? **B** Frothy, bubbly, bad smelling stools? **C** Stools like rice water? **D** Green stools? **E** Stools with worms in them? (9.6)

19. NAMITALA (3 years, 12 kg, 39·5 °C) has had severe watery diarrhoea without blood or mucus for three days. Before her diarrhoea started she was well, and her growth curve had been rising. She is comatose, her eyes are deeply sunken, and her skin elasticity is severely reduced. Her diarrhoea is—

A—acute on chronic? **B**—chronic? **C**—acute? (9.12)

20. Her dehydration is—

B—mild? **C**—moderate? **D**—severe? (9:1)

21. She has—

A—dysentery? **B**—hyperpyrexia? **C**—hypothermia? **D**—malnutrition? **E**—probably gained weight because of her dehydration? (10.4)

22. If possible, she should be rehydrated—

A—orally? **B**—intragastrically? **C**—intraperitoneally? **D**—intravenously? (9.18)

23. If you have no sterile intravenous fluids, and a severely dehydrated child will not drink, you should try to rehydrate him—

A—nasogastrically? **B**—orally? **C**—subcutaneously? **D**—intraperitoneally? **D**—with coconut water? (9.24)

24. Which of these children is LEAST likely to have diarrhoea?

A ALPHA with tonsillitis **B** BETA with kwashiorkor **C** GAMMA with scabies without secondary infection **D** DELTA with otitis media **E** EPSILON with measles (9.9 to 9.14)

25. BWALYA is severely dehydrated and an intravenous drip has just been started. How would you give the fluid?

B As fast as possible until he has had all the fluid he needs **C** Slowly at first then faster **D** Fast at first, then more slowly **E** Slowly all the time (9.28)

FEVER B
Chapter 10: Code 3

1. A child with hyperpyrexia should—

A—be cooled so fast that he shivers? **B**—be covered with clothes so that he does not get cold? **C**—be warmed up? **D**—not be made wet with water? **E**—be cooled slowly with water or wet cloths? (10.4)

2. Which of these diseases is LEAST likely to present as fever?

A Measles **B** Malaria **C** Whooping cough **D** Typhoid (10.5)

3. We diagnose hyperpyrexia when a child's temperature is—

A—above 39 °C? **B**—above 40 °C? **C**—42 °C? **D**—below 37·5 °C? **E**—below 36 °C? (10.1)

4. Which of these children have the greatest difficulty keeping their body warm? Children with—

B—pneumonia? **C**—typhoid? **D**—malaria? **E**—severe malnutrition? (10.1)

5. MAX (3 years) has had fever and no other symptoms for 3 days. When you look for a cause you would get LEAST help by examining his—

A—ears? **B**—throat? **C**—tonsillar lymph nodes? **D**—stools? (10.10)

6. If a child's mouth temperature is 37 °C, his rectal temperature is—

B—36·5 °C? **C**—37·5 °C? **D**—37 °C? **E**—36 °C? (10.1)

7. The most useful treatment for an ordinary attack of measles is—

A—liquid foods only, and plenty of clothes? **B**—food, fluids, and treatment for fever? **C**—an antipyretic injection? **D**—antibiotics? **E**—promethazine? (10.6)

8. Which of these is NOT true?

A Malaria parasites live and multiply inside the red cells. **B** The measles rash comes on the 2nd day of the fever. **C** Measles is more serious in a malnourished child. **D** In severe measles the rash is a very dark red. **E** A newborn child is usually protected from measles for several months by natural passive immunity. (10.6)

9. In a clinic you should take the temperature of—

A—all children? **B**—'ill' children only? **C**—underweight children only? **D**—children coming to the clinic for the first time? **E**—children with any kind of symptom? (10.2)

10. JOSEFINA has had fever for several days. The weather is hot and there is falciparum malaria in the district. Which of these does she NOT need?

A Few clothes **B** Chloroquine **C** A saline mouth wash to remove the crusts on her lips **D** No food until she is well **E** Any food she can eat (10.3)

11. Which of these are LEAST likely to cause fever?

A Worms **B** Bacteria **C** Protozoa **D** Viruses (10.5)

12. TADASHI (3 years) has had a cough, fever, and red eyes for three days. Which of these would be most helpful in making the diagnosis?

A Testing his urine **B** Looking for meningeal signs **C** Looking inside his cheeks **D** Counting his pulse **E** Measuring his chest circumference (10.6)

13. Which of these diseases CANNOT yet be prevented by immunization?

A TB **B** Polio **C** Measles **D** Diphtheria **E** Diarrhoea (4.2)

14. Which of these vitamins may prevent one of the serious complications of measles?

A Vitamin B **B** Vitamin A **C** Vitamin E **D** Vitamin K **E** Vitamin C (10.6)

15. Chloramphenicol should NOT be used for treating—

A—whooping cough in babies? **B**—typhoid? **C**—upper respiratory infections? **D**—meningitis? (8.17, 10.6, 10.8, 15.6)

16. In a very malarious area a child is in the greatest danger from malaria—

A—after he is two years old? **B**—in the first nine months of his life? **C**—during his first year? **D**—between the age of three months and five years? (10.7)

17. AIDA (6 months) has had fever for 3 days. She had two fits this morning. You must not forget to examine her—

A—eyes? **B**—tongue? **C**—stools? **D**—fontanelle? **E**—lips? (10.10, 15.9)

18. ZEKE (4 years, 39 °C), probably has cerebral malaria. He has had two fits, and is vomiting. He is drowsy and will not drink but is not yet in coma. There are *P. falciparum* + + in his blood slide. He needs all these things EXCEPT—

A—intravenous fluids? **B**—pyrimethamine? **C**—a lumbar puncture? **D**—cooling with water? **E**—subcutaneous chloroquine? (10.7)

19. In a large town children start to get measles at the age of about—

A—3 months? **B**—18 months? **C**—6 months? **D**—two years? **E**—12 months? (10.6)

20. MERAJ (3 years, 15 kg) has measles. He needs penicillin for at least three days—

A—if he has a secondary infection of his ears or lungs? **B**—to kill the measles virus? **C**—to prevent secondary infection? **D**—if his rash is very dark? **E**—if he has diarrhoea? (10.6)

21. Which of these diseases is most likely to cause anaemia?

A Measles **B** Bronchitis **C** Pneumonia **D** Urinary infection **E** Malaria (10.7, 22.7)

22. When a child has his first attack of malaria you can feel his spleen—

A—soon after the mosquito has bitten him? **B**—as soon as the fever starts? **C**—only when he has been treated? **D**—only after he has had fever for several days? (10.7)

23. MUHARAMI (9 months) has fever. Which of these signs would make you think that his fever was caused by meningitis?

A Koplik's spots **B** A large spleen **C** Movement of his nose **D** Red watery eyes **E** A swollen fontanelle (10.10, 15.6)

24. Which of these is the most common cause of fever in young children?

A Colds **B** Measles **C** Otitis media **D** Pneumonia **E** Typhoid (8.7)

25. MIREILLE (5 years) has had fever for ten days. She is not eating or playing normally but has no other symptoms. You must not forget to examine her—

A—stools? **B**—urine? **C**—fontanelle? **D**—mastoids? **E**—nose? (10.10)

SKINS B
Chapter 11: Code 2

MATCH these diseases with the places where you find them—

1. Herpes simplex **2.** Scabies **3.** Herpes zoster **4.** Tinea pedis

A In a line half way round the body B On the scalp C Between the toes D On the lips E Between the fingers (11.15, 11.10, 11.17, 11.21)

5. Which of these is the most important cause of skin sepsis in a community?

A Lack of minerals B Lack of water C Specially dangerous bacteria D Bad latrines E Lack of health workers (11.1)

6. Which of these diseases makes a child most ill?

A Molluscum contagiosum B Kwashiorkor C Creeping eruption D Scabies E Tinea versicolor (11.21)

7. Which of these causes lesions which look most like the lesions caused by burning with boiling water?

A Pellagra B Tinea versicolor C Eczema D Kwashiorkor E Impetigo (11.22)

8. Scabies causes—

A—lesions on the palms of the hands in babies? B—wet lesions round the neck? C—large vesicles? D—pale hypopigmented lesions? E—lesions on the lips? (11.10)

9. Penicillin can cure—

A—ringworm? B—dry eczema? C—cellulitis? D—scabies (not secondarily infected)? E—urticaria? (11.3)

10. Wet lesions can be caused by—

A—molluscum contagiosum? B—tinea versicolor? C—leprosy? D—ringworm? E—eczema? (11.27)

11. Which of these diseases causes lesions which are different on the two sides of the body (asymmetrical)?

A Herpes zoster B Measles C Heat rash D Pellagra E Eczema (11.17)

12. Which of these itch most? The lesions of—

A—kwashiorkor? B—chronic ringworm? C—leprosy? D—scabies? E—measles? (11.10)

13. PECHI (2 years, 7·5 kg, 38 °C) has pyoderma and tender lymph nodes. She—

A—might die from septicaemia if she is not treated? B—is unlikely to die because pyoderma is only a skin disease? (11.3)

14. Impetigo—

A—is not infectious? B—is caused by a virus? C—is a disease to which newborn babies are immune? D—can be treated with penicillin? E—is most common on a child's arms and legs? (11.3, 11.4)

15. DILBAHADUR (1 year) has a small sore on his lips every time he has a fever. The organism which is causing his lesions—

A—often kills children? B—causes stomatitis in babies? C—is easily killed with antibiotics? D—stays inside him for a short time only? E—is a bacterium? (11.15)

16. MELISSA (6 years) has two large (5 cm) chronic patches on her legs. You should make sure she has NOT got—

A—molluscum contagiosum? B—kwashiorkor? C—leprosy? D—herpes zoster? E—creeping eruption? (11.28, 12.3)

17. A health centre laboratory can help in diagnosing—

A—a heat rash? B—urticaria? C—a drug rash? D—measles? E—ringworm? (11.13)

18. NARMAYA has a symmetrical rash of very many small red itchy papules. There are more lesions on her body than on her face and arms. She is well. These lesions—

A—should be treated with penicillin? B—should be treated by wearing more clothes? C—are caused by blocked sweat glands? D—are caused by measles? E—do not become secondarily infected? (11.26)

19. Chickenpox—

A—is caused by bacteria? B—causes fever for several days before the rash comes? C—often kills children? D—is caused by the same virus that causes herpes zoster? E—does not become secondarily infected? (11.16)

20. Head lice—

A—cause lesions which do not become secondarily infected? B—are seldom shared by the whole family? C—do not cause itching? D—lay eggs on the skin? E—can be treated with gammabenzine hexachloride diluted with water? (11.11)

21. Permanganate solutions are NOT helpful in treating—

A—secondarily infected ringworm? B—pellagra? C—pyoderma? D—impetigo? E—a secondarily infected heat rash? (11.19)

22. Which of these is NOT true?

A Boils should be squeezed to make the pus come out. B Warts are caused by viruses. C In hot weather too many clothes cause rashes in babies. D Large ulcers can be prevented by treating small lesions early. E Drugs can cause rashes. (11.1, 11.20, 11.5, 11.7, 11.25)

23. Scabies—

A—causes lesions on the soles of a baby's feet? B—can be treated in one day? C—can be cured by chloramphenicol? D—is not infectious? E—often kills children? (11.10)

24. HEMLATA (3 years) has an itchy snake-like lesion on her buttock. This lesion—

A—will probably kill her? B—can be treated with tiabendazole? C—is caused by bacteria? D—can be prevented by drinking boiled water? E—stays in the same place in the skin? (11.21)

25. Urticaria—

A—usually lasts many weeks? B—is usually very serious? C—often becomes secondarily infected? D—should be treated with penicillin? E—can be caused by drugs or insect bites? (11.24)

LEPROSY B
Chapter 12: Code 3

1. Which kind of leprosy may need to be treated for the whole of a child's life?

C Tuberculoid leprosy **D** Indeterminate leprosy **E** Lepromatous leprosy (12.4)

2. LALAGE (8 years) has several patches of tuberculoid leprosy on her body. She has been treated and they have now gone. She—

B—can now stop treatment? **C**—must go on with her treatment for 10 years? (12.4)

3. A skin scraping for leprosy should be taken from—
A—the edge of a lesion? **B**—the middle of a lesion? (12.3)

4. Leprosy is caused by—
A—fungi? **B**—protozoa? **C**—spirochaetes? **D**—cocci? **E**—bacilli? (12.1)

5. Leprosy causes the most serious harm to a child's—
A—muscles? **B**—heart? **C**—brain? **D**—nerves? **E**—skin? (12.1)

6. AAFB are LEAST likely to be found in scrapings from—
C—tuberculoid lesions? **D**—lepromatous lesions? **E**—borderline lesions? (12.3)

7. Which of these does NOT cause deformity?
A Leprosy **B** Malnutrition **C** Severe injury **D** TB of the spine **E** Polio (12.1)

8. Leprosy can cause anaesthesia in—
A—normal looking skin only? **B**—normal looking skin and skin lesions? **C**—skin lesions only? (12.3)

9. Anaesthesia is important in leprosy because—
A—it makes a child's muscles weak? **B**—he may injure himself without knowing? **C**—it causes pain? **D**—it stops him walking? **E**—it makes him scratch himself? (12.1)

10. If a child with a strong immunity gets leprosy, he gets—
B—borderline leprosy? **C**—lepromatous leprosy? **D**—tuberculoid leprosy? (12.2)

11. The first leprosy lesion a child has is usually—
A—indeterminate? **B**—lepromatous? **C**—borderline? **D**—tuberculoid? (12.2)

12. JANE has nodules on her ears. Her leprosy is probably—
A—indeterminate? **B**—tuberculoid? **C**—lepromatous? **D**—borderline? (12.2)

13. Which of these children has certainly NOT got leprosy?
A ELINA with an anaesthetic lesion. **B** ELENESTO with several large hypopigmented (pale) lesions. **C** EVELINA with several large chronic patches. **D** ESINET with tender thickened nerves. **E** ESPINA with a hot red swollen lesion. (12.3)

14. The most severe nerve lesions are caused by—
B—tuberculoid leprosy? **C**—borderline leprosy? **D**—indeterminate leprosy? **E**—lepromatous leprosy? (12.2)

15. Which of these lesions might be caused by leprosy?
A Pustules **B** Urticarial lesions **C** Large chronic patches **D** Vesicles **E** Very many small red itchy papules (12.3)

16. AMRITBHAI (5 years) has lepromatous leprosy. He has been given dapsone for six months. For the last three days he has had fever and body pains. This morning his sclerae are yellow and his urine is dark. His jaundice might be caused by—
A—leprosy? **B**—hepatitis? **C**—dapsone? **D**—hepatitis or dapsone? (3.24)

17. AAFB + + + in a skin scraping show that a patient has—
C—tuberculoid leprosy? **D**—lepromatous leprosy? **E**—TB? (12.3)

18. Some leprosy lesions are anaesthetic because organisms are growing in—
A—skin? **B**—nerves? **C**—muscles? **D**—the brain? (12.7)

19. Which of these children is most likely to have anaesthetic lesions?
A ALAIDA with lepromatous leprosy. **B** ANIMONI with indeterminate leprosy. **C** ASIMEDI with tuberculoid leprosy. **D** ADINES with borderline leprosy. **E** All of them. (12.2)

20. Most children with indeterminate leprosy get—
A—well by themselves? **B**—tuberculoid leprosy? **C**—lepromatous leprosy? **D**—borderline leprosy? (12.2)

21. Children with leprosy should be treated—
A—at home but be kept away from other children? **B**—in bed at home? **C**—in an ordinary hospital? **D**—in a special hospital? **E**—while living a normal life at home? (12.4)

22. Which of these drugs should be given in small doses to begin with?
A Niridazole **B** Isoniazid **C** Dapsone **D** None of them (3.24)

23. ANDRY is a week old. His mother has leprosy. What would you NOT tell her?
A 'He will probably not be harmed by leprosy if you take your tablets.' **B** 'He does not need leprosy tablets.' **C** 'He should be immunized with BCG.' **D** 'We must put him on our special-care register.' **E** 'A mother who is taking leprosy tablets must not breast-feed.' (26.66)

24. When a child is examined for anaesthesia he should—
A—be examined with a piece of cotton wool? **B**—have his eyes open? **C**—tell you where he has been touched? **D**—be touched on his lesions only? **E**—be touched on normal skin only? (12.3)

25. Which of these signs is NOT diagnostic of leprosy—
B—pale lesions? **C**—anaesthesia? **D**—AAFB in a skin scraping? **E**—tender thickened nerves? (12:1)

TB B
Chapter 13: Code 4

1. Penicillin—
A—cures TB? **B**—prevents TB? **C**—is sometimes

useful for diagnosing whether a child has TB or a septic infection? **D**—should never be given to a child with TB? **E**—makes TB bacilli become penicillin resistant? (3.12, 3.15)

2. TB is caused by—
A—viruses? **B**—fungi? **C**—lack of protein? **D**—lack of vitamins? **E**—bacilli? (13.1)

3. MIRANDA (2 years) has a cough, mild fever, and a falling weight curve. She has been given DPT vaccine only. Her uncle has TB. What would you give her?
A Streptomycin and isoniazid **B** Streptomycin **C** Isoniazid **D** Penicillin **E** Isoniazid and penicillin (13.6)

4. Which of these parts of a child is harmed by TB most often. His—
A—oesophagus? **B**—meninges? **C**—muscles? **D**—teeth? **E**—diaphragm? (13.2)

5. TB usually spreads—
C—from child to adult? **D**—from child to child? **E**—from adult to child? (13.3)

6. Children in towns are usually infected with TB—
B—earlier than children in villages? **C**—later than children in villages? (13.2)

7. You think GEORGETTE might have TB, but you are not sure. Which of these things would make you more sure?
A Diarrhoea **B** A chronic scaly rash **C** Abdominal pain **D** Some firm painless lymph nodes in her neck **E** Pale urine

8. Which of these kinds of TB is most dangerous—
C—primary TB? **D**—miliary TB? **E**—TB lymph nodes of the neck? (13.2)

9. TB more often causes lung cavities in—
B—adults? **C**—children? (13.3)

10. TB in children most often presents as—
A—wheezing? **B**—TB meningitis? **C**—a chronic cough with blood-stained sputum? **D**—bloody diarrhoea? **E**—a falling growth curve in an 'ill' child? (13:1)

11. Which of these children are most likely to have TB?
A The severely malnourished child **B** The severely jaundiced child **C** The child with leprosy **D** The anaemic child **E** The backward child (13:1)

12. SAMI has TB. Her uncle has a chronic cough with bloody sputum. He probably has—
A—chronic bronchitis? **B**—pneumonia? **C**—a TB cavity in his lung? **D**—miliary TB? **E**—TB of his lymph nodes? (13.3)

13. Examining the sputum is helpful for diagnosing TB in—
C—adults? **D**—young children? **E**—both of them? (13.3)

14. AUDHUMLA (1 year). Her uncle has TB. She has had no immunizations, and has no symptoms. What would you do?
A Give her DPT. **B** Give her isoniazid. **C** Give her isoniazid and streptomycin. **D** Give her BCG vaccine. (13.7)

15. The best way to be sure that an adult has TB is to—
B—find AAFB in his sputum? **C**—X-ray his lungs? **D**—do a tuberculin test? **E**—do a blood test? (13.3)

16. BCG gives a child—
B—a natural passive immunity? **C**—a natural active immunity? **D**—an artificial passive immunity? **E**—an artificial active immunity? (13.4)

17. Which of these would you use for treating TB?
A Streptomycin with isoniazid **B** BCG **C** Tuberculin **D** PPD **E** Streptomycin alone (13.6)

18. BCG does NOT—
A—cause a scar? **B**—cause fever for one or two days after it has been given? **C**—prevent TB in most children who are given it? **D**—prevent TB meningitis and miliary TB almost completely? **E**—cause lymphadenitis occasionally? (4.6, 13.4)

19. We can help to prevent a child's TB organisms becoming resistant by giving him—
A—one drug only at a time? **B**—drugs for a short time? **C**—more than one drug at the same time? **D**—large doses of drugs? **E**—drugs for a long time? (13.6)

20. NERO (3 years) has TB and is taking TB drugs. He now has measles. While he has measles he should—
A—go on taking his drugs? **B**—stop taking them completely? **C**—stop taking drugs until he is well? **D**—take a larger dose? **E**—change to a different TB drug? (13.6)

21. Which of these is the most important symptom of TB in a child?
A Coughing up bloody sputum **B** Chest pain **C** Insuction **D** A falling growth curve **E** Fast breathing (13.1)

22. A child with TB usually has—
A—cyanosis? **B**—insuction? **C**—an increased respiratory rate? **D**—stridor? **E**—none of these things? (13.7)

23. Which of these children are LEAST likely to have TB?
A DULCIE who has pneumonia which is not being cured by penicillin? **B** ELSIE who had measles 6 weeks ago and still ill with a cough and 'not eating'. **C** ELVIE with a cough and a falling growth curve. **D** STEVIE who has slowly become ill with meningitis during the last two weeks. **E** DAVIE with large purulent tonsils. (13:1)

24. Which of these things does NOT help to prevent TB? Making sure that—
A—infectious TB adults finish their treatment? **B**—children have rising growth curves? **C**—children are immunized with BCG? **D**—children drink boiled water? **E**—infectious adults swallow their sputum and do not spit it out? (13.4)

25. Which of these diseases often presents as a high fever? **A** TB **B** Thrush **C** Leprosy **D** Giardiasis **E** Malaria (10.7)

ACCIDENTS B
Chapter 14: Code 7

1. Young children are most often injured—
D—inside their homes? **E**—outside their homes? (14.1)

2. NOAH (6 years) was waiting in a queue and fell to the ground. You are also standing in the queue and examine him. He is pale and sweating. His pulse is weak and he is making no abnormal movements. The weather is very hot. He—
A—is dehydrated? **B**—has probably fainted? **C**—is shocked? **D**—has had a fit? **E**—is anaemic? (14.2)

3. Contractures can be caused by—
B—burns on the back? **C**—any severe burn across a joint? **D**—superficial burns? **E**—small full-thickness burns? (14.3)

4. FRANCESCA (2 years) has pulled a kettle of boiling water over herself. She has partial-thickness burns covering 20 per cent of her body. She is most likely to be killed by—
A—infection and fluid loss? **B**—infection and contractures? **C**—tetanus and contractures? **D**—contractures and fluid loss? **E**—tetanus and fluid loss? (14.3)

5. Burns sometimes have to be grafted because—
B—the blood vessels of the burnt skin have been completely destroyed? **C**—there are blisters (vesicles) on them? **D**—the child is losing too much fluid from a burn? **E**—the epidermis has been completely destroyed? (14.3)

6. BENDICO'S house has burnt down, and he has breathed much hot smoke. He might die from—
A—TB? **B**—tonsillitis? **C**—pneumonia? **D**—upper respiratory infection? **E**—asthma? (14.3)

7. All these girls were burnt yesterday. Who has a superficial burn?
B CAROLINE who has erythema only **C** CLARISSA who has erythema and blisters **D** CATERINIA who has a dull yellow-grey burn without blisters (14.3)

8. JULES has been burnt. The hair follicles and sweat glands in his burn are still alive, but the rest of the epidermis in his burn is destroyed. What kind of burn has he?
A Deep partial-thickness **B** Superficial partial-thickness **C** Superficial **D** A full-thickness burn (14.3)

9. A child who has swallowed poison should be made to vomit if—
A—he has swallowed kerosine? **B**—he swallowed poison more than four hours ago? **C**—he is unconscious? **D**—only if NONE of these things is true? (14.6)

10. Children may get tetanus from—
A—large dirty wounds? **B**—chronic otitis media? **C**—infection of the umbilicus? **D**—infected burns? **E**—all of these? (14.3)

**PLEASE DO NOT WRITE ON THESE
QUESTIONS SOMEONE ELSE MAY NEED
THEM**

---

11. GUISEPPE has cut his wrist on some broken glass. He cannot touch his thumb with his middle finger. He has cut—
A—his skin only? **B**—a bone? **C**—a nerve? **D**—a tendon? **E**—a nerve or a tendon? (14.4)

12. A new clean cut in which the skin edges are pulled apart should be—
B—sewn up tomorrow when the bleeding is less? **C**—left for a few days to see if it will heal by itself? **D**—sewn up now? **E**—left to heal by itself? (14.4)

13. FLIC (6 years). Three weeks ago a piece of bamboo went into his arm. His mother pulled it out and put a dressing on the wound. His arm is still swollen and tender. This is probably because—
A—there is still a piece of wood in his arm? **B**—he is getting tetanus? **C**—the wood was infected with TB bacilli? **D**—he is still bleeding into the wound? **E**—a nerve has been injured? (14.4)

14. Ipecacuanha should NOT be given to children who have swallowed—
A—poisonous plants? **B**—kerosine? **C**—ferrous sulphate? **D**—pyrimethamine? **E**—phenobarbitone? (14.6)

15. ROMERO has a dirty cut on his foot. He has never been immunized with DPT vaccine. His cut needs local treatment. Which of these does he also need?
A Tetanus antitoxin (ATS) only **B** DPT vaccine **C** Tetanus antitoxin and tetanus toxoid **D** Tetanus toxoid only (14.4, 18.16)

16. KERR (2 years) swallowed some detergent 48 hours ago. He seems well. What would you tell his mother?
A 'Don't worry.' **B** 'I will give him penicillin to stop him getting pneumonia.' **C** 'We must make him vomit as soon as possible.' **D** 'We must watch him carefully, he may have symptoms this evening or tomorrow.' (14.7)

17. LUNA (2½ years, 38 °C) swallowed some kerosine last night. She is coughing and will not eat. What would you tell her mother?
B 'Don't worry, she will soon get well.' **C** 'She needs penicillin. Then she should to to hospital.' **D** 'We must make her vomit the kerosine.' **E** 'I must give her a purge to remove the kerosine from her gut.' (14.8)

18. Blisters on a burn are a sign that—
D—the burnt skin is still alive? **E**—the burnt skin is dead? (14.3)

19. Which of these malaria parasites is most likely to cause coma?
B *P. falciparum.* **C** Other kinds of malaria parasite. (14.6)

20. Which of these drugs can be used for treating a disease which causes coma?
A Gamma benzene hexachloride **B** Piperazine **C** Tetrachlorethylene **D** Dapsone **E** Quinine (3.26, 14.6, 15.7)

21. Which of these is an important complication of burns?
A TB **B** Tetanus **C** Diphtheria **D** Measles **E** Polio (14.3)

22. ALICE's clothes are burning. The best thing her mother could do would be to—

C—try to take her clothes off? D—take her quickly to the nearest pond? E—wrap her quickly in a blanket? (14.3)

23. Which of these would you NOT use to make a child vomit?

A Very strong salty water B Your finger C A spatula D The rubber tube from a stethoscope (14.6)

24. Which of these is the LEAST useful way of preventing the harm caused by accidents?

A Taking dangers away from children B Teaching them to avoid danger C Making children strong and healthy so they are less harmed by accidents D Immunizing children with DPT vaccine E Teaching mothers how to care for children with burns and cuts (14.1)

25. TAGHI (4 years) is in coma and you do not know why. He needs all these things EXCEPT—

A—a lumbar puncture? B—a blood slide for malaria? C—to be nursed on his front or his side? D—intravenous fluids? E—an injection of pyrimethamine? (14.8)

FITS B
Chapter 15: Code 6

1. Fits are more easily recognized in—

C—an older child? D—a baby? (15.1)

2. OMAR is a week old. His mother is worried because he has attacks in which his eyes look up to his top of his head, and he goes blue and stiff after which he goes to sleep. What would you tell her?

A 'OMAR is having fits.' B 'These cannot be fits because he is not vomiting.' C 'These attacks are not fits because he does not bite his tongue.' D 'These are the spasms of tetanus.' (15.1)

3. Normal CSF has—

A—more than 40 mg/dl of protein in it? B—more than 5 white cells per microlitre? C—a pale yellow colour? D—a slightly cloudy look? E—no organisms in it? (15.2)

4. Meningitis more often causes neck stiffness and a positive Kernig's sign in—

A—young babies? B—older children? C—boys? D—girls? (15.6)

5. The best antiseptic for lumbar puncture is—

A—flavine? B—permanganate? C—iodine? D—hypochlorite? E—lysol? (15.3)

6. Lumbar puncture is easier in—

D—an adult? E—a young child? (15.3)

7. You have sterilized two lumbar-puncture needles by boiling. The safest place to keep them while you are getting ready for lumbar puncture is—

A—in the box they came in? B—in a small bowl of antiseptic solution? C—in any clean place? D—in the bottom of the pan in which they have been boiled? E—in a bowl of sterile water? (15.3)

8. PAPIO (2 years, 39·5 °C) is having a fit. You have pulled his tongue forward so that he breathes normally, and have given him paraldehyde. What would you do next?

A Give him phenobarbitone by mouth. B Cover him with blankets. C Give him intravenous fluids. D Cool him with water. E Measure his haemoglobin. (15.9)

9. KARIKO (2 years, 38·8 °C) has fits, vomiting, and a stiff neck. He cannot put his head between his legs. You have tried twice to do a lumbar puncture, but no CSF comes. The nearest hospital is 25 miles away up river by canoe. What would you do?

C Give him an injection of penicillin and send him home. D Go on trying to get CSF. E Stop trying to do a lumbar puncture and treat him for purulent meningitis. (15.6)

10. If a child's CSF looks very mildly turbid and is not blood-stained, you can be sure he has—

A—meningitis? B—more than 1000 pus cells in each microlitre of CSF? C—virus meningitis? D—TB meningitis? E—cerebral malaria? (15.3b)

11. Which of these diseases often presents as febrile convulsions—

A—amoebic dysentery? B—tonsillitis? C—pyoderma? D—marasmus? E—hookworm anaemia? (15.5, 15.9, 18.11)

12. JUSTINE (3 years) has been treated for febrile convulsions. What would you say to her mother?

A 'When she has fever again, keep her cool with cold sponging.' B 'She is cured now and will not get convulsions again.' C 'Put plenty of clothes on her when she next has a fever.' D 'Do not give her paracetamol when she has fever.' (15.5)

13. There are no causal drugs to treat—

C—TB meningitis? D—pyogenic meningitis? E—virus meningitis? (15.6)

14. ALIREZA (4 years, 38·8 °C) has had two fits and is drowsy. *P. falciparum* in the district is resistant to chloroquin. He needs—

A—resochin? B—camoquin? C—quinine or sulphadoxine with pyrimethamine? D—pyrimethamine alone? E—primaquin? (3.25, 15.7)

15. SERAPHINA has had mild fever and a cough for several weeks. Two days ago she had her first fit. She has also been losing weight and not eating. She has meningeal signs. Her meningitis is most likely to be caused by—

B—fungi? C—cocci? D—AAFB? E—viruses? (15.6)

16. BERNARD ($2\frac{1}{2}$ years, 38 °C) has not been well for several days and has just had two fits. Does he need a lumbar puncture?

B Yes **C** No (15.9)

17. KWALAHO (6 years, 37 °C) has epilepsy. He had another fit an hour ago and is now normal. Does he need a lumbar puncture?

A Yes **B** No (15.9)

18. EDGAR (2 years) has had a fit. His neck is stiff and he is unable to put his head between his legs. Does he need a lumbar puncture?

C Yes **D** No (15.9)

19. MARLENE has had two fits. Kernig's sign is positive. She has '*P. falciparum* + +' in her blood. Does she need a lumbar puncture?

D Yes **E** No (10.7, 15.9)

20. Fits are most likely to harm a child's brain if—
A—they last too long? **B**—the child is very young? **C**—the child does not have a lumbar puncture? **D**—they are caused by hyperpyrexia? **E**—they are caused by pneumonia or tonsillitis? (15.9)

21. In meningitis a swollen fontanelle is—
B—an early sign? **C**—a late sign? (15.6)

22. BOGOT (10 months) has meningitis. He has also been vomiting and is dehydrated. Will this vomiting make his fontanelle—
D—swell more? **E**—swell less? (5.6)

23. Lumbar puncture should be done in a health centre—
A—so that meningitis can be treated? **B**—so that meningitis can be diagnosed and the children with meningitis sent for help? **C**—because lumbar puncture stops fits? **D**—because lumbar puncture cures headache? (15.3)

24. SIEGRIED (2 years, 39 °C) has had two fits. He is drowsy and has vomited. His CSF is clear. Pandy's test is negative. He has 4 cells in a microlitre of CSF. His blood slide is negative. Which of these diseases is he most likely to have?

B Virus meningitis **C** TB meningitis **D** Febrile convulsions **E** Pyogenic meningitis (15.6, 15.7)

25. Which of these diseases does NOT cause fits?

A Dehydration **B** Meningitis **C** Epilepsy **D** Hookworm infection **E** Falciparum malaria (15.4)

EYES B
Chapter 16: Code 6

1. The thin wet mucosa that covers the white parts of the eyes and the insides of the eyelids is called the—

A—sclera? **B**—cornea? **C**—conjunctiva? **D**—retina? **E**—iris? (16.2)

2. The retina is—
A—the part of the eye which sends messages to the brain? **B**—the white part of the eye? **C**—made of smooth muscle? **D**—a circle of blue or brown tissue? **E**—the gland which makes tears? (16.2)

3. Which of these diseases would you treat with fluorescein?

A Xerophthalmia **B** Corneal ulcer **C** Acute conjunctivitis **D** Trachoma **E** None of them (16.2)

4. Trachoma is—
A—an acute purulent conjunctivitis? **B**—an important cause of blindness in some countries? **C**—a common complication of measles? **D**—easily prevented with vitamin A? **E**—a late stage of xerophthalmia? (16.9)

5. The best way to let pus out of a stye is to—
C—pull out the eyelash in the middle of it? **D**—open it with a scalpel? **E**—squeeze it? (16.3)

6. Signs in a child's eye are helpful in diagnosing—
A—meningitis? **B**—malaria? **C**—typhoid? **D**—chickenpox? **E**—measles? (16.4)

7. Foreign bodies inside the ball of the eye—
A—always cause blindness immediately? **B**—usually come out by themselves in a few days? **C**—always leave a hole that is easy to see? **D**—often become infected and cause blindness? **E**—can easily be removed in a health centre? (16.5)

8. When ointment is put into a child's eyes it should be put onto his—
B—cornea? **C**—upper eyelids? **D**—lower eyelids? (16.2)

9. When an eye is stained with fluorescein corneal ulcers stain—
C—blue? **D**—red? **E**—green? (16.7)

10. PRISCA (5 years) has got bleach (or any other harmful liquid) in her eyes. Her mother should immediately—
A—wash her eyes with plenty of water? **B**—wipe out the bleach with a cloth? **C**—put oil in her eyes? **D**—put antibiotic ointment in her eyes? **E**—wash her eyes with salt water? (16.6)

11. Corneal ulcers—
A—are easily seen? **B**—may only be seen after staining? **C**—cause no changes in the sclera? **D**—cause most redness away from the cornea? **E**—are always in both eyes? (16.7)

12. Trachoma is caused by —
A—organisms half way between viruses and bacteria? **B**—venereal disease? **C**—lack of vitamin A? **D**—bacterial infections? **E**—viruses? (16.9)

13. Acute conjunctivitis is mostly spread by—
A—droplets? **B**—infected dust? **C**—flies? **D**—washing in dirty water? **E**—contact from patient to patient through infected towels, fingers, etc.? (16.8)

14. Which of these diseases causes blindness most rapidly?

A Allergic conjunctivitis **B** Vitamin B deficiency **C** Keratomalacia **D** Trachoma **E** Phlyctenular conjunctivitis (16.8)

15. LO'ONO (6 years) has several attacks of sore red eyes, usually at the same time each year. Her sclerae are dark. There are some follicles under her upper lids, but no pannus. She probably has—

A—trachoma? **B**—acute conjunctivitis? **C**—vitamin A deficiency? **D**—allergic conjunctivitis? **E**—corneal ulcers? (16.10)

16. If you think of the eye as a clock where would you expect to see pannus?

B 12 O'clock **C** 3 O'clock **D** 9 O'clock **E** 6 O'clock (16.9)

17. MARCELLO (15 years) has had red watery eyes for many years. The underneath of his eyelids is scarred and there are a few pinkish-grey follicles. There is much pannus. He has—

A—xerophthalmia? **B**—third or fourth stage trachoma? **C**—vitamin A deficiency? **D**—allergic conjunctivitis? **E**—phlyctenular conjunctivitis? (16.9)

18. MELODIA (2 years) has keratomalacia in both eyes. She can just see enough to count your fingers when you ask her to. Vitamin A will—

C—probably stop her blindness getting worse? **D**—make her see normally again? (16.13)

19. PADDY has a 1 mm yellow–grey swelling at the outer side of his cornea close to his sclera. He needs treatment with—

A—vitamin A? **B**—scopolamine eye ointment? **C**—chlortetracycline eye ointment? **D**—isoniazid? **E**—penicillin? (16.11)

20. Which of these are in the right order from the most mild to most severe?

A Night-blindness, xerophthalmia, keratomalacia **B** Xerophthalmia, night-blindness, keratomalacia **C** Keratomalacia, xerophthalmia, night-blindness. (16.13)

21. Bitot's spots are a sign of—

A—phlyctenular conjunctivitis? **B**—vitamin B deficiency? **C**—xerophthalmia? **D**—keratomalacia? **E**—night-blindness? (16.13)

22. Very large doses of vitamin A cause—

A—no symptoms? **B**—vomiting? **C**—itchy, peeling skin? **D**—swelling of the fontanelle? **E**—any of these symptoms? (16.14)

23. Which of these foods is LEAST good at preventing xerophthalmia?

A Eggs **B** White polished rice **C** Papaya **D** Cassava leaves **E** Liver (16.13)

24. LORENZO (2 years) has severe conjunctivitis with much swelling of his eyelids. His mother needs to be told all these things EXCEPT—

A 'Give him his own towel until he is well.' **B** 'Put this ointment (chlortetracycline) in three times a day.' **C** 'Wash his eyes carefully in the way I am going to show you.' **D** 'This disease does not spread to other children.' **E** 'Bring him daily for penicillin injections.' (16.8)

25. Which of these children most needs vitamin A by injection?

A KINO (1 year) who is having vitamin A capsules every six months **B** BILL with night-blindness **C** VANES with xerophthalmia **D** TOM with xerophthalmia and a small lesion on his cornea **E** FRED who has been blind with scarred eyes for several years (16.15)

EARS B
Chapter 17: Code 6

1. The meatus is—

A—a bone in the ear? **B**—the skull behind the ear? **C**—the hole in the outer ear? **D**—a part of the middle ear? **E**—a part of the inner ear? (17.2)

2. Otitis externa is a disease of the—

A—outer ear? **B**—middle ear? **C**—inner ear? **D**—the Eustachian tube? (17.2)

3. The quickest way to sterilize an ear swab is to—

B—dip it in antiseptic solution? **C**—heat it in a pressure cooker? **D**—boil it? **E**—flame it? (17.5)

4. The bone in the ear drum is called the—

A—mastoid? **B**—maleus? **C**—incus? **D**—stapes? (17.2)

5. The middle ear is filled with—

A—bone? **B**—the mastoid air spaces? **C**—air? **D**—fluid? **E**—the nerves of hearing? (17.2)

6. Which of these children is LEAST likely to have acute otitis media?

A LITETA with fever **B** LUAMPA with fits **C** LUKULU with severe ear pain **D** LUAPULA with a swollen ear-drum **E** LUKULANYA with a discharging ear for three years (17.9)

7. Which of these is LEAST useful for treating an acute septic ear infection?

A Penicillin **B** Sulphadimidine **C** Chloramphenicol **D** Tiabendazole **E** Ampicillin (17.9)

8. If the ear of a child with chronic otitis media is swabbed with dirty cotton wool he is in danger from—

A—diphtheria? **B**—pneumonia? **C**—pharyngitis? **D**—tetanus? **E**—TB? (17.5)

9. The only way to know that an ear is clean is to—

C—syringe it? **D**—swab it? **E**—look into it? (17.6)

10. Which of these can cause ear pain but not ear discharge?

A Carious teeth **B** Foreign body **C** Otitis externa **D** Acute otitis media with a perforated drum **E** Chronic otitis media (17.8)

11. QUEENIE (18 months, 38·2 °C) woke up in the night crying and rubbing her ear. Her ear-drum and the deeper part of the meatus near it are red and dull. She has—

A—a foreign body in her ear? **B**—acute otitis media? **C**—chronic otitis media? **D**—otitis externa? **E**—carious teeth? (17.9)

12. Otitis media should be treated—

A—as soon as you diagnose it? **B**—only when it has begun to discharge pus? **C**—after the drum has started swelling? **D**—after the drum has perforated? **E**—only if it is causing pain? (17.9)

13. When you examine a child for deafness you should—

A—examine both his ears together? **B**—leave both his ears open? **C**—speak loudly all the time? **D**—let him see your lips? **E**—examine one ear and block the other one? (17.7)

14. MEROPI (3 years, 37·8 °C) has had a discharge from his left ear for three months. His drum is perforated. Sometimes the discharge stops. At other times it is very severe and he has pain. Which of these is true?

A He has acute otitis media. **B** He can be cured easily and quickly. **C** Antibiotics may help his symptoms. **D** He needs ear-drops only. **E** He probably has otitis externa. (17.10)

15. The first sign of otitis media is—

A—a perforated drum? **B**—a swollen drum? **C**—a fixed drum? **D**—a red drum? (17.9)

16. The way to examine a child for mastoiditis is to see if he is tender by pressing—

A—his ear lobe? **B**—behind his ear? **C**—above his ear? **D**—below his ear? **E**—in front of his ear? (17.11)

17. HERMIA (5 years, 38·6 °C) has had a discharge from her right ear since she was three. She vomited several times yesterday and this morning she had a fit. She says she feels giddy. The diagnosis that would best explain these symptoms is—

A—otitis externa? **B**—brain abscess? **C**—septicaemia? **D**—mastoiditis? **E**—tetanus? (17.11)

18. Ears should be syringed with—

A—cold water? **B**—cold saline? **C**—water at body temperature? **D**—hot water? **E**—hot saline? (17.6)

19. A foreign body in the ear which cannot be removed with a syringe may be removed with—

A—a needle? **B**—a straight wire? **C**—a thin stick? **D**—a bent wire? **E**—a pair of forceps? (17.13)

20. Which of these children has mastoiditis?

A NANO with a warm welling behind his ear pushing it forwards. **B** PICO with swellings below and in front of both his ears for one week. **C** FEMTO with a swollen ear drum and ear symptoms for three days. **D** ATO with a painful swelling in his meatus. (17.11)

21. The deafness caused by chronic ear infection—

A—stops if the ear stops discharging? **B**—cannot be prevented? **C**—is difficult to cure? **D**—slowly cures itself? **E**—is easily cured with penicillin? (17.10)

22. Which of these children would you NOT expect to have a discharging ear?

A THINKWELL with a chronically infected foreign body. **B** LIVEWELL with mastoiditis. **C** STANDWELL with otitis externa. **D** LOVEWELL with chronic otitis media. **E** DANCEWELL with a dull mildly swollen ear-drum, who is being given daily injections of procaine penicillin. (17.9, 17.10)

23. ADETOKUNBO (4 years) has acute otitis media. His ear-drum has just perforated. Now, most probably, his—

A—pain will get less? **B**—pain and fever will get less? **C**— fever will get less? **D**—pain and fever will get worse? **E**—fever will get worse? (17.9)

24. Which of these is the LEAST likely way for acute otitis media to present?

A A discharging ear **B** Vomiting **C** A child rubbing and pulling his ear **D** Cough **E** Pain (17.9)

25. Which of these is NOT true? The swelling caused by mastoiditis—

A—pushes the ear forwards? **B**—is caused by acute infection and inflammation? **C**—is tender? **D**—can be moved over the bone under it? **E**—is behind the ear? (17.11)

MOUTH AND THROAT B
Chapter 18: Code 2

1. In young children acute sore throats may present with any of these symptoms EXCEPT—

A—fits? **B**—abdominal pain? **C**—vomiting? **D**—being unable to pass urine? **E**—coughing? (18.1)

2. A young child's throat should be examined—

A—at the beginning of the examination? **B**—while he is lying on his back? **C**—while he is standing up? **D**—while his mother is out of the room? **E**—while he is sitting firmly held on his mother's lap? (18.2)

3. A spatula for examining the throat—

A—should be boiled between one child and the next? **B**—must be completely sterile? **C**—need only be sterilized after every ten children? **D**—need not be sterilized? **E**—can be safely kept in an antiseptic solution? (18.2)

4. A child's tonsils are—

A—at the sides of his neck? **B**—in front of his ears? **C**—at the sides of his throat? **D**—on his tongue? **E**—on his palate? (18.2)

5. Which of these diseases can you prevent in a child by immunizing his mother?

A Measles **B** Tetanus **C** Malaria **D** Diphtheria **E** Thrush (18.16)

6. Which of these diseases most often causes lesions in a child's mouth and on his skin?

A Scabies **B** Measles **C** Tonsillitis **D** Pharyngitis **E** Heat rash (18.3)

7. Which of these diseases does NOT make a child's mouth sore?

A Thrush **B** Herpes stomatitis **C** Cancrum oris **D** Herpes zoster **E** Vincent's stomatitis (18.3)

8. The organism which causes one of these diseases can live in a child for the rest of his life and cause lesions on his lips whenever he has a fever. Which disease is it?

A Herpes stomatitis B Vincent's stomatitis C Chicken-pox D Diphtheria E Tonsillitis (18.6)

9. RASHA (3 months) has thrush. What would you tell her mother?

A 'This is a serious disease.' B 'Scrape the lesions of her mouth like this ...' C 'Put this medicine (gentian violet) on her lesions.' D 'Penicillin cures thrush.' E 'If she cannot suck, express your milk and throw it away.' (18.5)

10. Which of these diseases causes small painful round yellow-grey ulcers in a child's mouth?

A Vitamin A deficiency B Vitamin B deficiency C Vincent's stomatitis D Thrush E Herpes stomatitis (18.6)

11. Which of these diseases is most likely to be complicated by cancrum oris if you do not treat it early?

A Vincent's stomatitis B Herpes stomatitis C Thrush D Diphtheria E Tonsillitis (18.7, 18.8)

12. Herpes stomatitis does NOT—

A—stop a child eating? B—cause swelling of his lips and tongue? C—cause swelling of the lymph nodes under the jaw? D—cause laryngeal obstruction? E—cause fever and make a child ill? (18.6)

13. Which of these diseases causes severe deformity of a child's face?

A Cancrum oris B Vincent's stomatitis C Herpes stomatitis D Thrush E Diphtheria (18.8)

14. Large tender lymph nodes at the angles of a child's jaws show that he has—

A—tonsillitis? B—diphtheria? C—herpes stomatitis? D—an infection of his throat or tonsils? E—Vincent's angina? (18.9)

15. JILL has an infection of her upper respiratory tract. The most important question to decide is whether she—

A—has lymphadenitis or not? B—needs an antibiotic or not? C—has 'URI' or pharyngitis? D—has pharyngitis or tonsillitis? E—has fever or not? (18.11)

16. A child CANNOT get tetanus from—

A—a small cut? B—chronic otitis media? C—breathing in an infected droplet? D—a burn? E—a dirty syringe and needle? (18.16)

17. Tetanus bacteria—

A—infect the meninges? B—grow in the blood? C—spread all over the body? D—grow in the nerves? E—stay in the local lesion and make toxin? (18.16)

18. A child with a sore throat—

A—always needs an antibiotic? B—should have his throat painted with gentian violet? C—sometimes needs penicillin? D—never needs an antibiotic? E—should be given chloramphenicol? (18.11)

19. KANTHUNKAKO (6 years) is very ill. He has a cough, and pain when he swallows. There is dirty-grey membrane on his tonsils and on his pharynx. His neck is very swollen. He probably has—

A—Vincent's angina? B—herpes stomatitis? C—tonsillitis? D—diphtheria? E—bronchitis? (18.12)

20. A membrane in a child's mouth is probably caused by thrush if it is—

A—causing fever? B—obstructing his larynx? C—making him very ill? D—a dirty yellow-grey? E—on his tongue and inside his cheeks? (18.5)

21. An important complication of diphtheria is obstruction of a child's—

A—bronchi? B—larynx? C—nose? D—pharynx? E—Eustachian tubes? (18.12)

22. Tetanus of the newborn usually presents as—

A—the baby who stops sucking? B—vomiting? C—spasms? D—cyanotic attacks? E—sepsis of the umbilical cord? (18.16)

23. Tetanus and meningitis both make a child bend backwards, but in meningitis he does NOT have—

A—spasms? B—a stiff neck? C—fits? D—a swollen fontanelle? E—a positive Kernig's sign? (18.16)

24. Tetanus bacteria spread—

A—by contact from child to child? B—by infected dust or earth getting into a wound? C—in infected droplets from adult carriers? D—as a faeces to mouth infection? E—in unboiled water? (18.16)

25. An acute infection of the throat is LEAST likely to present as—

A—fever? B—the ill child who does not eat? C—fits? D—vomiting? E—loss of weight? (18.11)

SWELLINGS B
Chapter 19: with revision: Code 7

1. SPYROS has a painful tender swelling over his right cheek. Under the swelling is a painful carious tooth. What would you say to his mother?

A 'We must drain the abscess and then remove the tooth.' B 'The tooth will fall out by itself soon.' C 'We must take the tooth out now.' D We must give him penicillin first and then somebody must take out the tooth.' (19.5)

2. Hernias can cause swellings—

A—over a bone? B—in the groin? C—over the whole abdomen? D—near the spine? E—in the eyelids? (19.9, 20.5)

3. A common place for oedema to cause swelling is—

A—in the groin? B—in the middle of the neck? C—over the feet? D—at the umbilicus? E—behind the ear? (19.8)

4. Swellings almost anywhere in the body can be caused by—

A—acute septic infections? B—mumps? C—goitre? D—diphtheria? E—hernias? (19.1)

5. Neck swellings may be a presenting symptom in all these diseases EXCEPT—

A—tonsillitis? B—goitre? C—mumps? D—TB? E—sickle cell anaemia? (19.2)

6. MIRAN has some mildly enlarged painless lymph nodes in his groin. They are probably caused by—

A—tumours? B—acute septic infection? C—chronic septic infection? D—TB? (19.2)

7. MIRAN probably needs—
A—an antibiotic? B—no treatment? C—isoniazid? D—an operation to remove the infected nodes? (19.2)

8. TB lymph-nodes are most commonly seen and felt—
A—at the sides of the neck? B—in the lungs? C—in the abdomen? D—in the axillae? E—at the back of the neck? (19.3)

9. One way to find out if enlarged lymph-nodes in the neck are caused by chronic sepsis or TB is to give a child a drug and examine him a few weeks later. Which drug would you give?
B Streptomycin C Penicillin and streptomycin D Penicillin E Isoniazid (19.3)

10. Mumps is caused by—
A—lack of iodine? B—fungi? C—protozoa? D—bacteria? E—a virus? (19.4)

11. When goitres are common in a community people need more—
A—iron? B—fluorine? C—salt? D—vitamins? E—iodine? (19.6)

12. ALI has swollen eyelids and pus discharging from his eyes. His swollen eyelids are caused by—
A—the nephrotic syndrome? B—kwashiorkor? C—severe anaemia? D—conjunctivitis? E—acute nephritis? (19.8)

13. Swelling of the eyelids and ankles can be caused by disease of the—
A—kidneys? B—spleen? C—ureter? D—urethra? E—stomach? (19.7)

14. ANNA-MARIA has swollen eyelids and ankles. You examine her urine and find protein + + +. She probably has—
A—schistosomiasis? B—the nephrotic syndrome? C—a urinary infection? D— lymphadenitis and cellulitis? E—kwashiorkor? (19.7)

15. Lymph-nodes can be found in all these places EXCEPT—
A—in the groins? B—behind the ear? C—at the umbilicus? D—in front of the ear? E—under the angles of the jaw? (2–5, 19–1)

16. Tenderness in a lymph-node is a sign that it is caused by—
A—acute infection? B—chronic infection? C—TB? D—a tumour? (19.2)

MATCH these treatments with the children who need them—
17. Dapsone **18.** Penicillin **19.** Gentian violet **20.** More protein and energy food.
A The child with an umbilical hernia B The child with thrush C The child with a chronic anaesthetic skin lesion D The child with a discharging ear for one week E The child with oedema of the feet and flaking paint rash (19.6, 17.9, 18.7, 11.22 (Revision))

MATCH these children with the things you would say to their mothers—
21. SATURN is newborn. His mother has lepromatous leprosy. **22.** VENUS (5 years) has severe hookworm anaemia. **23.** URANUS (3 years) has severe diarrhoea. **24.** PLUTO has pyoderma.
A 'Give him plenty of fluids. Give him food as soon as he can eat.' B 'Breast-feed him.' C 'Wash him well with soap and water.' D 'Here is some benzoic acid ointment for him.' E 'Wearing shoes prevents this.' (2.7, 9.31, 11.6, 26.66 (Revision))

25. CELESTE (9 years) has TB lymph-nodes in her neck. She might have been infected—
C—by inhaling infected droplets of sputum? D—by drinking infected milk? E—in either of these ways? (19.3)

ABDOMINAL PAIN B
Chapter 20: with revision: Code 3

1. The roof of the abdominal cavity is formed by—
A—the pelvis? B—the heart? C—the stomach? D—the liver? E—the diaphragm? (20.1)

2. Which of these children is most likely to have an acute abdomen?
A TATSUO with abdominal pain and severe diarrhoea for one day. B SITI with abdominal pain and mild diarrhoea for three months. C SIBYL with abdominal pain and vomiting for one day. D SAM with swollen abdomen for two months. (20.2.)

3. When we examine a child's abdomen with our hand we can find out—
A—how big his liver is? B— if his kidneys are working normally? C—if he lacks vitamins? D—if he has worms? E—if he is malnourished? (20.3)

4. Enlarged lymph nodes in the groin are usually caused by—
A—TB? B—acute septic infection? C—worms? D—urinary infections? E—chronic septic lesions on the legs? (20.5)

5. Which of these does NOT cause vomiting?
A Whooping cough B Meningitis C Gut infections D Hookworm infection E Ipecacuanha (20.14)

6. Which of these is a sign of a healthy abdomen?
A Rigidity B Tenderness C Softness D Guarding (20.3)

7. An enlarged spleen is usually caused by—
A—measles? B—malaria? C—chickenpox? D—hookworms? E—infective hepatitis? (20.3)

8. TOM has abdominal pain. When you take your hand away from his abdomen after examining it, he feels a sharp pain. He has—
A—guarding? B—rebound tenderness? C—rigidity? D—gut obstruction? (20.3)

9. Which of these is NOT true. An inguinal hernia—
A— becomes larger and smaller quickly? B—usually

cures itself in a few months? **C**—may go away when a child lies down? **D**—gets bigger when a child coughs, cries, or runs about? **E**—may become strangulated? (20.4)

10. A child with abdominal swelling should go to hospital if—

A—he has passed worms? **B**—he has had the swelling for more than a month? **C**—he has a very large spleen? **D**—he also has abdominal pain, vomiting, and tenderness? **E**—the swelling is caused by malnutrition? (20.8)

11. If a hernia becomes painful and tender and cannot be made to go away when a child lies down it is—

A—strangulated? **B**—obstructed? **C**—reduced? **D**—chronic? **E**—infected? (20.6)

12. MACHIKO (3 years) has a painful inguinal hernia. It cannot be made to go away when he lies down. He has vomited twice. What are you going to tell his mother?

A 'He needs glucose saline.' **B** 'We must go on pressing it until it goes away.' **C** 'He needs an operation in hospital immediately.' **D** 'Penicillin for three days will cure him.' **E** 'He will recover by himself in about a week.' (20.5)

13. Which of these is a cause of acute abdominal swelling?

A Malnutrition **B** A large spleen **C** A large liver **D** Hookworm infection **E** Gut obstruction (20.8)

14. Which of these does NOT cause vomiting?

A Whooping cough **B** Ringworm **C** Meningitis **D** Urinary infection **E** Gut infection (20.14)

15. A child with abdominal pain should go to hospital if he has—

A—malaria? **B**—tonsillitis? **C**—signs of an acute abdomen? **D**—diarrhoea? **E**—had pain for more than a month? (20.11)

16. Which of these is most important when you examine a child's abdomen?

A To examine him from the left **B** To lift up his clothes **C** To examine his abdomen first before doing anything else **D** To let him stand or lie quiet and relaxed **E** To examine him with only the tips of your fingers touching his abdomen (20.3)

17. Which of these does NOT cause abdominal pain?

A Urinary infection **B** Pneumonia **C** Malaria **D** Malnutrition **E** Diarrhoea (20.11)

18. Which of these shows that a child's abdominal pain is probably not serious?

A Vomiting and constipation **B** Several attacks like this before from which he recovered **C** Looking 'ill' **D** Severe pain for more than four hours **E** Abdominal rigidity (20.13)

19. Which of these would make you think that a child's vomiting was caused by gut obstruction?

A Worms in his vomit **B** White vomit **C** Vomit which looks like stools **D** Yellow vomit **E** Diarrhoea with the vomiting (20.14)

20. Which of these diseases usually needs an operation quickly?

A Acute abdomen **B** Umbilical hernia **C** Hydrocoele **D** Acute septic lymphadenitis **E** A large fontanelle (20.2)

21. The best symptomatic treatment for vomiting is—

A—diphenoxylate ('Lomotil')? **B**—promethazine? **C**—an antihistamine? **D**—aspirin? **E**—fluids? (20.15)

22. Rebound tenderness is a sign of—

A—hepatitis? **B**—dehydration? **C**—gasteroenteritis? **D**—inflammation of the peritoneum? **E**—gut obstruction? (20.3)

23. Which of these is LEAST likely to cause diarrhoea in a young child?

A Heavy *Trichuris* infection **B** Dirty feeding-bottles **C** Tonsillitis **D** Malnutrition **E** Scabies (9.5 (Revision))

24. Glucose–salt solution contains—

A Potassium chloride? **B** Ordinary sugar? **C** Sodium carbonate? **D** Sodium citrate? **E** Potassium bicarbonate? (9.21 (Revision))

25. LEVI is vomiting. Which of these would make you think that he had meningitis?

A Diarrhoea? **B** A stiff neck? **C** Constipation? **D** Tender lymph-nodes in his neck? **E** Shock? (15.6, 20.15 (Revision))

WORMS B
Chapter 21: with revision: Code 7

MATCH these children with the treatment they need.

1. KULYANI who has just been given a penicillin injection which caused shock and wheezing. **2.** RAM with several chronic thickened anaesthetic patches on his skin. **3.** RANI who has a long itchy lesion on her lower leg like a worm under her skin. **4.** HARI who keeps scratching his anus.

A Piperazine **B** Dapsone **C** Thiabendazole **D** Adrenalin **E** Bephenium (21.5, 12.3, 11–15, 3.2 (Revision))

MATCH these with the places where you would find them.

5. The axilla **6.** The spleen **7.** The meninges **8.** The uvula

A In the throat **B** Around the brain **C** On the left side of the abdomen **D** In the ear drum **E** Under the shoulder (17.7, 15.2, 20–4, 1–7 (Revision))

9. Which of these worms has to go through a cow before it can infect a child?

A *Ascaris* **B** *H. nana* **C** *T. solium* **D** *T. saginata* **E** *Strongyloides* (21.4)

10. A child is most likely to have many worms inside him if he is infected by—

C—*T. solium*? **D**—*T. saginata*? **E**—*H. nana*? (21.4)

11. Which of these can we use to treat the most kinds of worm?

A Tetrachlorethylene **B** Piperazine **C** Niclosamide **D** Metrifonate **E** Pyrantel pamoate (3:1b)

12. Which of these worms are you most likely to see crawling out of a child's anus?

A Hookworms **B** *Ascaris* **C** Schistosomes **D** Threadworms (21.5)

13. Which of these is most likely to cause acute septic infection?

A Bacteria **B** Worms **C** Protozoa **D** Viruses **E** Fungi (21.3)

14. LEELA has pulled a worm out of her nose. It is most likely to be—

A—*H. nana*? **B**—*Ascaris*? **C**—a threadworm? **D**—a hookworm? **E**—a tapeworm? (21.3)

15. Which of these spreads from one person's faeces to another person's mouth?

A Hookworms **B** *Strongyloides* **C** *Ascaris* **D** *Schistosoma haematobium* (21.1)

16. Which of these spreads from faeces to skin?

A Hookworms **B** *Trichuris* **C** Tapeworms **D** Threadworms **E** *Schistosoma haematobium* (21.1)

17. Which of these CANNOT be caused by worms?

A Creeping eruption **B** Abdominal pain **C** Tonsillitis **D** Loss of weight **E** Blood and mucus in the stool (21.1)

18. Which of these children most needs to have his stools examined?

A GUSTAV with a respiratory rate of 60. **B** GEORGES with itchy lesions on his hands. **C** GILES with jaundice. **D** GORDON with a haemoglobin of 5 g/dl. **E** GODFREY with a temperature of 39·5 °C. (22.5)

19. MIRA has 10 hookworm ova in a standard faecal smear. She has got a—

A—moderate load? **B**—light load? **C**—heavy load? (21.1)

20. A child most often infects himself with hookworms by—

A—sucking toys which have fallen on infected ground? **B**—eating food which flies have walked on? **C**—scratching his anus and sucking fingers? **D**—drinking dirty water? **E**—walking or playing on ground where an infected person has passed his faeces? (21.1)

21. Which of these worms is most likely to obstruct a child's gut?

A *Strongyloides* **B** *Ascaris* **C** *Trichuris* **D** Tapeworms **E** Hookworms (21.3)

22. KUMAR has a heavy load of *Ascaris* and hookworms. He should be given—

B—tetrachlorethylene only? **C**—piperazine only? **D**—tetrachlorethylene first then piperazine? **E**—piperazine and tetrachlorethylene together? (21.3)

23. Which of these worms can spread from one child to another by faeces-to-mouth infection?

A *H. nana* **B** Hookworms **C** *T. saginata* **D** *T. solium* **E** *Schistosoma haematobium* (21.4)

24. In which of these infections can a child make his worm load heavier by infecting himself with his own faeces on his own hands?

A *T. saginata* **B** *Schistosoma haematobium* **C** Threadworms (21.1)

25. Niclosamide is used for treating—

A—all kinds of worms? **B**—roundworms? **C**—hookworms? **D**—threadworms? **E**—tapeworms? (21.4)

ANAEMIA AND JAUNDICE B
Chapter 22: Code 7

1. Haemoglobin is—

A—a plasma protein? **B**—iron dissolved in the plasma? **C**—part of the lymph? **D**—the red substance inside red cells? **E**—the white substance inside white cells? (22.1)

2. Where is the pallor of anaemia MOST easily seen?

A On the nose **B** In the conjunctivae **C** In the ears **D** In the skin **E** In the throat (22.1)

3. Which of these diseases causes painful lesions in the hands and feet, and in the long bones of the arms and legs?

A The sickle-cell trait **B** Hookworm anaemia **C** Sickle-cell anaemia **D** Malaria **E** Infective hepatitis (22.8)

4. Which of these people would you expect to have the highest haemoglobin?

A A full-term newborn baby **B** A two-months-old child **C** An adult man **D** An adult woman **E** A premature baby (22.2)

5. Severe hookworm anaemia may present as swelling of the—

A—hands? **B**—thyroid? **C**—parotid? **D**—abdomen? **E**—feet? (22.1)

6. Haemoglobin is measured as the number of grams of it that there are in—

A—a centilitre of blood? **B**—a litre? **C**—a decilitre? **D**—a millilitre? **E**—a microlitre? (22.2)

7. VIRTUE is newborn. Her haemoglobin is 18·5 g/dl. She—

A—has too much haemoglobin? **B**—is normal? **C**—is mildly anaemic? **D**—is severely anaemic? (22.2)

8. DILLIP is a year old. His haemoglobin is 9 g/dl. Is he—

A—mildly anaemic? **B**—moderately anaemic? **C**—normal? **D**—severely anaemic? (22.2)

9. When you are using a weight chart to draw a child's haemoglobin curve, where would you draw a red line?

B On the 8 kg line **C** On the 14 kg line **D** On the 10 kg line **E** On the 12 kg line (22–3)

10. Anaemia can be caused by lack of—

A—citric acid? **B**—iodine? **C**—vitamin D? **D**—vitamin A? **E**—folic acid (22.3)

11. Anaemia can be caused by—

A—dehydration? **B**—tonsillitis? **C**—leprosy? **D**—*Ascaris* infection? **E**—chronic septic infection? (22.3)

12. Which of these is NOT a cause of anaemia?

A Lack of the nutrients that the body needs to make haemoglobin **B** Destruction of red cells in the blood **C**

Bleeding outside the body **D** Drinking too much water **E** Not enough red cells being made (22.3)

13. Which of these children is NOT losing iron from his body?

A FERDINAND with malaria. **B** FENELLA with schistosomes in her bladder. **C** FERNANDA with a heavy hookworm infection. **D** FREDERICO with many nose bleeds. (22.3, 23.8)

14. An anaemic child has—

A—too little blood in his blood vessels? **B**—too little haemoglobin in his blood? **C**—too many white cells? **D**—no red cells? **E**—too little protein in his plasma? (22.3)

15. Which of these is NOT true? A young child can get iron deficiency anaemia because—

A—he has bled into a cephalhaematoma? **B**—there is too little iron in his food? **C**—he is destroying iron in his body? **D**—he was given too little iron by his mother while he was in the womb? **E**—he has bled from his umbilicus? (12.4, 26.4)

16. Breast-milk from a healthy mother contains—

A—enough iron for a normal baby? **B**—too much iron? **C**—enough iron for a preterm baby? **D**—enough iron for both these babies? (22.4)

17. Which of these children most needs 'Children's iron mixture', either now or later?

A PRITHNA who has jaundice. **B** JOKO who has sickle-cell anaemia. **C** NIGHTY (7 days) who is preterm. **D** SENKUBA who has malaria. **E** MOWGLI (2 months) who is breast-fed but is given no other food. (22.4)

18. When a severely anaemic child is given the right treatment his haemoglobin rises about one gram—

B—each day? **C**—each month? **D**—each week? (22.4)

19. Bilirubin is made from—

A—broken-down white cells? **B**—broken-down haemoglobin? **C**—food which is not wanted by the body? **D**—dead liver cells? **E**—iron? (22.7)

22. Which of these leaves contains folic acid and vitamin A?

A Pumpkin leaves **B** Cassava leaves **C** Spinach **D** Cabbage leaves **E** All of them (22.6)

21. If you want to see whether a child has jaundice you should look at—

A—his conjunctivae? **B**—his sclerae? **C**—the inside of his lower lip? **D**—his skin? **E**—the palms of his hands? (22.10)

22. Which of these is NOT a symptom of hepatitis?

A Pale stools **B** Vomiting **C** Not eating **D** Jaundice **E** Cough (22.11)

23. Which of these diseases CANNOT be caused by an infection with a dirty syringe?

A Sickle-cell anaemia **B** Septicaemia **C** Tetanus **D** Hepatitis **E** Malaria (22–7)

24. Which of these children is LEAST likely to have sickle-cell anaemia?

A MWAMI with a large spleen. **B** MINGA with mild

jaundice. **C** MUKINGE with a haemoglobin of 15 g/dl. **D** MANGANGO (5 years) with pains in his bones. **E** MWEWA (18 months) with swollen painful fingers. (22.8)

25. JIM'S mother says that the medicine he has been given makes his stools black. What drug does this?

A Tetrachlorethylene **B** Pyrimethazine **C** Piperazine **D** Folic acid **E** Iron (22.4)

URINOGENITAL B
Chapter 23: Code 8

1. WILFRED passes urine about every 20 minutes. He has—

A—incontinence? **B**—dysuria? **C**—haematuria? **D**—frequency? **E**—dyspepsia? (23.1)

2. Infections of the urinary tract are usually caused by—

A—bacteria? **B**—viruses? **C**—fungi? **D**—protozoa? **E**—worms? (23.1)

3. Which of these things would you expect to find in healthy urine?

A Red cells **B** Pus cells **C** Protein **D** Sugar **E** None of them (23.3)

4. Haematuria means—

A—bile in the urine? **B**—haemoglobin in the urine? **C**—red blood cells in the urine? **D**—dark urine? **E**—white cells in the urine? (23.1)

5. JANE has not been well for several days. Today she is passing smoky red urine. She has not had a sore throat for several months, but she has got secondarily infected scabies. This might be causing—

A—schistosomiasis? **B**—acute nephritis? **C**—the nephrotic syndrome? **D**—a urinary infection? **E**—jaundice? (23.7)

6. ABU has 3 pus cells in a microlitre of his urine. This is—

B—normal? **C**—abnormal? (23.2)

7. Passing very little urine, difficulty breathing and fits are danger signs to watch for in a child with—

A—acute nephritis? **B**—kwashiorkor? **C**—a hydrocoele? **D**—a urinary infection? **E**—schistosomiasis? (23.7)

8. Which of these causes mistakes in examining a child's urine?

A Taking only the middle part of the stream. **B** Examining it too soon after it was passed. **C** Leaving the specimen too long before examining it. **D** Drinking water before taking the specimen. **E** Taking the specimen in a sterilized jar. (23.2)

9. What happens to the specimen if you make the mistake in Question 8?

A All the bacteria die. **B** The white cells grow. **C** The white cells are destroyed. **D** Many bacteria grow in the specimen. **E** Both C and D happen. (23.2)

10. LOLOMA-MANYINGA (1 year). His mother says that

the hole in his foreskin is too small. Which of these questions would you say to her?

A 'Is his father circumcised?' **B** 'Does he pass blood in his urine?' **C** 'This is very serious.' **D** 'Does his foreskin swell when he passes urine?' **E** 'He needs penicillin.' (23.11)

11. Whose urine would it be most helpful to examine for pus cells?

A AMBROSE with anaemia. **B** AGUSTIN with vomiting and a stiff neck. **C** AYAR with diarrhoea and dehydration. **D** ADI with a cough and stridor. **E** ADENAN who vomited this morning and has had fever for five days. (23.4)

12. Which of these is the LEAST useful drug for treating urinary infections?

A Penicillin **B** Sulphadimidine **C** Tetracycline **D** Chloramphenicol (23.4)

13. Acute urinary infections should be treated because they—

A—cause severe dehydration? **B**—spread to the peritoneal cavity? **C**—easily cause septicaemia? **D**—may become chronic and destroy the kidneys? **E**—often kill children quickly? (23.4)

PLEASE DO NOT WRITE ON THESE QUESTIONS SOMEONE ELSE MAY NEED THEM

---

14. ANEKA has been treated for a urinary infection. Her symptoms have gone. She—

A—now has a strong natural active immunity? **B**—should be observed carefully because she may get further attacks? **C**—is still infectious? **D**—is more likely to get infections in other parts of her body? **E**—should drink fluid as little as possible? (23.4)

15. A child with an acute urinary infection needs treatment for—

A—3 days? **B**—one week? **C**—at least two weeks? **D**—one year? **E**—two years? (23.4)

16. Which of these symptoms CANNOT be caused by a urinary infection?

A Cough **B** Fever **C** Vomiting **D** Abdominal pain **E** Loin pain (23.4)

17. An increased number of pus cells in the urine is useful for diagnosing—

A—anaemia? **B**—schistosomiasis? **C**—acute nephritis? **D**—the nephrotic syndrome? **E**—urinary infections?

18. PRISCILLA has a normal urine. Which of these diseases could she have?

A The nephrotic syndrome **B** Marasmus **C** Urinary infection **D** Schistosomiasis **E** Acute nephritis (23.7)

19. Which of these diseases sometimes follows about two weeks after a child has had a sore throat?

A Kwashiorkor **B** Urinary infection **C** Acute nephritis **D** The nephrotic syndrome **E** Schistosomiasis (23.7)

20. *Schistosoma haematobium* usually goes into a child through—

A—his lungs? **B**—the water he drinks? **C**—the food he eats? **D**—his skin? **E**—insects which bite him? (23.8)

21. FATIMA (3 years) has a gonoccoccal infection. She was probably infected from—

A—dirty water? **B**—her parents? **C**—sitting on infected soil? **D**—not using a latrine? **E**—other children? (23.10)

22. When you examine a child to see if she has a foreign body in her vagina, you should put a finger into her—

C—urethra? **D**—rectum? **E**—vagina? (23.10)

23. When gonoccocci infect a two-year-old girl they usually cause sepsis in her—

A—vulva and vagina? **B**—vulva? **C**—vagina? **D**—cervix? **E**—Fallopian tubes? (23.10)

24. Which of these is NOT a complication of circumcision?

A Sepsis **B** Septicaemia **C** Meningitis **D** Tetanus **E** Severe bleeding (23.1)

25. Which of these is true?

A Boys have urine infections more often than girls. **B** Babies don't get urine infections. **C** Boys and girls get urine infections equally often. **D** Girls have urine infections more often than boys. (23.4)

NOT WALKING B
Chapter 24: Code 1

1. A child who walks normally and then stops—

A—has a different disease from the child who walks late? **B**—probably has cerebral palsy? **C**—must be backward? **D**—usually has a hereditary disease? **E**—probably has Down's syndrome? (24.1)

2. CHITOKOLOKI's left leg is weak. The best way to see if it is also wasted is to—

B—examine each leg by itself? **C**—compare CHITOKOLOKI with another child of the same age? **D**—pinch CHITOKOLOKI's muscles? **E**—compare his left leg with his right leg? (24.2)

3. XIMENES (16 months) started walking when he was a year old but has not walked for two days. His LEAST likely diagnosis is—

A—an acute infection? **B**—malaria? **C**—cerebral palsy? **D**—an injury during the last few days? **E**—poliomyelitis? (24.1)

4. BASIR (4 years) has begun walking with a limp. This might be caused by—

A—TB of his hip? **B**—Down's syndrome? **C**—cretinism? **D**—cerebral palsy? **E**—some other disease which causes backwardness? (24.1)

5. HOK (3 years) has not walked for the last 3 days. He should be examined for—

A—anaemia? **B**—signs of Down's syndrome?

C—deafness? D—weakness of his legs? E—signs that show he is spastic? (24.2)

6. Which of these causes of a child not walking can be prevented by immunization?

A Down's syndrome B Malnutrition C Osteomyelitis D Polio E Cerebral palsy (24.4)

7. Polio is caused by—

A—lack of the right vitamins? B—bacteria? C—viruses? D—protozoa? E—fits? (24.4)

8. The organisms which cause polio spread in the same way as the organisms which cause—

A—TB? B—diarrhoea? C—malaria? D—anaemia? E—scabies? (24.4)

9. Which of these may help to cause paralysis in a child who has been infected by the polio virus?

A Lack of fluids B Malnutrition C Injections D Resting in bed E Treatment started too late (24.4)

10. Acute polio causes—

A—hypoglycaemia? B—cough? C—wasting? D—contractures? E—tender muscles? (24.4)

11. MASUD (4 years) had severe polio three months ago. His right leg is already thin. He is starting to have difficulty straightening his knee. What would you say to his mother?

A 'It is too late for a splint to help him.' B 'Put his leg through all its movements five times a day.' C 'Keep him sitting down so that his leg does not bend any more.' D 'Disabled children should not go to school.' E 'His leg will recover by itself.' (24.4)

12. BENEDICT (20 months, 37·2 °C) was normal yesterday, but today he will not move his right arm. Otherwise he has no signs. He most probably has—

A—polio? B—TB of his arm bone? C—pyomyositis? D—a minor injury? E—osteomyelitis? (24.7)

13. Wasted muscles are a sign of—

A—Down's syndrome? B—chronic polio? C—acute polio? D—iodine embryopathy? E—backwardness? (24.4)

14. HOEK (2 years) has had a mild fever and has not been well for three days. When he woke this morning he could not move his left leg because it was weak. There is no wasting, and moving his leg doesn't hurt him. He probably has—

A—chronic polio? B—meningitis? C—acute polio? D—cerebral palsy? E—kwashiorkor? (24.4)

15. Contractures in an arm or leg can be prevented by—

A—giving the child special injections? B—keeping it still? C—moving it once a week? D—moving it several times a day? E—letting the child move it as much as he wants to? (24.4)

16. Most backward children have—

A—a disease we cannot diagnose? B—Down's syndrome? C—cerebral palsy? D—chronic polio? E—iodine embryopathy? (24.9)

17. Contractures are LEAST likely to happen in children who have—

A—polio? B—severe burns of their arms and legs? C—had a fracture? D—tuberculoid leprosy? E—severe malnutrition? (24.7)

18. TAN is late starting to walk. This could NOT be caused by—

A—cretinism? B—living in a children's home where nobody talks to him or plays with him? C—pneumonia? D—protein energy malnutrition? E—cerebral palsy? (24.12)

19. Which of these questions would be LEAST helpful in finding out why a child of 21 months has not begun to walk?

A 'Was his birth normal?' B 'Has he ever had an illness with fits?' C 'Is he below the road to health?' D 'Has he got a rash on his feet?' E 'Has he had much diarrhoea or other infections?' (24.10)

20. Which of these backward children has Down's syndrome?

A KEIZO who is cold, constipated, and still. B JOSEF who has one fold on the palms of his hands. C ALY whose mother has goitre. D NOURI who had febrile convulsions lasting 45 minutes. E SABIH who had meningitis which was treated late. (24.13)

21. Penicillin does NOT help—

A—acute septic lymphadenitis? B—cellulitis? C—septic arthritis? D—osteomyelitis? E—polio? (24.4)

22. NGO (2 years) is late walking. When he was born his muscles were hypotonic. As he has got older their tone has increased. His legs now cross one another like a pair of scissors. His arms make slow twisting movements. He may be late walking because his mother—

A—had a difficult labour so that he had a birth injury? B—was over 40 when he was born? C—does not love and play with him? D—does not give him enough protein and energy food? E—lacked iodine during pregnancy? (24.15)

23. Ninety-seven per cent of children are able to walk by the age of—

A—6 months? B—18 months? C—22 months? D—28 months? (24:1)

24. None of these children can walk. Which of them might be helped by a splint now?

A HO with chronic polio. B GO with acute polio. C SO with Down's syndrome. D LO with cretinism. (24–5)

25. Backwardness can be caused by—

A polio? B—bad behaviour? C—meningitis that has been treated too late? D—fluorine deficiency? E—calcium deficiency? (24.12)

SOME OTHER SYMPTOMS B
Chapter 25: with revision: Code 6

1. Which of these diseases can cause a blood-stained discharge from one side of the nose?

A Tetanus **B** Herpes **C** Diphtheria **D** Thrush
E Whooping cough (25.11)

2. Frequent tantrums are a child's way of saying that he
is—
A—unhappy? **B**—not well? **C**—malnourished? **D**—
anaemic? **E**—in pain? (25.2)

3. A baby who only passes a stool once every two or
three days is probably—
C—infected with worms? **D**—malnourished? **E**—normal? (25.1)

MATCH these side effects with the drugs that cause
them.
4. Yellow teeth **5.** Harm to the white cells of the blood
6. A rash, fever, and anaemia **7.** Shock, wheezing,
cyanosis
A Children's cough mixture **B** Tetracycline **C** Chloramphenicol **D** Penicillin **E** Dapsone (3.17, 3.18, 3.24, 3.15
(Revision))

MATCH these presenting symptoms with the worms
that cause them.
8. Vomiting a worm **9.** Anaemia **10.** Itching anus **11.**
Bloody diarrhoea. (21.3, 22.5, 21.5, 21.7, 21.4 (Revision))
A Threadworms **B** *Trichuris* (heavy load) **C** *Taenia*
D *Ascaris* **E** Hookworms

MATCH these diseases with the signs they cause.
12. Cerebral palsy **13.** Down's syndrome **14.** Polio
15. Meningitis
A Hypertonic muscles and 'scissors legs'. **B** Swollen
parotid glands. **C** Paralysis of the diaphragm. **D** Swollen
fontanelle. **E** One fold on the palms of the hands. (24.15,
24.13, 24.4, 23.5 (Revision))

16. Which of these causes diarrhoea WITHOUT blood
in the stools?
A *H. nana* (heavy load) **B** Malnutrition **C** Amoebae
D Severe measles **E** *Trichuris* (heavy load) (9.4, 0.12, 10.6,
21.4, 21.7 (Revision))

17. YOLANDE (3 years, 10 kg). He has a red ulcerated
swelling which came out of his anus two days ago. There
are some small worms on the swelling. His mother needs
to be told all these things EXCEPT—
A 'Let me show you how to push the swelling back
inside him.' **B** 'The swelling will not come back again.'
C 'He is frightened, this injection will make him sleepy
while we put back the swelling.' **D** 'He needs plenty of
protein and energy food.' **E** 'The worms need treating.'
(25.7)

18. Which of these signs needs the most urgent
treatment?
A A respiratory rate of 44 per minute **B** Itchy lesions
between the fingers and on the palms of the hands
C A temperature of 41 °C **D** White, milky lesions on the
tongue and inside the cheeks **E** A weight of 10 kg at the
age of one year (8.9, 11.10, 10.4, 7–1 (Revision))

19. Anal fissures are more likely to be caused by—
A—worms? **B**—scratching? **C**—diarrhoea? **D**—constipation? **E**—eating something hard which has torn the
anus? (25.6a)

20. TALIB (3 years) has been 'clean' for the last year.
During the last week he has been dirtying his trousers
with faeces. Otherwise he has been normal. This is most
probably happening because—
A—there is a ball of hard faeces in his rectum? **B**—he
has diarrhoea? **C**—he has an anal fissure? **D**—he has an
anal fistula? **E**—he has a rectal prolapse? (25.6)

21. CHIAN's nose is bleeding. What would you ask him
to do?
A Put his head back. **B** Keep swallowing. **C** Hold the
soft part of his nose shut with his fingers. **D** Blow his nose
as often as he can. **E** Lie down. (25.10)

22. Which of these drugs can be used to prevent travel
sickness?
A Phenobarbitone **B** Paracetamol **C** Pyrimethamine
D Paraldehyde **E** Promethazine (25.8)

23. A foreign body is most serious if it gets into a
child's—
B—larynx? **C**—ear? **D**—nose? **E**—gut? (25.4)

24. SOETOMO (3 years) has been passing soft stools
mixed with blood and mucus for two weeks. He is mildly
ill and is not dehydrated. He probably has—
A—haemorrhagic disease? **B**—anal fissure? **C**—bacillary dysentery? **D**—amoebic dysentery? **E**—malaria?
(25.7b)

25. Which of these symptoms needs the most urgent
treatment?
A A large spleen **B** Abdominal swelling **C** An umbilical
hernia **D** Inflammation round the umbilicus of a
newborn baby **E** A hydrocoele (25.1, 26.36 (Revision))

NEWBORN BABY B
Chapter 26: First part: Code 5

1. A normal baby one hour old—
B—has floppy arms and legs? **C**—'grunts' when he
breathes? **D**—has a pulse of less than 100? **E**—has a pink
face and body? (26.1)

2. SUNNY (4 months) is bottle-fed. How many feeds a
day would you tell his mother to give him?
A Three **B** Four **C** Five **D** Seven or eight **E** As many
feeds as she wishes (26.15a)

3. The hypochlorite solution used to sterilize a baby's
feeding bottle—
A—must not be diluted? **B**—can be used for several
weeks before it is changed? **C**—should be boiled? **D**—can
be made from ordinary household bleach? **E**—needs to
be changed at each feed? (26.14)

4. A useful way to help prevent anaemia in a newborn
baby is to hold him for a few minutes before his cord is
cut—
A—above his mother? **B**—below his mother? (26.2)

5. If a mother's liquor smells bad her baby should be
given—
B—sulphadimidine? **C**—tetracycline? **D**—chloramphenicol? **E**—penicillin and streptomycin? (26.2)

6. A baby's cord should be tied—
C—as close to his umbilicus as possible? **D**—5 cm from his umbilicus? **E**—10 cm from his umbilicus? (26.2)

7. When you resuscitate a baby mouth-to-mouth you should—
A—blow from your lungs? **B**—blow in and out strongly? **C**—blow 40 times a minute from your cheeks only? **D**—be sure his nose is open? (26.3)

8. Caput (succedaneum) is the name for—
A—the swelling on the part of a baby's head which comes out first during labour? **B**—bleeding under the cover of one of his skull bones? **C**—a change in shape of his skull? **D**—a hard scaly rash on a baby's head? (26.4)

9. ABDUL was born yesterday. When you lower him quickly as if he was being dropped, he reaches out his arms as if he were going to catch something. This is a sign that he—
B—is normal? **C**—has a damaged brain? **D**—is hypoglycaemic? **E**—has tetanus? (26.4)

10. The vernix (grease) which covers a newborn baby should be—
A—left to go by itself? **B**—washed off on the first day of his life? (26.5)

11. A newborn baby should sleep—
A—on his front or side? **B**—on his back? (26.4)

12. Badly-managed bottle feeding may cause—
A—meningitis? **B**—marasmus? **C**—diphtheria? **D**—pharyngitis? **E**—worms? (26.15a)

13. A newborn baby should be put to the breast—
A—after four days? **B**—after 6 hours? **C**—after two days? **D**—after 12 hours? **E**—as soon as possible (26.7)

14. A baby should be breast fed—
A—4 times a day? **B**—5 times a day? **C**—whenever he feels hungry? **D**—in the day only? **E**—every 4 hours exactly? (26.7)

15. If a mother has had to use nipple shields with her first child she will probably—
D—not have to use them again? **E**—have to use them with all her children? (26.9)

16. KABALENGE (1 week) is too weak to suck. Which of these could his mother use to feed him?
A A cotton wick **B** A plastic tube **C** A dropper **D** None of them **E** All of them (26.18)

17. JAMES's mother has had an engorged breast for the last two days. Her temperature is normal and she has no tender swellings in her axilla. What would you tell her?
A 'Let him suck as much milk as possible, then press out the mild that is left like this ...' **B** 'Don't let him suck until the swellings have gone.' **C** 'The milk from your sore breast will not be good for him.' **D** 'Some penicillin injections will help.' **E** 'He must suck less so that less milk will come.' (26.10)

18. What would you say to the mother of a one-month old baby who says that he cries immediately after a bottle-feed?

B 'He is probably not getting enough milk.' **C** 'Start giving him porridge.' **D** 'Let the air out of his stomach like this.' **E** 'Put him to sleep on his back.' (26.14)

19. Which of these is LEAST good for making artificial feeds?
A Full-cream milk powder **B** Sweetened, condensed milk **C** Evaporated milk **D** Fresh cow's milk **E** Goat's milk (26.14)

20. A child is LEAST likely to get diarrhoea if he is fed from—
A—a bottle? **B**—a cup and spoon? **C**—the breast? **D**—a jug? **E**—a cotton wick? (26.7)

21. PETER (2000g) is newborn. He has creases in the skin over his heels. His breasts are about 1 cm in diameter and there is cartilage in his ears. He is—
C—small-for-dates? **D**—preterm? (26.22)

22. Fruit juice is needed by all babies—
A—at the age of 1 month? **B**—at the age of 3 months? **C**—who are breast-fed? **D**—when they start eating porridge? **E**—who are bottle-fed? (26.15a)

23. An 1800 g newborn baby should be given—
A—his first feed when he is about 2 hours old? **B**—iron mixture when he is two days old? **C**—half a mixed vitamin tablet when he is six months old? **D**—four feeds a day? (26.22)

24. During the first few days of life healthy babies—
B—may lose up to 25 per cent of their body weight? **C**—usually gain weight? **D**—may lose up to 10 per cent of their body weight? (26.21)

25. When a newborn baby fails to gain weight after two weeks the first question to ask is—
A Is he given other foods? **B** Is he getting enough milk? **C** Has he got a congenital abnormality? (26.21)

NEWBORN BABY B
Chapter 26: Second part: Code 2

1. Severe jaundice is dangerous because it may harm a baby's—
A—lungs? **B**—liver? **C**—skin? **D**—brain? **E**—heart? (26.23)

2. Physiological (normal) jaundice usually comes—
B—at any time? **C**—on the first day of life? **D**—after the fifth day? **E**—between the second and the fifth day? (26.23)

3. Pyloric stenosis—
A—can be treated by a surgical operation? **B**—causes diarrhoea? **C**—causes fever? **D**—is most common in the first two weeks of life? **E**—can be treated by oral rehydration? (26.27)

4. Which of these is NOT a sign of septicaemia?
A Vomiting **B** Cyanotic attacks **C** Constipation **D** Sucking weakly **E** Fits (26.24)

5. Septicaemia is most common—

A—during the first two days of life? B—during the first month of life? (26.24)

6. SONJIWE (1 week). His mother has infectious TB and is breast-feeding him. Which of these things would you NOT do?

A Treat his mother with isoniazid and streptomycin B Give him BCG and isoniazid now C Give him isoniazid until she is sputum negative D Tell his mother to go on breast feeding him E Put him on the special care register (26.66)

7. MARY JANE brings up a milky fluid and wind after she has fed from the breast. She has no other symptoms and is gaining weight. She is—

D—posseting? E—vomiting? (26.27)

8. MARIE-VERGINE (2 days) has vomited yellow fluid several times since she was born. She has not passed meconium and her abdomen is distended.

A She probably has an obstruction in her gut. B Her diesase is probably not serious. C You can easily treat her yourself. D She needs a purgative. E She has a gut infection. (26.27)

9. A newborn baby needs vitamin K if he vomits—

A—bile? B—faeces? C—blood? D—meconium? E—much fluid? (26.33)

10. Blood-stained vomit is most likely to be serious if it happens—

D—in the first 24 hours? E—after the second day? (26.28)

11. MARY-LOU (3 months) is bottle-fed. Her mother is worried because her stools are very hard. What is the best advice to give her?

A 'Give her a little soft mashed fruit.' B 'Feed her more often.' C 'Give her more water.' D 'Give her this laxative medicine.' E 'Give her sugar.' (26.30)

12. Haemorrhagic disease of the newborn usually causes bleeding—

C—on the first day of life? D—between the second and the fifth day? E—after the fifth day? (26.33)

13. You have examined both these new born children for jaundice. Which of them is most severely jaundiced?

A TOSIN who is jaundiced including his feet? B TAMSIN whose head only is jaundiced? (26.23)

14. Tetanus of the newborn usually presents as—

A—swelling of the fontanelle? B—fits? C—spasms? D—'not sucking'? E—a sticky, septic umbilicus? (26.27)

15. Which of these diseases would you most expect to see during the first two days of life?

A Tetanus B Gonococcal conjunctivitis C Pyloric stenosis D TB E Septicaemia (26.40)

16. CHARLES (7 days) makes sudden movements of parts of his body. He stops breathing for a minute or two, goes blue and his eyes look up to the top of his head. Making a noise or moving him does not bring on these movements. He has—

C—fits? D—the spasms of tetanus? (26.42)

17. Teething can cause—

A—rashes? B—ear rubbing? C—diarrhoea? D—not sucking? E—none of these things? (26.65)

18. ROHINI is 2 days old. His mother says that when he feeds milk comes down his nose. His face looks normal and he has passed meconium. What is his diagnosis?

A Vomiting B Hiatus hernia C A cleft palate D Posseting E Gut obstruction (26.51)

19. Paronychia is the name for—

B—a medicine for fits? C—a fungus infection of the skin? D—a septic infection beside a baby's fingernail? E—a congenital abnormality of a baby's umbilical cord? (26.48)

20. TOMMY is three days old. He was born one week late. His skin is peeling over most of his body. He has—

A—kwashiorkor? B—pellagra? C—a fungus infection? D—eczema? E—none of these things? (26.44)

21. The baby you have just delivered has a small extra finger on his left hand. There is no bone it it. How would you treat it?

A Send him to hospital. B Tie a cotton thread soaked in iodine round it. C Cut it off now. D Cut it off in a month's time. (26.54)

22. EITHNE has not passed any urine since she was born 24 hours ago. This is—

A—normal? B—abnormal? (26.57)

23. STIJN (3 days) passes urine which stains his nappies lightly red-brown. What would you tell his mother? This is—

A—normal and will soon stop? B—caused by acute nephritis? C—caused by schistosomes? D—a congenital abnormality? E—caused by jaundice? (26.58)

24. All these children were injured in some way during birth. Which of them may be helped by their mother doing something special for them?

A AMETHYST with a facial palsy. B PEARL with Erb's palsy. C RUBY with a broken clavicle (collar bone). D SAPPHIRE with a cephalhaematoma. E ONYX with caput (succedanem). (26.61)

25. These children were injured during birth. Which of them should be treated in hospital?

A MANFRED with a broken clavicle. B MANSOOR with Erb's palsy. C MEHITABEL with a broken leg. D MAXIMILIAN with a broken arm. E None of them. (26.63)

SELF EVALUATION MULTIPLE-CHOICE QUESTIONS OF THE 'SICK CHILDREN SERIES', ONE TO EIGHTEEN.

SICK CHILDREN ONE
Code 1

RUDI (2 years, 38·5 °C) has had a cold for a few days. Now he has a dry cough and his nose moves when he breathes. He has severe inspiratory stridor, and gross insuction. He is breathing 50 times a minute. His tonsillar lymph-nodes are mildly enlarged and tender. He has been immunized with DPT vaccine. There is no membrane in his throat. What is probably his diagnosis?

1. A Obstructive laryngitis (croup) **B** Bronchitis **C** Diphtheria **D** Bronchiolitis **E** Asthma

IDA (5 years, 20 kg) has had red, watery eyes for several years. Underneath her upper eyelids there are many small blood-vessels and some small pink lumps. The edges of her corneae are grey and there are some small blood-vessels in them. What is her diagnosis?

2. A Acute conjunctivitis **B** Third-stage trachoma **C** Allergic conjunctivitis **D** Keratomalacia **E** Second-stage trachoma

3. What would you give IDA?

A Procaine penicillin once a day for for three days **B** Sulphadimidine tablets for two weeks **C** Chlortetracycline eye ointment twice a day for five days each month for six months **D** Vitamin A, 100 000 units once a week for three weeks

4. Which of these is most important to tell IDA's mother?

A 'Wash her eyes carefully in the way I am going to show you.' **B** 'Give her plenty of protein food, such as beans.' **C** 'She needs plenty of green vegetables and yellow fruits.' **D** 'She may become blind quickly, so take her to hospital immediately.'

GUSTAVO (13 months, 11 kg) has had ten liquid stools since yesterday morning. He is 'floppy' (hypotonic), his skin elasticity is normal, his eyes are moderately sunken and his mouth is dry. His respirations are 28 and his pulse is 108. He sucks from his feeding-bottle. Which of these would be best for him?

5. A A mixture of neomycin and kaolin **B** Penicillin **C** Salt-and-sugar water in his feeding-bottle **D** Glucose–salt solution in his feeding bottle **E** Tetracycline mixture

IJEBU (53 months, 8 kg) has been brought to the clinic because his left leg is thin. Last year he was ill for a few days with fever and a stiff neck. After the illness his leg was weak, and in the months that followed it became thin. He walks with a stick, his left leg is thinner than his right leg, and he cannot straighten it. He has no skin lesions, thickened nerves, or anaesthesia. Why is his leg thin?

6. A Malnutrition **B** Leprosy **C** Chronic osteomyelitis **D** Polio **E** A complication of meningitis or cerebral malaria

FLORES (37 months, 13 kg, 38·4 °C) cries with pain and rubs her vulva when she passes urine. She passes urine very often and sometimes she wets herself although she used to be 'dry'. She has 'protein + pus cells + + +' in her urine. Her vulva looks normal. Why is passing urine painful for her?

7. A Threadworms **B** Nephritis **C** Urinary infection **D** Stone **E** Nephrotic syndrome

8. Which of these would you give FLORES?

A Penicillin injections **B** Sulphadimidine for at least two weeks **C** Sulphadimidine for three days **D** Chloramphenicol

JEROME (24 hours) passed meconium while he was being born. His mother is worried because he has not passed any more meconium. What are you going to tell her?

9. A 'I am going to pass a rubber tube into his anus to see if it is blocked.' **B** 'Don't let him suck yet.' **C** 'Don't worry, this is normal.'

ENA (7 days, 37·2 °C) vomited three times in the last 24 hours and has passed two watery stools. Her cord has just dropped off. Her umbilicus is sticky and the skin round it is red. She is not sucking. Which of these would best explain all her symptoms?

10. B Gut infection and septic umbilicus **C** Gut infection only **D** Septic umbilicus **E** Septic umbilicus and septicaemia

11. Which of these would you give ENA?

A Penicillin injections **B** Penicillin and streptomycin injections **D** Streptomycin **D** Chlortetracycline ointment on her umbilicus **E** Penicillin ointment on her umbilicus

12. How would you feed ENA?

A From her mother's breast **B** From a bottle **C** From a jug **D** Down a nasogastric tube until she begins to suck

13. What would you give ENA?

A SGM (an infant food made of sugar, dried skim milk, and oil) **B** Expressed breast milk **C** Full-cream dried milk **D** Salt-and-sugar water only **E** Dried skim milk

CHRISTINE (15 months, 9 kg, 38·5 °C) has had fever for three days and vomited once last night. Last week she had a cold. Yesterday she kept rubbing her right ear. Her right ear-drum is red, dull, and swollen. Her ear is not painful when it is moved. Her nose and throat are normal. What is her diagnosis?

14. A Acute otitis media which has perforated **B** Chronic otitis media **C** Acute otitis media **D** Otitis externa **E** Foreign body in her ear

15. Which of these would be best for CHRISTINE?

B Ephedrine nose drops **C** Streptomycin **D** Penicillin and sulphadimidine **E** Penicillin ear drops

Which of these is the MOST PROBABLE complication of CHRISTINE's disease?

16. A Chronic otitis media **B** Septicaemia **C** Otitis externa **D** Mastoiditis **E** Meningitis

HENK (1 day) has broken the upper bone (femur) in his left leg during birth. His skin has not been broken. What are you going to do?

17. B Put his leg in plaster. **C** Put his left leg through its full movements several times a day. **D** Send him for help. **E** Bandage his leg to a simple splint and treat him at home.

ROSARIO (3 years, 18 kg, 37·4 °C). For the last few weeks he has had several yellow liquid stools each day. They are frothy with bubbles of gas and have an abnormal smell. There is no blood in his stools. He is mildly ill and is not dehydrated. Unfortunately your clinic has not got a microscope to examine his stools. What is his probable diagnosis?

18. A Bacillary dysentery **B** Amoebic dysentery **C** Giardiasis **D** The chronic diarrhoea of malnutrition

19. Which of these would be the best treatment for him?

A Sulphaguanidine **B** Chloramphenicol **C** Tetracycline **D** Metronidazole

JURG (2 years, 12 kg, 37·2 °C, Hb 13 g/dl) has had severe diarrhoea for three days and has been treated at home. He is moderately dehydrated and is breathing deeply 50 times a minute. He is not coughing, his nose is not moving, and he has no stridor or insuction. He is too weak to drink. What is his probable diagnosis?

20. A Pneumonia **B** Acidotic breathing **C** Gross anaemia **D** Asthma

21. HASSAN (1 year) is recovering from measles and diarrhoea. He should—

A—be given an antibiotic? **B**—not be given milk? **C**—be given no food except milk until his diarrhoea has stopped? **D**—be given diphenoxylate ('Lomotil')? **E**—be breast-fed often?

22. PRAMILA (5 years, 39·2 °C) has had fever for 3 days. She has mild jaundice and an enlarged spleen. She is not vomiting and has no other symptoms. She comes from a district where the malaria parasites are resistant to chloroquine. Which of these would you give her?

A Sulphadoxine with pyrimethamine **B** Pyrimethamine only **C** Metrifonate **D** Clofazimine **E** Promethazine

ROBIALE (18 months) pulled a pot of hot water over herself last night. The skin of part of her right arm is red. There are blisters on it. She has had three injections of DPT. Her burnt skin is—

23. A—dead? **B**—still alive and able to recover?

24. What would you do?

A Put vaseline gauze on ROBIALE's burn. **B** Give her tetracycline. **C** Send her for help. **D** Put her arm into cold water immediately.

DEMISSIE (6 years). Her mother is worried because her new front teeth are yellow. She had jaundice when she was five and has had many attacks of bronchitis since she was a year old. During these attacks she was given penicillin, chloramphenicol, tetracycline, and sulphadimidine. Which of these could have made her teeth yellow?

25. A Jaundice **B** Penicillin **C** Tetracycline **D** Chloramphenicol **E** Sulphadimidine

---

SICK CHILDREN TWO
Code 2

JON is three days old. His mother has lepromatous leprosy and is being treated. The family are very poor. What would be best for him?

1. B Artificial feeding in another family **C** Going to live with his grandmother in a different house **D** Breast feeding by his mother **E** Artificial feeding by his mother

2. Which of these would you give him?

B Clofazimine **C** Isoniazid **D** Dapsone **E** BCG

KADAR (27 months, 7·5 kg) has had swelling of his ankles for a few days, cough for one week, and mild diarrhoea for two months. He has been brought to the clinic by his grandmother. His mother ran away from his father when he was 9 months old. His father works in a factory a long way from the village and only comes back to visit him sometimes. His grandfather is a farm labourer and only has rice for a short time after the harvest. So KADAR has mostly been fed on sweet tea from a bottle, cassava from the small garden round the house, and green leaves. His arm circumference is 11·3 cm and he does not walk. His skin has some septic scabies lesions only. His eyelids are not swollen and there is no protein in his urine. His diarrhoea is probably caused by—

3. A—the same disease that is making his ankles swell? **B**—dysentery? **C**—too many green leaves? **D**—worms? **E**—lack of vitamins?

He should be examined for signs of lack of—

4. A—vitamin C? **B**—vitamin D? **C**—vitamin A? **D**—iodine? **E**—calcium?

What would KADAR's arm circumference be if he was healthy?

5. A 10—11 cm **B** More than 14 cm **C** 11—12 cm **D** 11—14 cm **E** more than 20 cm

Which of these would you expect to see on KADAR's skin if he is not treated soon?

6. A Urticaria **B** A 'flaking paint rash' **C** A rash of fine macules **D** A petechial rash **E** Some large anaesthetic patches

SIGRID (8 days, 3·5 kg, 37·5 °C). His mother thinks he is not breathing normally. He was born at 41 weeks. His respirations are 40 per minute and irregular. There is no grunting, insuction, or cyanosis. He is sucking well and gaining weight. What is his diagnosis?

7. A 'Ordinary pneumonia' **B** 'Pneumonia of prematurity' **C** Asthma **D** 'Worried mother' **E** Bronchiolitis

TRAN (26 months, 12 kg) cannot walk, and does not say any words. He started to sit up when he was 14 months old. The bridge of his nose is flat. He keeps his mouth open and his tongue sticks out. He has swollen eyelids, and thick dry skin and hair. There is no fold of skin joining his eyelids. There are two creases on the palms of his hands. He is constipated and moves very little. His muscle tone is normal. His mother was 21 when he was born, and labour was normal. He is—

8. A—a cretin? **B**—a child with Down's syndrome? **C**—malnourished? **D**—a backward child we cannot diagnose? **E**—a child with cerebral palsy?

HOPE (1 month, 4 kg) is her mother's first child. She is given nothing except breast milk. The family have a weighing scales at home and weigh her every week. Her mother is worried because she is only gaining about 175 grams each week, and does not pass stools every day. What are you going to say?

9. A 'Hope needs a feeding bottle.' **B** 'You have not got enough milk.' **C** 'She is normal.' **D** 'Give her some rice porridge after she has fed from the breast.' **E** 'She is probably constipated.'

MEAVE (1900 g) was born a few minutes ago. Her mother is well. She is pink, she moves her arms and legs, and she cries loudly. She should be put to the breast—

10. B—after 12 hours? **C**—after 24 hours? **D**—after 2 hours? **E**—now?

AMMON (7 years) scratches his scalp and says it itches. There are small white swellings fixed to the hairs of his head and some very small insects in his scalp. Which of these would you give him?

11. A Gammabenzine hexachloride **B** Benzyl benzoate **C** Penicillin **D** Potassium permanganate soaks **E** Hypochlorite

SCHOLASTICA (2 years) has about 10 small (5 mm), red, itchy, papules on the uncovered parts of her body. Some of them are starting to become yellow in the middle. They are probably—

12. A—urticaria? **B**—ringworm? **C**—varicella (chickenpox)? **D**—insect bites? **E**—scabies?

KEES (1 day) broke the middle of his upper arm (humerus) during birth. His skin is not broken. What are you going to do?

13. A Bandage it to his body. **B** Put his arm in traction. **C** Put him in a plaster splint. **D** Send him for help.

PAISA (9 years) has had some scaly patches on his body for several months. They started as round papules with raised edges. Some of the papules have now healed in the middle and are spreading as curved lines. They are not anaesthetic and they itch occasionally. They are the lesions of—

14. A—scabies? **B**—leprosy? **C**—eczema? **D**—ringworm? **E**—molluscum contagiosum?

MARCHANAH (3 years, 37·2 °C) has had difficulty breathing out for three days. Each time she breathes out she make a wheezing noise. She coughs, is restless, and has a nasal discharge. She breathes 46 times a minute. Her lips are blue. This is her third attack like this during the last year. She has—

15. A—pneumonia? **B**—asthma? **C**—bronchiolitis? **D**—whooping cough? **E**—an upper respiratory infection?

Which of these drugs would help MARCHANAH LEAST?

16. A Ephedrine tablets **B** An adrenaline injection **C** Aspirin tablets

LUPERCIO (6 years) cut the palm of his hand on some broken glass. There is not much bleeding, but he cannot touch the end of his middle finger with his thumb. What would you do?

17. A Stitch him up yourself. **B** Pull the edges of his cut together with adhesive tape. **C** Put on a tourniquet. **D** Put on vaseline gauze and send him home. **E** Send him for help.

DARLENE (3 years, 14 kg, 37 °C) has had some painless swellings in both her groins for several months. They are about the size of a bean and the skin moves easily over them. They do not get bigger when she coughs or cries. When she lies down they do not go away. There are several healing sores on her lower legs, but no other signs. What is causing her swellings?

18. A Acute septic lymphadenitis **B** Hernias **C** Chronic septic lymphadenitis **D** TB lymphadenitis **E** Hydrocoeles

What would you say to her mother?

19. A 'Darlene needs penicillin injections.' **B** 'She needs an operation.' **C** 'I want to make some small cuts in the swellings to let out the pus.' **D** 'She needs no treatment, try to keep her legs clean.' **E** 'These tablets (isoniazid) will help her.'

LWA (18 months, 8 kg) has failed to gain weight for several months. He was given some dried skin milk in the clinic but his mother says this gives him diarrhoea. What are you going to tell her?

20. A 'This kind of milk never causes diarrhoea.' **B** 'Add plenty of water and give it to him in a feeding bottle.' **C** 'It won't cause diarrhoea if you boil it first.' **D** 'He has lactose intolerance, he must not have any kind of milk.' **E** 'Try adding a spoonful of milk to all the porridge you give him.'

ROBIAH (19 months, 37·8 °C) has been coughing for two months. She often wakes the family at night with her cough. She has a purulent nasal discharge and breathes with her mouth open. Her nose is obstructed, and pus drips down the back of her pharynx. Sometimes she has fever. She is not ill. She has been gaining weight normally during the last few months. What is her diagnosis?

21. A Whooping cough **B** Chronic upper respiratory infection **C** Acute pharyngitis **D** Acute tonsillitis **E** TB

Your procaine penicillin is finished, so which ONE of these would you give ROBIAH?

22. A Sulphadimidine tablets **B** Benzyl penicillin once a day **C** Ephedrine tablets **D** Tiabendazole **E** Phenobarbitone

RON (30 months, 11½ kg) has not begun to talk. He makes sounds with his mouth, but does not say any words. He sat up when he was five months old, and started to walk when he was eleven months old. Which of these examinations would be most useful?

23. A Testing his hearing **B** Looking at his ears with an auriscope **C** Examining his throat **D** Looking at his tongue to see if he has tongue tie **E** Testing his sight

JAIME (8 months, 38 °C) has been coughing and wheezing for four days. His lips are blue. He is breathing 58 times a minute and there is insuction. He is sucking weakly. He has—

24. A—an upper respiratory infection? **B**—bronchiolitis? **C**—whooping cough? **D**—asthma? **E**—measles?

You cannot send JAIME to hospital. What would you do?

25. A Give him adrenalin **B** Give him cough mixture **C** Give him ephedrine **D** Give him aminophylline **E** Treat him as if he had pneumonia

---

SICK CHILDREN THREE
Code 3

KAIMU (33 months, 10 kg) has had diarrhoea on many days for several months. Occasionally she has fever, and there is sometimes blood and mucus in her stool. The laboratory report on her stool shows *Ascaris* ova +, hookworm ova +, *Strongyloides* larvae + + + +. The laboratory assistant says he has looked hard and cannot find any amoebae. She should be treated with—

1. A—niclosamide? **B**—TCE (tetrachlorethylene)? **C**—one dose of piperazine? **D**—piperazine every day for a week? **E**—tiabendazole?

UNG (6 years) has many small (5 mm) round hard swellings on his face, neck, and thighs. They have come during the last three weeks. In the middle of each swelling there is dark spot and a small hole. He is otherwise well. He has—

2. A—warts? **B**—boils? **C**—molluscum contagiosum? **D**—herpes? **E**—chickenpox?

3. His lesions are caused by—
A—viruses? **B**—protozoa? **C**—bacteria? **D**—fungi? **E**—insects?

GEMMA (37·2 °C, Hb 10 g/dl) was born last night. This morning her eyes, face, and body are yellow. She probably has—

4. A—sickle-cell anaemia? **B**—physiological or normal jaundice? **C**—septicaemia? **D**—hepatitis? **E**—a serious haemolytic anaemia?

EDDY (7 years) often has mildly red watery eyes, usually at the same time each year. His mother is worried that he may go blind. The only abnormal signs are pinkish grey swellings under his upper eyelids. His corneae are normal and there is no pannus. He probably has—

5. A—second-stage trachoma? **B**—vitamin A deficiency? **C**—gonococcal conjunctivitis? **D**—allergic conjunctivitis? **E**—first-stage trachoma?

WOLF (3 months) has an umbilical hernia. What would you tell his mother?

6. A 'He needs an operation soon, because his hernia might strangulate.' **B** 'It will stop getting bigger if you put plaster over it like this ...' **C** 'It will probably go as he grows older.' **D** 'He needs an operation now.'

VAN (47 months, 15 kg, haemoglobin 4 g/dl) has swollen feet. His face and his tongue and his conjunctivae are very pale. His face, especially his eyelids, and his feet are swollen also. There are 58 hookworm ova and 5 *Ascaris* ova in a standard faecal smear. He has no skin lesions and there is no protein in his urine. His feet are probably swollen because he has—

7. A—the nephrotic syndrome? **B**—hookworm anaemia? **C**—cellulitis? **D**—kwashiorkor? **E**—a heavy load of *Ascaris* worms.

His parents cannot pay for hospital care, so which of these would you give him FIRST?

8. A Penicillin **B** An injection of iron dextran **C** Children's iron medicine **D** TCE **E** Vitamin B tablets

TEMBO (3 years, 13 kg, 36·8 °C) has a warm red 1 cm swelling on the back of his neck. Yesterday the skin in the middle of the swelling became yellow. Today the skin over it broke and pus is coming out. He is 'well' and the redness is becoming less. There is no cellulitis. What would you tell his mother?

9. A 'Remove the organisms in his lesion by squeezing out the pus.' **B** 'A dry dressing is all he needs.' **C** 'We must give him pencillin.' **D** 'Don't wash his lesion, because this will spread organisms over his skin.' **E** 'Chloramphenicol will help him.'

ERASMUS (4 months, 4 kg, 38·4 °C) has been vomiting since yesterday. He has several septic skin lesions on his legs and there is a spreading swelling and redness round one of them. His mouth is dry and he is thirsty. His last two stools have been watery. He is breast-fed and is not sucking well. He probably has—

10. B—skin sepsis only? **C**—skin sepsis and a gut infection? **D**—skin sepsis and septicaemia?

11. ERASMUS needs—
A—a broad spectrum antibiotic and glucose–salt solution? **B**—a broad spectrum antibiotic? **C**—glucose–salt solution? **D**—streptomycin and kaolin?

LEN (4 years, 38·6 °C) has had pain in his abdomen since yesterday and has vomited twice. He has large tonsils with pus on them and large tender tonsillar lymph nodes. His abdomen shows no tenderness, rigidity, or guarding. His spleen is not enlarged, and his blood slide is normal. There are three hookworm ova and one *Ascaris* ovum in a standard stool smear. There is no protein or pus cells in his urine. His abdominal pain is probably caused by—

12. A—an acute abdomen? **B**—*Ascaris* infection? **C**—tonsillitis? **D**—malaria? **E**—a urine infection?

13. LEN needs—

A—an operation in hospital? **B**—piperazine? **C**—chloroquine by mouth? **D**—chloroquine by injection? **E**—procaine penicillin?

MARIJKE was born last week. Her mother is coughing up blood-stained sputum which is AAFB positive. She is being given INH and streptomycin. The family are very poor. MARIJKE should be—

14. A—bottle-fed by her mother? **B**—breast-fed by her mother? **C**—sent to a home for children? **D**—bottle-fed by her aunt?

15. MARIJKE should be given—

A—BCG and isoniazid now? **B**—BCG now and isoniazid when she is six months old? **C**—isoniazid until her mother is sputum negative? **D**—streptomycin and isoniazid for six months? **E**—dapsone only now?

CARLO (10 months, 38 °C) has just had several fits. He has had diarrhoea and vomiting for several days. He is bottle fed. His eyes and his fontanelle are deeply sunken. His mouth is dry and his skin elasticity is severely reduced. His skin, throat, and ears are normal. His blood slide and his CSF are normal. His fits are probably caused by—

16. A—fever? **B**—epilepsy? **C**—meningitis? **D**—hypernatraemic dehydration?

HSU (36 months, 13 kg). His mother is worried because he is not saying any words. He sat up when he was a year old and walked when he was 30 months old. His eyes are far apart, there are folds across the inner ends of his eyebrows and one fold across the palm of each of his hands. His muscles are hypotonic. His tongue sticks out a little. His mother is 42, and he is her 11th child. What is his diagnosis?

17. A Deafness **B** Poliomyelitis **C** Cerebral palsy **D** Down's syndrome **E** Iodine embryopathy

18. What are you going to tell HSU's mother?

A 'I am going to give you some injections which will make him talk.' **B** 'We cannot cure him, but if we teach him carefully we can help him a lot.' **C** 'He needs an operation on his tongue.' **D** Some weeks of hospital treatment may help him.' **E** 'He needs plenty of protein food and vitamin A.'

KEITH is one day old. His breasts are large, and a few drops of milk are coming out of them. What are you going to tell his mother?

19. A 'This is serious, he will have large breasts when he is a man.' **B** 'Squeeze all the milk out of his breasts three times a day.' **C** 'Don't worry, his breasts will be normal in a few weeks.' **D** 'Your milk is causing this. Give him a bottle.'

KHY (3 months, 38 °C) has a sore mouth. There are round yellow–grey ulcers on his tongue and on the mucosa inside his cheeks. His lips are swollen. His mouth does not smell bad and his gums are not bleeding. He is not sucking well. His mother had a cold sore on her lips a few days ago. He has—

20. A—herpes stomatitis? **B**—thrush? **C**—Vincent's stomatitis? **D**—vitamin B deficiency? **E**—cancrum oris?

TOJIB (4 days) has some large (1 cm) vesicles on his skin. The skin around them is red. Some of them are already becoming pustules and crusts. He is sleepy and is not sucking well. He has—

21. A—chickenpox? **B**—milk rash? **C**—smallpox? **D**—boils? **E**—impetigo of the newborn?

22. What are you going to tell TOJIB's mother?

A 'These vesicles will go by themselves in a few days.' **B** 'Don't worry, he will not infect your other children.' **C** 'You must stop breast-feeding.' **D** 'This is a dangerous disease, he needs penicillin.'

LONG (17 months, 8 kg, 38 °C) had left ear pain and fever four months ago. After he had been ill for three days his ear started to discharge. Now his mother is worried because his ear is still discharging. His left ear-drum is abnormally red and there is a perforation in it. Pressing his left mastoid does not hurt him. He has—

23. A—acute otitis media? **B**—external otitis? **C**—mastoiditis? **D**—a foreign body in the ear? **E**—chronic otitis media?

One of these could NOT be a complication of his disease. Which one?

24. A Measles **B** Deafness **C** Meningitis **D** Mastoiditis **E** Tetanus

25. Which of these would you give him?

A Penicillin for 3 days **B** Penicillin and sulphadimidine for 10 days **C** Antibiotic ear drops for two weeks **D** Sulphadimidine for 3 days

SICK CHILDREN FOUR
Code 7

DIMITRI (10 days) has white patches, like little pieces of white cloth, on the inside of his cheeks and on his tongue. He has—

1. A—Vincent's stomatitis? **B**—diphtheria? **C**—milk curds in his mouth? **D**—thrush? **E**—herpes stomatitis?

JUFIE (3 years, 10 kg, 38 °C). Both her eyes are grossly swollen and are discharging pus. She cries when you try to open them, but you can open them enough to see that her conjunctivae are very red. Her eyes started to hurt two days ago. Her grandmother brought her to the health centre yesterday and eye ointment was put into them once. Nobody else in the family has had red eyes. She has—

2. A—allergic conjunctivitis? **B**—acute conjunctivitis?

C—keratomalacia? D—xerophthalmia? E—phlyctenular conjunctivitis?

The most serious cause of her symptoms might be—
3. A—TB bacilli? B—fungi? C—gonococci? D—viruses? E—vitamin A deficiency?

ULLI (4 years) cannot open his mouth. His muscles are stiff and painful. Sometimes they contract so much that his head and body bend backwards. When this happens he does not become unconscious and he cries with pain. He has no skin lesions and no ear discharge? He has—
4. A—tetanus? B—mumps? C—meningitis? D—cerebral malaria? E—febrile convulsions?

His symptoms are caused by—
5. A—a toxoid? B—viruses? C—fungi? D—protozoa? E—a toxin?

FAISAL (3 years). His mother says that every time he has fever pus comes out of his left ear. This first happened a year ago. He probably has—
6. A—impetigo in his ear? B—a foreign body in his ear? C—acute on chronic otitis media? D—external otitis? E—acute otitis media?

OLOF (6 years, 13 kg, haemoglobin 9 g/dl). His mother is worried, because his abdomen has been swollen for several months. Sometimes he has abdominal pains. His spleen is very large and there are very many *Ascaris* ova in his stool. He is thin and mildly anaemic but has no oedema. He has some scabies lesions. His swelling is probably caused by—
7. A—malnutrition only? B—malnutrition, *Ascaris,* and malaria? C—*Ascaris* only? D—malaria, malnutrition, *Ascaris,* and scabies? E—an acute abdomen?

GREET is 3 days old. A few drops of blood are coming from her vagina. What are you going to tell her mother?
8. A 'This is not serious. Her bleeding will stop in a few days.' B 'This injection (vitamin K) will cure her.' C 'She has a tumour in her uterus.' D 'Give her this iron medicine.'

FADJAR (two weeks). Both his breasts are abnormally large. During the last few days his left breast has become red, tender, and painful. Pus is coming from his left nipple. His breast is not yet fluctuant. What are you going to tell his mother?
9. A 'Squeeze the pus out of the abscess in his breast like this ...' B 'He needs an operation.' C 'Put hot compresses on both his breasts.' D 'He needs penicillin injections.'

YOYO (2 months, 4 kg, 37·2 °C) is not sucking well and cries more than usual. His nose is obstructed and discharging. He is wide awake and looking around. His sclerae are normal and his fontanelle is not swollen. His respiratory rate is 44. He has no stridor or insuction. He is not sucking well because he has—
10. A—a cleft palate? B—pneumonia? C—meningitis? D—allergy to breast milk? E—a cold?

What would you tell his mother?
11. A 'Stop breast-feeding him.' B 'Feed him with a bottle.' C 'He needs to be fed with a tube.' D 'He needs penicillin.' E 'Keep his nose clear like this ...'

MOAMMER (22 months, 8 kg). His right eye has been mildly painful and red since yesterday. The redness is most severe close to the cornea. Both his corneae look dry and are not shining normally. There are Bitot's spots in both eyes. When you stain his eyes with fluorescein you can see a green lesion in his right cornea. It is—
12. A—a Bitot's spot? B—pannus? C—a follicle? D—a corneal ulcer? E—a phlycten?

If he is not treated quickly he will—
13. A—get keratomalacia? B—get night blindness? C—get septicaemia? D—get acute conjunctivitis? E—recover by himself?

He needs—
14. A—vitamin A capsules by mouth? B—an injection of water-soluble vitamin A? C—penicillin eye-drops? D—sulphadimidine tablets? E—treatment for TB?

ADE (15 months, 9 kg) has been taken off his mother's back now that his younger brother has been born. He crawls about the family compound. Sometimes he eats earth. Dogs, chickens, and children pass faeces on this earth and everyone spits on it. He is thin and irritable, his abdomen is swollen, and he has abdominal pains. Which of these deseases will he NOT get by eating infected earth?
15. A *Ascaris* infection B *Trichuris* infection C Malaria D TB E Diarrhoea

Which of these diseases will he NOT get by sitting on infected earth?
16. A Measles B Hookworm infection C *Strongyloides* infection D Creeping eruption

SURAH (18 months) swallowed about half a cupful of kerosine an hour ago. She has no symptoms yet. You should—
17. A—wash out her stomach? B—give her ipecacuanha? C—give her procaine penicillin? D—make her vomit by putting a spatula down her throat? E—send her home and tell her mother not to worry about her?

THANOM (6 years) has round smooth swellings on both sides of his face in front of and under his ears. The swelling is larger on the right than on the left. He has had mild fever for three days. Opening his mouth hurts. His throat is normal. Several of his friends have had the same disease. He has—
18. A—mastoiditis? B—goitre? C—lymphadenitis? D—mumps? E—tooth abscesses?

KASIMUN (18 months) has a chronic, symmetrical, dry, red, scaly, itchy rash. It is worse on the front of his elbows and the back of his knees. Sometimes the rash gets worse and becomes wet. He has—
19. A—a heat rash? B—eczema? C—scabies? D—pellagra? E—ringworm?

When he is older he is more likely than other children to get—

20. A—measles? **B**—bronchitis? **C**—whooping cough? **D**—pneumonia? **E**—asthma?

RENE (4 years) has a small (1 cm) tender swelling behind her left ear. It has come in the last few days and can easily be moved over her skull. She has several septic lesions on her scalp. Both her ears are normal and she looks 'well'. She has—

21. A—chronic septic lymphadenitis? **B**—acute septic lymphadenitis? **C**—mumps? **D**—TB lymphadenitis? **E**—mastoiditis?

SONNY (2 years, 37·8 °C) has had mild fever for two days and has passed two liquid stools. His mouth is wet, he is not thirsty, and his skin elasticity is normal. He needs—

22. A—Vibramycin? **B**—'Lomotil'? **C**—an antibiotic mixture? **D**—an antipyretic injection? **E**—none of these things?

LOUISE (3 weeks) has a small ($\frac{1}{2}$ cm), red, wet swelling on her umbilicus which is healing very slowly. What are you going to tell her mother?

23. A 'Keep it clean and dry. It will probably heal slowly. We may have to treat it (cauterise it) later.' **B** 'An injection (vitamin K) will help.' **C** 'She needs penicillin.' **D** 'She has a hernia, but it will go by itself as she grows older.' **E** 'This sulphur ointment will make it heal quickly.'

SUPRATI (2 years) has mildly red watery eyes, a cough and nasal discharge. He has had fever for three days. There are small white spots inside his cheeks. He has—

24. A—bacterial conjunctivitis? **B**—vitamin A deficiency? **C**—measles? **D**—trachoma? **E**—thrush?

OLIPA (14 months, 10·5 kg, 38·5 °C) has had severe bloody diarrhoea for two days. She is breast-fed, but she also has a bottle. She is restless, her skin elasticity is reduced, and her eyes are moderately sunken. Her mouth is dry, and she drinks thirstily. Her blood slide and her ear-drums are normal. There are red cells and pus cells in her stools, but no parasites. Her MOST URGENT need is—

25. A—a penicillin injection? **B**—neomycin suspension? **C**—intravenous fluids? **D**—an amidopyrine injection? **E**—oral rehydration?

SICK CHILDREN FIVE
Code 6

BARNEY (3 years, 38·6 °C) has had fever and a cough for three days. He has a nasal discharge, red watery eyes, and some small white spots on the inside of his cheeks. His nose is not moving and he has no stridor or insuction. His respirations are 40 and you can just feel his spleen. He probably has—

1. A—tonsillitis? **B**—bronchitis? **C**—measles? **D**—bacterial conjunctivitis?

2. Which of these would you give BARNEY?

A Chloroquine **B** Penicillin **C** Measles vaccine **D** Streptomycin **E** Tetracycline

REMO (3 years, 37·2 °C) has had a cough for two days. He has no nasal discharge and his nose is not moving. He has no stridor, or insuction. His ear drums are normal. His throat is abnormally red but his tonsillar lymph nodes are not enlarged. His respirations are 40. He probably has—

3. A—a lower respiratory infection? **B**—tonsillitis? **C**—bronchiolitis? **D**—malaria? **E**—an upper respiratory infection?

4. What are you going to give REMO?

A Chloroquine **B** Nothing or cough mixture **C** Depot penicillin **D** Procaine penicillin **E** Tetracycline

ENELA (10 years) has a sore on the same place on her upper lip whenever she gets a cold or malaria. This starts as a macule and then becomes a papule, a vesicle, and a pustule. She has—

5. A—herpes zoster? **B**—impetigo? **C**—herpes simplex? **D**—molluscum contagiosum? **E**—pyoderma?

6. Her lesions are caused by—

A—protozoa? **B**—insects? **C**—bacteria? **D**—fungi? **E**—viruses?

ZVI (4 years, 39·2 °C, haemoglobin 8 g/dl) has had fever and sweating for four days. He is weak, and you can easily feel his spleen. His respirations are 32. He is not vomiting. His fever is probably caused by—

7. A—typhoid? **B**—a urinary infection? **C**—an upper respiratory infection? **D**—malaria? **E**—anaemia?

8. What are you going to give ZVI?

A Intramuscular chloroquine **B** Chloramphenicol **C** Benzyl penicillin **D** Chloroquine by mouth **E** Procaine penicillin

9. What are you going to tell ZVI's mother?

A 'We must send him to hospital quickly.' **B** 'Put plenty of clothes on him, especially a woolly hat and socks.' **C** 'Give him as little fluid as possible.' **D** 'Don't give him any solid food until his fever has gone.' **E** 'We must cool him with water quickly like this ...'

BENEDICT (2 days) has a swelling in his scrotum. The light from a torch shines through it easily and it does not get larger when he cries. He has—

10. A—a hydrocoele? **B**—an inguinal hernia? **C**—a scrotal abscess? **D**—inguinal lymphadenitis? **E**—phimosis?

What are you going to tell his mother?

11. A 'Swellings of this kind seldom cure themselves. He needs an operation.' **B** 'He needs no treatment because his swelling will probably be gone by the time he is a year old.' **C** 'Some penicillin injections will cure him.' **D** 'Here is some chloramphenicol for him.'

IRAWAN (two years, 38·4 °C) has had fever for 4 days, and a cough for 2 days. Since yesterday he has eaten nothing and vomited twice. He is ill, his throat is red, his tonsils are large, and there is pus on them. His tonsillar lymph nodes are large and tender. He has never had any fits. His fever and cough are caused by—

12. A—tonsillitis? B—diphtheria? C—malaria? D—a lower respiratory infection?

Which of these does he need?

13. A Covering with warm clothes B Vitamin B tablets C Phenobarbitone tablets D Antitoxin E Plenty of fluids and as much food as he will eat.

He should be given—

14. B—benzyl penicillin once a day for three days? C—one injection of depot penicillin (benethamine penicillin)? D—one injection of procaine penicillin? E—chloramphenicol four times a day for 3 days?

The organisms in his throat are LEAST likely to harm his—

15. A—joints? B—heart? C—kidneys? D—liver?

DIDIER (2 years, 38 °C) has had a cough and fever for three days. He has a nasal discharge but no other signs. He has—

16. A—tonsillitis? B—a cold? C—measles? D—a chronic upper respiratory infection? E—whooping cough?

He needs—

17. A—penicillin? B—aspirin? C—tetracycline? D—chloramphenicol?

BABA (2 years) has had severe diarrhoea for four days. Which of these would be LEAST helpful in deciding how to manage him?

18. A 'Has he been vomiting.' B 'Let us see if he can drink.' C 'We must test his urine for protein.' D 'Let me look at his throat.' E 'Let me take his temperature.'

Fortunately, you are able to treat BABA with an oral rehydration fluid. When you send him home his mother should watch for the danger signs of dehydration. Which of these is NOT one of the signs she should watch for?

19. A Vomiting B Not drinking C Diarrhoea becoming worse D Pale urine E Sunken eyes

ELVIS (3.5 years, 39·5 °C) is in coma. He has just had a fit. During the last three days he has had fever and vomiting. He is moderately anaemic and you can just feel his spleen. His CSF is clear and Pandy's test negative. The health centre has no laboratory, so you cannot do any more tests on his CSF, or test his urine, or examine a blood slide. There are a few cases of malaria in the village. There is no chloroquine resistance in the district. He must be treated now for—

20. A—cerebral malaria? B—ordinary malaria? C—meningitis? D—typhoid? E—anaemia?

He needs URGENTLY—

21. A—chloroquine by mouth? B—subcutaneous quinine? C—subcutaneous chloroquine? D—chloramphenicol by injection? E—large doses of benzyl penicillin?

He should he be nursed—

22. D—lying on his back? E—lying on his side or on his front?

He needs—

23. A—fluids by intragastric tube? B—fluids by intravenous drip? C—no fluids until he is conscious and can drink again?

PRIMROSE (4 years, 38·5 °C) has had fever for ten days. She does not eat her food and she does not want to play. Otherwise she has no symptoms. Her throat and her eardrums are normal. You cannot feel her spleen. She has no meningeal signs. There are a few hookworm ova in her stool and 'protein +' and 'pus cells + +' in her urine. She has a few septic scabies lesions. Her blood slide is negative and she is not anaemic. Her fever is caused by—

24. A—her hookworm infection? B—malaria? C—secondarily infected scabies? D—a urinary infection? E—an upper respiratory infection?

She needs—

25. A—sulphadimidine four times a day for three days? B—one injection of benzathine penicillin? C—procaine penicillin daily for two weeks? D—sulphadimidine four times a day for at least two weeks? E—none of these things?

SICK CHILDREN SIX
Code 4

LONG (5 years, 17 kg) wets his bed at night. Until a few weeks ago he was dry at night. His father and mother used to fight, so his mother has now married another man. He has no frequency, dysuria, or fever. There is no protein or pus in his urine. What is his diagnosis?

1. A Urinary infection B Nephritis C Unhappy child D Schistosomiasis E Stone

What would you tell his mother?

2. A 'These injections will help.' B 'Punish him whenever he wets his bed.' C 'Here are some tablets which will cure him.' D 'He needs an operation in hospital.' E 'Be kind to him, punishing will not help.'

EDDY (14 months, 5·5 kg, arm circumference 10 cm) is the son of a school teacher and a laboratory assistant. His mother went off to work in another district and left him with his aunt who does not love him. His ankles are swollen with oedema and the skin is peeling off both his legs. His hair is pale and straight. He is apathetic and will not eat. He has chronic diarrhoea. What is his diagnosis?

3. A Marasmic kwashiorkor B Pellagra C Dysentery D Marasmus E Kwashiorkor

What does he need most?

4. A Penicillin B Protein, energy food, and loving care C More protein food D Vitamin B E Glucose–salt solution?

JIGAL was born last night. His left foot is bent inwards. You can easily bend his foot so that the outer side of his foot touches the outer side of his lower leg. He has—

5. D—true talipes? E—false talipes?

What would you tell his mother?

6. A 'We must tie up his foot with strapping.' B 'His foot will grow normally by itself. He needs no treatment.'

C 'His foot must go into plaster.' D 'He needs hospital treatment.' E 'There was too much water in your uterus.'

RAMON (1 year, 10 kg, 37·0 °C, haemoglobin 13 g/dl) has just started walking. Is he—

7. A—underweight? B—backward? C—feverish? D—normal? E—anaemic?

CARLOS (one week) has a red swelling beside his right thumb nail. He has—

8. A—a congenital malformation? B—haemorrhagic disease of the newborn? C—scabies? D—paronychia? E—impetigo of the newborn?

CYRUS (4 days) has passed some bright blood with his stools. He probably has—

9. A—amoebic dysentery? B—haemorrhagic disease? C—intussusception? D—a prolapsed rectum? E—bacillary dysentery?

He needs—

10. A—vitamin A? B—an operation? C—glucose–salt solution? D—metronidazole? E—vitamin K?

MARY LOU (3·7 kg, 2 days) has mildly red eyes. When she was born drops of 1 per cent silver nitrate were put into them. She has—

11. A—a mild chemical conjunctivitis? B—gonococcal conjunctivitis? C—ophthalmia neonatorum? D—trachoma? E—xerophthalmia?

What are you going to tell MARY LOU's mother?

12. A 'She may have caught this disease from you. You and your husband need treatment.' B 'She may go blind.' C 'This is probably not serious, her eyes will soon recover, but we must watch her carefully.' D 'She needs vitamin A.' E 'She is dangerously infectious.'

ALAIN (5 years, 18 kg) has many attacks of loud crying. He lies on the floor and beats it angrily with his feet (tantrums). His mother and father are clever busy people with good jobs and are away from home most days. They have little time to care for ALAIN, his brother, and his two elder sisters, so they are looked after by servants who do not love them. ALAIN behaves like this because he is—

13. A—backward? B—sick? C—unhappy? D—deaf? E—underweight?

DADANG (1 year, 10 kg, 38·5 °C) has had fever, a cough, and a nasal discharge for four days. His throat, tonsillar lymph-nodes, and ear-drums are normal. His breathing is normal. You can just feel his spleen. There is malaria in the village. He probably has—

14. A—pneumonia? B—measles? C—tonsillitis? D—a cold? E—typhoid fever?

What are you going to give him?

15. A Chloramphenicol B Chloroquine C Procaine penicillin D Depot penicillin E An antihistamine

MAYONDO (4 years) has many hard, smooth, round, solid papules on her skin. They are about 3 mm across. There is a small dark spot in the middle of each papule. At first she only had one or two papules. Now she has many. She has—

16. A—leprosy? B—warts? C—chickenpox? D—herpes zoster? E—molluscum contagiosum?

How are you going to treat them?

17. A Leave them to go by themselves. B Paint them with gentian violet. C Inject penicillin. D Put benzoic acid ointment on them. E Rub them with sulphur ointment.

CORDELL (4 years, 13 kg) has slowly been getting ill for three weeks. At first he would not eat or play. Then he had fever and vomited. Yesterday he had a fit. Today he has a stiff neck and a positive Kernig's sign. He probably has—

18. A—pyogenic meningitis? B—TB meningitis? C—cerebral malaria? D—viral meningitis? E—epilepsy?

ANDREAS (52 months, 38·6 °C) has had a firm tender 3 cm swelling in his left groin for three days. There are several septic lesions on his left leg. The swelling does not get bigger when he coughs, and does not go when he lies down. He has—

19. A—an inguinal hernia? B—a TB lymph-node? C—acute septic lymphadenitis? D—a hydrocoele? E—chronic septic lymphadenitis?

ANNA-MAGDALENA (18 months) is your own little girl and is choking. A sweet has stuck in her throat. She is unable to breathe, and is cyanosed. You should—

20. A—pick her up by the ankles and hit her on her back? B—give her ipecacuanha? C—look down her throat with a torch to see if you can see the sweet? D—try to get out the sweet with your finger? E—put your finger down her throat to make her vomit?

ULA (2 years, 11 kg, 38 °C) has had ten liquid stools since yesterday and has vomited twice this morning. She is very drowsy, her mouth is dry, her skin elasticity is severely reduced, and her eyes are severely sunken. Her pulse is 150 and her respirations are 38. She will not drink. She needs—

21. A—sulphaguanidine? B—chloramphenicol? C—penicillin? D—intravenous Darrow's solution? E—oral glucose–salt solution?

Unfortunately you have not got any of these drugs, or any sterile fluids, so you will have to treat her in some other way. Which of these would be the best for her?

22. A Kaolin and opium mixture B Streptomycin injections C Oral rehydration with salt-and-sugar water D Intragastric rehydration with salt-and-sugar water E Intragastric rehydration with glucose–salt solution

PRISCA was delivered 36 hours ago by a traditional midwife. She now has red swollen eyes which are discharging pus? She probably has—

23. A—mild conjunctivitis? B—dacrocystitis? C—trachoma? D—allergic conjunctivitis? E—gonococcal conjunctivitis? She needs—

24. A—penicillin eye ointment only? B—streptomycin eye ointment? C—silver nitrate eye drops? D—freshly made penicillin eye drops and penicillin injections? E—penicillin injections only?

What would you say to her mother?

25. A 'This disease is not infectious.' B 'You need

treatment also.' C 'All the family need treatment.'
D 'There is no danger of PRISCA going blind.' E 'Both you
and your husband need treatment.'

SICK CHILDREN SEVEN
Code 6

GENE is 24 months old. Yesterday, while she was eating
some groundnuts she started to cough severely. Her lips
became blue and her mother thought she was going to die.
Since then she has had several more severe attacks.
Sometimes there is an hour or more between them.
During these attacks she wheezes and there is severe
insuction. She probably has a groundnut in her—

1. A—larynx? **B**—stomach? **C**—bronchi? **D**—lungs?
E—throat?

She should be—

2. A—sent to hospital quickly? **B**—treated with
antibiotics to prevent infection while the groundnut
dissolves? **C**—made to vomit? **D**—given cough mixture?

ERIK (1 year, 39·4 °C) had two fits during the night. He
has had severe watery diarrhoea and mild fever for three
days. He has only been given a little tea to drink. His eyes
are sunken and his skin elasticity is severely reduced. His
throat and ear drums are normal and he has no meningeal
signs. He will not drink. His fits could be caused by—

3. A—meningitis? **B**—cerebral malaria? **C**—fever?
D—dehydration? **E**—any of these things?

HAN (1 month, 3 kg) has lesions inside his cheeks and
tongue like small pieces of white cloth. They are difficult
to wipe off. He sucks well and has no other signs. His
lesions are caused by—

4. A—diphtheria? **B**—thrush? **C**—Vincent's stomatitis? **D**—herpes stomatitis? **E**—milk curds?

WALTER is 2 days old. His urine stains his nappies a pale
red–brown. What are you going to tell his mother?

5. A 'I must give him an injection of vitamin K.' **B** 'He
has a stone in his bladder.' **C** 'This is normal, his urine will
soon go yellow.' **D** 'He may have a disease of his kidneys.'
E 'Take him to hospital.'

CHING (11 months, 7 kg.) His mother says that he will
not eat solid food and will only suck breast-milk. What
are you going to tell her?

6. A 'Try to make him eat porridge when he is full of
milk after he has fed from the breast.' **B** 'Stop breast-
feeding him so that he will start eating porridge.' **C** 'Go on
breast-feeding him and give him a feeding-bottle also.' **D**
'He needs vitamin-injections.' **E** 'Give him porridge when
he is hungry before he feeds from the breast.'

KHALID (19 months, haemoglobin 13 g, 37·7 °C). His
mother thinks he is not eating enough. He looks well and
has no symptoms. There are three hookworm ova in a
standard stool smear. Last month he weighed 10·5 kg.
Today he weighs 11 kg. What is the diagnosis?

7. A Fever **B** Malnutrition **C** Hookworm anaemia **D**
'Worried mother' **E** TB

SOPHIE (3 weeks, 35·5 °C) has had several liquid stools
during the last few days. She has vomited twice and is
pale, mildly yellow, sleepy and is not sucking well.
Sometimes she goes blue and does not breathe for several
minutes. She probably has—

8. A—anaemia? **B**—lactose intolerance? **C**—a gut
infection? **D**—septicaemia? **E**—tetanus?

AGATHA (6 years) has swallowed a small coin. What are
you going to tell her mother?

9. A 'This is dangerous. Take her to hospital quickly.
She needs an operation.' **B** 'Here is some medicine which
will help the coin to go through her gut quickly.' **C** 'Let
me put a finger down her throat to make her vomit.' **D**
'This ipecacuanha will make her vomit up the coin.' **E**
'Don't worry, it will probably go through her safely. Bring
her back if she has pain or vomiting.'

MARIA (2 years, 7 kg, 38 °C) is thin and small, and lies
frightened in her mother's arms. She has had mild
diarrhoea for several months. During the last three days
her diarrhoea has got worse, so her mother has brought
her to see you. She is restless, her skin elasticity is severely
reduced, and her eyes are moderately sunken. Her
corneae are dry, but not yet ulcerated. Her respirations
are 38, her mouth is dry, and her pulse is 130. She drinks
thirstily, passes little urine, and is not vomiting. What
kind of diarrhoea has she got?

10. A Acute-on-chronic **B** Acute **C** Chronic

Her skin elasticity reduced because of—

11. A—malnutrition only? **B**—dehydration and malnutrition? **C**—dehydration only?

She does NOT need—

12. A—sulphadimidine? **B**—more energy food?
C—oral rehydration? **D**—more protein food? **E**—a
capsule of vitamin A?

VALERIAN (3 days) looks normal, but when he feeds,
milk comes down his nose and he coughs. He—

13. A—has a cleft lip? **B**—is posseting? **C**—is vomiting?
D—has a hiatus hernia? **E**—has a cleft palate?

He is in special danger from—

14. A—gut obstruction? **B**—meningitis? **C**—malnutrition? **D**—diarrhoea?

ISAU (5 years, 14 kg, 37 °C) has had yellow frothy
diarrhoea for several months. His eyes, throat, and ear-
drums are normal. His mouth is wet. He is not thirsty, and
his skin elasticity is normal. His respirations are 25, and
his pulse is 95. There are many *Giardia lamblia* and a four
hookworm ova in a standard stool smear. He is—

15. C—mildly dehydrated? **D**—not dehydrated?
E—moderately dehydrated?

He should be treated with—

16. A—chloramphenicol? **B**—metronidazole? **C**—tetracycline? **D**—tiabendazole?

KEUKY (40 months, 9 kg) started to get a sore mouth

about three weeks ago. He will not eat. His mouth smells bad. There are large grey ulcers on his gums and on the inside of his cheeks. One of these ulcers has spread through to his face and is starting to make a hole in his cheek. He has—

17. A—Vincent's stomatitis? B—cancrum oris? C—thrush? D—herpes stomatitis? E—vitamin B deficiency?

MARCELLO (5 weeks, 3·5 kg). He weighed 3·2 kg when he was born. His mother is worried because he is not growing. She saw an advertisement in the clinic saying that bottle-feeding makes babies grow strong and healthy. So he has been bottle-fed since he was two weeks old. She feeds him six times a day. She adds three level teaspoonfuls of full-cream milk powder to a cupful of water. She sterilizes his bottle in hypochlorite. He is not growing because his mother—

18. A—started bottle feeding too late? B—does not feed him often enough? C—makes his feeds too weak? D—sterilizes his bottle in hypochlorite? E—uses full-cream milk powder?

EMILIO (9 months, 5 kg, 34 °C) has had mild diarrhoea for several months, but during the last few days it has become more severe, and he has vomited twice. He is given a feeding-bottle because his mother thinks that this is the 'modern way'. She is too poor to buy enough milk and she has not got enough time or fuel to sterilize his bottle. She is not giving him porridge. He is drowsy. His skin elasticity is severely reduced, his eyes are severely sunken, and his mouth is dry. He has no skin rash or oedema. His corneae look dry but there are no Bitot's spots. There are no red blood cells or parasites in his stools, his blood slide and his ear-drums are normal. His diarrhoea is—

19. B—acute? C—chronic? D—acute-on-chronic?

EMILIO has NOT got—

20. A—kwashiorkor? B—marasmus? C—hypothermia? D—signs of vitamin A deficiency?

What would you NOT say to his mother?

21. A 'We must give him fluids through a tube into his arm.' B 'When he recovers he should eat plenty of green vegetables.' C 'Bottle-feeding is enough by itself for a child of Emilio's age.' D 'Give him food as soon as he can eat.' E 'We must warm him.'

PANI (4 years, 37·8 °C) has had pain and discharge from his ear for two days. His meatus is red and swollen. His ear-drum is difficult to see but looks normal. His ear hurts when it is moved. He is not deaf and his mastoids are not tender. He has—

22. A—acute otitis media? B—mumps? C—chronic otitis media? D—mastoiditis? E—otitis externa?

Which of these would you give him?

23. A Streptomycin B Penicillin C Ephedrine nose-drops D Antibiotic ear-drops E Promethazine

SASHA is three hours old and does not move one side of her face. She had a difficult birth, and forceps were used.

What are you going to tell her mother?

24. A 'Her face will be paralysed all her life.' B 'Her face will be normal tomorrow.' C 'Move her mouth three times a day to stop it getting a contracture.' D 'Her face will recover in a few weeks.' E 'Let her sleep on her normal side.'

FRANCOIS (35 months, 10 kg, 37·2 °C) has been brought to see you because he has sores at the corners of his lips. The inside of his mouth, tongue and tonsils are normal. He probably has—

25. A—vitamin A deficiency? B—fever? C—thrush? D—vitamin B deficiency? E—Vincent's stomatitis?

SICK CHILDREN EIGHT
Code 4

PETER (2 years, 38·8 °C, haemoglobin 12 g/dl) has been ill with a cough and fever for three days. He is drowsy, and has vomited twice. His neck is stiff, and Kernig's sign is positive. His throat is normal. You cannot feel his spleen. The microscope is broken, so you cannot look at a blood slide. His CSF is clear to look at, but Pandy's test is 'positive + +'. There is falciparum malaria in the district. He probably has—

1. A—upper respiratory infection? B—typhoid? C—meningitis? D—cerebral malaria? E—bronchitis?

GUY (18 months, 38·2 °C) woke up in the night crying and rubbing his ear. This morning he vomited. His throat and tonsillar lymph-nodes are normal. His right ear-drum is swollen, red, and dull. He vomited because he has—

2. A—chronic otitis media? B—otitis externa? C—an ordinary vomiting attack? D—an upper respiratory infection? E—acute otitis media?

3. Which of these would you give him?

A Penicillin and sulphadimidine B Aspirin C Chloramphenicol D Ephedrine nose-drops E Antibiotic ear-drops

JON (7 years). During the last six months a large (3 cm) pale lesion has slowly grown on his left leg. When you touch it with a piece of cotton wool, JON feels nothing. The nerve on the inside of his right elbow (ulnar nerve) is thicker than normal and the muscles of his right hand are thinner than those of his left hand. His face and ears are normal. He probably has—

4. A—borderline leprosy? B—tuberculoid leprosy? C—polio? D—lepromatous leprosy? E—indeterminate leprosy?

5. Which of these special tests could you expect to be positive?

A A skin scraping for AAFB B A skin scraping for fungi C Sputum for AAFB D All of them E None of them

6. What would you start treatment with?

A Isoniazid B Dapsone C Streptomycin and isoniazid D Clofazimine and dapsone E Clofazimine

7. He will need treatment for—

A—a few weeks? **B**—one year? **C**—the rest of his life? **D**—more than two years? **E**—two years only?

KORESI (19 months, 9·5 kg, haemoglobin 9 g/dl) sits quietly in his mother's arms. Pieces of skin are peeling off his lower legs. His ankles are swollen with oedema, his hair is paler than normal, and he is miserable. His face is round and fat. He has—

8. A—the nephrotic syndrome? **B**—pellagra? **C**—marasmus? **D**—kwashiorkor? **E**—leprosy?

SHINTA (36 months, 13 kg, 38·0 °C) has had a cough, and a discharge from her nose for two days. She puts a finger into her throat and says it hurts. Her throat and tonsils are red, but they are not enlarged and there is no membrane. Her tonsillar lymph-nodes are tender. She is 'well' and lives 1 km away in a malarious district. She probably has—

9. A—diphtheria? **B**—an upper respiratory infection? **C**—measles? **D**—herpes stomatitis? **E**—thrush?

10. What would you give her?

A Aspirin and cough mixture **B** Chloramphenicol **C** Tetracycline **D** Sulphadimidine **E** Procaine penicillin

11. If she is not treated, she will probably—

A—recover by herself in a few days? **B**—have these symptoms for a long time? **C**—get worse slowly? **D**—die? **E**—get serious complications?

12. Which of these things would you NOT tell her mother?

A 'Let her eat whatever foods she likes.' **B** 'Don't put too many clothes on her.' **C** 'She has hyperpyrexia, we must cool her with water quickly.' **D** 'Give her plenty of fluids.' **E** 'There is much malaria in the district, she needs chloroquine tablets also.'

JUMBE (4 years, 37·2 °C) has symmetrical dry itchy lesions between his fingers and toes, round his wrists and along the folds of his axillae. Most lesions are papules, but there are some small pustules. His itching is so severe that he cannot sleep. He has—

13. A—impetigo? **B**—ringworm? **C**—scabies? **D**—eczema? **E**—molluscum contagiosum?

14. He should be treated with—

A—potassium permanganate soaks? **B**—gamma-benzene hexachloride not diluted with water? **C**—gentian violet? **D**—benzyl benzoate diluted with water? **E**—benzoic acid ointment?

15. What would you NOT tell his mother?

A 'We must treat his brothers and sisters also.' **B** 'Treatment for one day is enough.' **C** 'When you have put on this medicine don't wash it off until next day.' **D** 'Keep the medicine away from his eyes.' **E** 'Wash all your clothes and blankets.'

CAMILLA (1 month) has vomited once. She has not been well for three days, and is pale and sleepy. Yesterday she sucked weakly. Today she has stopped sucking. Her stools are liquid, and she is mildly jaundiced. This morning she went blue for a few minutes. Her mouth is wet and her skin elasticity is normal. She probably has—

16. A—pneumonia? **B**—bronchitis? **C**—gastroenteritis? **D**—gut obstruction? **E**—septicaemia?

Besides treatment for her disease, she need fluids. How much fluid does she need every day for each kilo she weighs?

17. A 150 ml **B** 250 ml **C** 100 ml **D** 300 ml **E** 75 ml

FULVIO (19 months, 9 kg, 38 °C) is breast-fed. He has had 'hotness of the body' for two days. He will drink fluids, but does want to eat. He has no cough, no diarrhoea, no rash, no urinary symptoms, and no neck stiffness. His throat and ears are normal. His respirations are 48. He does not look ill. There is no malaria in the district. Which of these is probably causing his fever?

18. A Pneumonia **B** Some mild infection we cannot diagnose **C** Tonsillitis **D** Mengingitis **E** Typhoid

He lives near the health centre and has a sensible mother. How would you manage him?

19. A Send him for help. **B** Give him penicillin. **C** Give him paracetamol and ask him to come again tomorrow. **D** Do a lumbar puncture. **E** Give him chloramphenicol.

IMAM (2½ years) has been unconscious for 5 minutes. His arms and legs are moving, his muscles are contracting tightly, and his eyes are looking upwards. His lips are blue and blood is coming from a bite on his tongue. He feels hot. This is the second time that he has had an attack like this today. There is chloroquine-resistant malaria in the district. He needs all these things EXCEPT one immediately. Which one?

20 A Subcutaneous chloroquine **B** Turning him onto his front **C** Putting something between his teeth to stop him biting his tongue again **D** Intravenous quinine **E** Cooling with water

Ten minutes later his arms and legs are still moving. Which ONE of these drugs would you give him?

21. A Phenobarbitone by mouth **B** Penicillin **C** Adrenalin by injection **D** Paraldehyde or phenobarbitone by injection

His movements have now stopped. Which of these things would be LEAST useful?

22. A Lumbar puncture **B** Looking for signs of dehydration **C** A blood slide for malaria parasites **D** Taking his temperature **E** Examining his stools for ova

YAROSLAV (1 day, 1500 g) makes sudden short movements with his arms and legs. He stops breathing for a minute or two, he goes blue, and his eyes look up to the top of his head. He is not sucking and needs an intragastric drip. What would you put down the tube first?

23. A Boiled water **B** His mother's milk **C** Cow's milk **D** Glucose saline **E** 7 per cent glucose solution

HEDA (3 years, 38 °C) has been ill for five days. She has several round, tender, 1 cm swellings under the angles of her jaw. Her tonsils are enlarged and there is pus on them. She has a cough and a sore throat. What is causing her swellings?

24. A Diphtheria **B** Acute lymphangitis **C** Goitre **D** Acute lymphadenitis **E** TB lymphadenitis

KADI (3 years) became ill about a week ago with nasal discharge, fever, and a cough. During the last ten days his cough has got worse. It now comes in spasms and makes him vomit. After a spasm of coughing he makes a loud noise in his throat as he breathes in. Between these coughing attacks his breathing is normal. KADI has a younger brother called PAUL who is four months old. PAUL became ill with cough and fever soon after KADI did. Sometimes PAUL stops breathing for a minute or two, becomes cyanosed, and vomits. Which of these does PAUL need?

25. A Chloroquine **B** Penicillin **C** Cough mixture **D** DPT vaccine **E** Chloramphenicol or tetracycline

---

SICK CHILDREN NINE
Code 4

KEN (10 years) has many 1–2 cm painless skin lesions on his face and body. They have grown slowly for several months. They are paler than his normal skin. Some lesions are flat and other lesions are raised. They do not itch. They are not anaesthetic, and his nerves are not thickened. There are several small nodules on the lobes of his ears. He probably has—

1. A—ringworm? **B**—tinea versicolor? **C**—lepromatous leprosy? **D**—indeterminate leprosy? **E**—tuberculoid leprosy?

Which of these special tests is going to be most useful?
2. B Measuring his haemoglobin **C** Sputum for AAFB **D** A skin scraping for fungi **E** A skin scraping for AAFB

What would you give him?
3. A Dapsone and clofazimine **B** Isoniazid **C** Benzoic acid ointment **D** Vitamin B **E** None of these things

He needs treatment for—
4. A—3 days? **B**—at least ten years? **C**—3 weeks? **D**—at least one year? **E**—3 months?

ARIATI (20 months, 7 kg). His mother is worried because he only says a few words, and he has not yet started to say any sentences. He sat up at five months and walked at 10 months. What are you going to tell her?

5. A 'He has Down's syndrome.' **B** 'I am sorry, he is backward.' **C** 'He is normal.' **D** 'I am sorry, he is deaf.' **E** 'He is not backward, but he is underweight.'

ONG (7 years) has a bleeding nose. What would you say to him?

6. A 'Lie down, we are going to put some ice on your forehead.' **B** 'Sit still, put your head forward, and pinch your nose.' **C** 'I am going to put some of this wet gauze into your nose.' **D** 'Let me see if I can see where the blood is coming from.' **E** 'You need an injection of vitamin K.'

LAMEK (12 years) has many 1–2 cm macules across on the skin of his back and chest. They are many different sizes and shapes. Some are nearly white, others are brown. His lesions are not itchy, or anaesthetic. He probably has—

7. A—ringworm? **B**—herpes zoster? **C**—scabies? **D**—tinea versicolor? **E**—leprosy?

If you looked at a scraping from the lesion with a microscope you would find—
8. A—bacteria? **B**—insects? **C**—viruses? **D**—fungi? **E**—none of these?

ABDUL (3 years) has had a blood-stained discharge from one side of his nose for several days. Otherwise he is well. He has probably got—

9. A—an upper respiratory infection? **B**—a foreign body in his nose? **C**—a cold? **D**—an ordinary nose bleed? **E**—diphtheria?

WONG (5 years, 38 °C) has had about 15 stools since yesterday. At first they were like the stools of ordinary diarrhoea. Now there is no faeces in them. They look like dirty water. His skin is cold and he is comatose. His skin elasticity is much reduced. His eyes are deeply sunken. His mouth is dry and his lips are cyanosed. The last dot on his weight chart was at 20 kg, but today he weighs 17·5 kg. His mother thinks he is going to die. He probably has—

10. A—amoebic dysentery? **B**—giardiasis? **C**—'ordinary diarrhoea'? **D**—bacillary dysentery? **E**—cholera?

Besides intravenous rehydration he needs—
11. A—tetracycline? **B**—sulphadimidine? **C**—penicillin? **D**—streptomycin? **E**—metronidzaole?

NATIMIN (5 years) passes hard stools every two or three days. He has no abdominal swelling, or vomiting. Sometimes he has mild abdominal pain before he passes these hard stools. He never passes blood and his anus is normal. What are you going to tell his mother?

12. A 'give him more water to drink.' **B** 'He probably has worms.' **C** 'Don't worry. Teach him to go to the latrine regularly. Give him more vegetables and fruit.' **D** 'He needs an enema.' **E** 'It is very serious for a child not to pass faeces every day.'

TITUS (5 years, 13 kg). His parents are so poor that maize porridge is almost his only food. He has a symmetrical dark scaly rash, round the lower part of his neck, on the backs of his hands, and on the front of his lower legs. He has—

13. A—eczema? **B**—scabies? **C**—pellagra? **D**—a drug rash? **E**—kwashiorkor?

He needs—
14. A—tiabendazole? **B**—plain ointment? **C**—benzyl benzoate? **D**—vitamin B tablets? **E**—vitamin A capsules?

ADINAS (4 years) has a long (6 cm) thin, itchy, snake-like swelling which is slowly moving up her leg. She has—

15. A—molluscum contagiosum? **B**—creeping eruption? **C**—tapeworms in her skin? **D**—scabies? **E**—lymphangitis?

She needs—
16. A—sulphur ointment? **B**—tetracycline? **C**—gentian violet? **D**—benzyl benzoate? **E**—tiabendazole?

SANCHA (3 weeks, 3·7 kg, 38·0°C) is breathing 104 times a minute. Her lips and fingers are blue. There is grunting and insuction. This morning she will not suck. Pregnancy lasted 39 weeks. She has been well until this illness started two days ago. She has—

17. A—pneumonia? B—asthma? C—bronchitis? D—breathing difficulties because of prematurity? E—septicaemia?

What would you give her?

18. A Streptomycin B Penicillin and streptomycin C Chloramphenicol D Sulphadimidine E Isoniazid

INEZ (4 days, 2·5 kg) will not suck. She has been sleeping in a cot by herself with no blanket. When her temperature is taken with an ordinary thermometer, the mercury does not get to the bottom of the scale. She is her mother's 13th child. Pregnancy lasted 38 weeks. Birth was normal She has—

19. A—a cold? B—septicaemia? C—hypothermia? D—hypoglycaemia? E—hypotonia?

She needs all these things EXCEPT one. Which one?

20. A Chloramphenicol B Warmth C Expressed breast-milk D Penicillin E Streptomycin

TORBEN (3 years, 38·6 °C). His mother says that for four days she has noticed that his body has felt hot. Since yesterday he has not been eating. He has a 'wet' cough, mild stridor, and mild insuction. His nose is not moving. His respirations are 84. His ears and throat are normal. He has—

21. A—tonsillitis? B—diphtheria? C—asthma? D—pneumonia? E—whooping cough?

OSCAR (2 years) has faeces which are hard and painful to pass. During the last two days there has been blood in them. There is a small sore at the side of his anus. He has—

22. A—amoebic dysentery? B—intussusception? C—an anal abscess? D—anal prolapse? E—an anal fissure?

What would you tell his mother?

23. B 'Give him very little food for a few days. He will pass less stools which will let his sore heal.' C 'Here is some benzoic acid ointment to put on his sore.' D 'He needs an operation in hospital.' E 'Give him some of this liquid paraffin. It will keep his stools soft and help his sore to heal.'

DEWI (4 days, 4·2 kg) is her mother's third child. Her first child was normal and is still alive. Soon after the birth of her second child both her nipples became severely cracked and sore. So she stopped breast-feeding and gave the child a bottle. This caused such severe diarrhoea that the child was sent to hospital. After a week in hospital the child died. Now with DEWI her nipples are sore again after only four days' sucking and both her breasts are engorged. All these things would help DEWI and her mother EXCEPT one? Which one?

24. A—using a breast pump? B—using a nipple shield? C—expressing her breast-milk? D—giving DEWI artificial feeds? E—feeding DEWI with a spoon?

HUGO (3 years, 10 kg, 38 °C) has had a painful red swelling on his right leg for several days. During the last two days the swelling has been growing much faster and red lines are spreading up his leg. There are some tender swellings in his right groin. He has NOT got—

25. A—cellulitis? B—acute septic lymphadenitis? C—lymphangitis? D—signs of malnutrition? E—signs of a virus disease?

SICK CHILDREN TEN
Code 7

LEONORA (4 years, 39·2 °C) had fever yesterday and a fit last night. This morning she vomited. Her left ear-drum is red, dull, fixed, and swollen. She has no meningeal signs. There is malaria in the district. She has—

1. A—gastroenteritis? B—cerebral malaria? C—otitis externa? D—acute otitis media? E—meningitis?

2. She needs all these things EXCEPT one. Which one?

A Penicillin and sulphadimidine B Chloramphenicol C Cooling with water D Paracetamol E Chloroquine tablets

MUSA (6 years) has many itchy papules all over his body. The middle of each papule is pale and around it there is a red ring. His mother says he gets a rash like this each time he eats fish. He has—

3. A—pellagra? B—tinea versicolor? C—urticaria? D—molluscum contagiosum? E—miliaria?

SAK (3 years) has a painful discharging left ear. When you have swabbed away some of the pus you can see a small red bead. Which of these would you use FIRST to try to remove the bead from his ear?

4. A An ear syringe B A special hook or bent paper-clip C Forceps D An applicator stick

KOZO (13 months). His mother is worried because she cannot pull back his foreskin. It does not swell up when he passes urine. The urine comes in a good stream. What will you tell her?

5. B 'Pull back his foreskin every day.' C 'He needs a small operation (circumcision).' D 'Put this ointment on it.' E 'Don't worry, his foreskin is normal.'

HEM (20 months, 8 kg, 37·1 °C) has a very sore mouth which smells very bad. There are deep grey ulcers on his gums and the inside of his cheeks. He is breast-fed and is given some other food. His sore mouth is probably caused by—

6. A—herpes stomatitis? B—thrush? C—Vincent's stomatitis? D—diphtheria? E—vitamin B deficiency?

7. What complications would you be most frightened of?

A Pneumonia B Cancrum oris C Tonsillitis D Otitis media E Heart failure

8. What would you NOT tell HEM's mother?

A 'You have breast-fed him for too long.' **B** 'He is not growing, you must feed him often.' **C** 'We must give him penicillin.' **D** 'He needs this mouth wash (hydrogen peroxide).'

HANG (7 years, 36·8 °C) has come to the clinic because he has sores on his face. While you are looking at him you see he has a discharging right ear. His mother says it has been discharging for several years. There is a large perforation in his right ear-drum. His drum and meatus are not inflamed. He has no pain. His right mastoid is not tender. He has—

9. B—otitis externa? **C**—acute otitis media? **D**—chronic otitis media? **E**—mastoiditis?

His ear disease is most probably caused by—

10. A—fungi? **B**—worms? **C**—protozoa? **D**—viruses? **E**—bacteria?

11. At any time he might get any of these complications EXCEPT one. Which one?

A Mastoiditis **B** Meningitis **C** Deafness **D** Tetanus **E** Tonsillitis

12. Which of these vaccines would help to prevent one of these complications?

A Measles **B** BCG **C** Polio **D** DPT

JUANITA is seven months old and weighs 6 kg. When she was six months old she weighed 5·5 kg. When she was five months old she weighed 5 kg. She is given rice and beans after she has fed from the breast. Her growth curve is—

13. A—below the road to health but rising well enough? **B**—on the road to health and rising? **C**—flat? **D**—falling? **E**—Rising too slowly?

14. What are you going to tell her mother?

A 'JUANITA is very well nourished.' **B** 'She is smaller than other children, but she is growing well.' **C** 'She needs artificial feeds.' **D** 'She is seriously underweight and needs hospital treatment.' **E** 'Stop breast-feeding and give her more rice.'

TOFIBA (4½ years, 38·8 °C). She seems to be asleep but her mother cannot wake her up. She has had fever for three days and has been getting more and more drowsy since yesterday morning. You can just feel her spleen. Yesterday she had a fit. The nearest hospital is 10 hours away by horse and cart. Falciparum malaria is common in the district. She has no meningeal signs. She most probably has—

15. A—TB meningitis? **B**—ordinary malaria? **C**—cerebral malaria? **D**—epilepsy? **E**—pyogenic meningitis?

16. TOFIBA does NOT need—

A—promethazine? **B**—a lumbar puncture? **C**—subcutaneous chloroquine? **D**—intravenous fluids? **E**—nursing on her front with her head on one side?

NIRUBA (6 years, 37·2 °C) has fallen down unconscious several times during the last six months. During these attacks her arms and legs shake, and she sometimes bites her tongue. The attacks last a few minutes. Then she wakes up and in a few hours she is completely well again. She has—

17. A—cerebral malaria? **B**—meningitis? **C**—epilepsy? **D**—fainting attacks? **E**—tetanus?

18. These attacks could be prevented by—

A—penicillin? **B**—promethazine? **C**—chloroquine? **D**—phenobarbitone? **E**—paracetamol?

KOAM (5 years, 38·2 °C) has had fever and a cough for about 3 days. He looks very ill. There is a noise in his throat as he breathes, and there is some insuction. His neck is swollen. His throat is sore and he can only swallow with difficulty. His mouth smells bad. There are lesions which look like dirty pieces of grey cloth fixed to his tonsils and pharynx. He probably has—

19. A—tonsillitis? **B**—diphtheria? **C**—pharyngitis? **D**—thrush? **E**—bronchitis?

20. His disease is—

A—caused by viruses? **B**—very common? **C**—not serious? **D**—caused by fungi? **E**—infectious?

21. Which of these complications would you LEAST expect?

A Obstruction of his larynx **B** Mastoiditis **C** Paralysis of his palate **D** Sudden death

22. His disease could have been prevented by—

A—tonsillitis vaccine? **B**—BCG vaccine? **C**—nutrition education? **D**—boiling his drinking water? **E**—DPT vaccine?

MARGOT (14 years) has a smooth painless swelling over the front of the lower part of her neck. Each time she swallows it moves up and down. She has—

23. A—goitre? **B**—septic lymphadenitis? **C**—TB lymphadenitis? **D**—a dangerous tumour? **E**—mumps?

MWIKALI (5 years, 16 kg) has been passing pieces of flat, white worm in her faeces. The longest piece was about 40 cm. They move slowly and are made of many smaller pieces joined together. What kind of worm are they?

24. A *Ascaris* **B** Hookworms **C** *Taenia* **D** *H. nana* **E** *Strongyloides*

She needs—

25. A—tiabendazole? **B**—niridazole? **C**—metrifonate? **D**—metronidazole? **E**—niclosamide?

SICK CHILDREN ELEVEN
Code 7

LOGAWARA (5 years, 38·8 °C) has had fever for 20 days. He has had a few liquid stools during this time, but the rest of the time he has been constipated. He is very 'ill', drowsy, and coughs sometimes. He is anaemic, and you can just feel his spleen. His throat and ear-drums are normal. He has no neck stiffness. His respirations are 48. There are a few ova of *H. nana* in his stool. His blood slide is negative. There is no protein or pus cells in his urine. His fever is probably caused by—

1. A—urinary infection? **B**—*H. nana?* **C**—pneumonia? **D**—typhoid? **E**—malaria?

He needs—

2. **A**—sulphadimidine? **B**—chloramphenicol? **C**—chloroquine? **D**—niclosamide? **E**—pyrimethamine?

ADORA (5 years, 20 kg, 39·6 °C) has had fever and pain in her left leg for four days. She has cried a lot and would not eat or play. For the last two days she has not been able to walk because her leg hurts. The bone below her left knee is tender and painful. Bending her knee makes her cry with pain. She also has severe secondarily infected scabies. She probably has—

3. **A**—TB of the bone? **B**—cellulitis? **C**—acute osteomyelitis? **D**—polio? **E**—pyomyositis?

LATIM (8 months, 9 kg) had diarrhoea. A health worker told his mother to stop breast-feeding. This caused breast engorgement and did not cure the diarrhoea. LATIM is mildly dehydrated. He has stopped breast-feeding but he wants to suck. What would you NOT say to LATIM's mother?

4. **A** 'Give him an artificial feed.' **B** 'Give him glucose–salt solution.' **C** 'Cure the engorgement by letting him suck.' **D** 'Express your breasts like this.' **E** 'Breast-feeding very seldom causes diarrhoea.'

MALINI (4 years, 16 kg) is still breast-fed sometimes. What would you say to her mother?

5. **B** 'She is malnourished.' **C** 'Breast feeding as long as this is bad for her teeth.' **D** 'You must stop.' **E** 'Go on longer if you want to.'

RAMCHANDRAN (4 years, 37·0 °C). Ten days ago he trod on a sharp piece of wood and it went into his foot. A health worker tried to remove the wood, but today RAMCHANDRAN's foot is still tender and swollen. For the last two days he has not been able to open his mouth, and has spasms of his muscles. His inguinal lymph-nodes are normal. Which of these has he NOT got?

6. **A** Signs of a foreign body in his foot **B** Signs of local infection **C** Signs of septicaemia **D** Signs of tetanus **E** A virus disease

PIERIES (4 years, 18 kg). His mother says he is not eating enough. She is a midwife and is always anxious about him. He is taller than other children his age. What would you tell her?

7. **A** 'This iron tonic will help him.' **B** 'Don't worry, forget about his eating.' **C** 'He is malnourished.' **D** 'He needs more vitamins.' **E** 'He needs more protein and energy food.'

KOKOI (20 months, 8·5 kg) is not eating normally and often has mild diarrhoea. He is not dehydrated. He is still breast-fed. What would you NOT say to his mother?

8. **A** 'Breast-feed him and give him a bottle.' **B** 'Try to feed him at least four times a day.' **C** 'Give him plenty of protein and energy food.' **D** 'His growth curve should climb up this chart.' **E** 'He needs your breast milk.'

MAUARKUAR had a fit late last night. His mother said he felt very hot indeed. She cooled him with water. An hour later he had fits again. Only his right arm and the right side of his face moved. His temperature is now 37·8 °C. He needs—

9. **A**—more cooling with water? **B**—paracetamol? **C**—intramuscular chloroquine? **D**—a lumbar puncture? **E**—promethazine?

SANDRA (3 weeks, 36°C) has almost stopped sucking. She is sleepy, she has vomited twice, and passed two watery stools. Two hours ago she had a fit. She is pale and slightly yellow. All this would be explained by a diagnosis of—

10. **A**—jaundice? **B**—febrile convulsions? **C**—septicaemia? **D**—meningitis? **E**—septicaemia or meningitis?

PETER (1 month). His mother is worried because his tongue is tied to the floor of his mouth by a fold of mucosa. She is frightened that he may not be able to speak as he grows older. What are you going to tell her?

11. **C** 'He needs a small operation to cut his tongue from the floor of his mouth.' **D** 'Take him to hospital.' **E** 'Don't worry, he will be able to speak normally.'

AUGUSTIN was delivered by a traditional midwife yesterday. He did not pass any meconium during birth and has not passed any since. What are you going to do first?

12. **B** Give him a drug to make him pass faeces. **C** Send him for help. **D** Look at his anus to see if it is normal. **E** Tell his mother he is normal.

RANYAN (18 months) has been passing watery stools for three days. His eyes are sunken, his skin elasticity is reduced, and his mouth is dry. He is not vomiting. He will drink but he will not eat. He needs—

13. **A**—glucose–salt solution? **B**—papaverin to stop the diarrhoea? **C**—sulphaguanidine tablets? **D**—penicillin injections? **E**—streptomycin injections?

SURINDER (4 months, 6 kg) is breast-fed. His mother is also giving him skimmed milk in a bottle to make him fat. He has had mild diarrhoea for two days, but is not dehydrated. What would you tell her?

14. **A** 'Stop breast-feeding him and give him the bottle only.' **B** 'Stop giving him the bottle but go on breast-feeding.' **C** 'Stop breast-feeding him until his diarrhoea has stopped.' **D** 'Here are some sulphadimidine tablets for him.' **E** 'Give him this medicine (neomycin suspension).'

TARUN (4 years, 40 °C) has just had a rigor during which he felt very cold. This has now stopped and he feels warmer. You have taken his temperature. What would you do FIRST?

15. **A** Wrap him in warm clothes. **B** Give him an injection to lower his fever. **C** Cool him with water. **D** Inject penicillin. **E** Examine his throat.

JAN (2 weeks) has a round swelling in his scrotum which makes one testicle look larger than the other. When light from a torch shines through the swelling his testicle makes a shadow at one side of it. The swelling does not get larger when he coughs or cries. You cannot push it back into his abdomen. He has—

16. A—a hydrocoele? B—lymphadenitis? C—TB lymph nodes? D—an inguinal hernia? E—an umbilical hernia?

WAHEED (14 months) has had fever for two days. Since this morning he will not eat, and has vomited once. His throat is red, but his tonsillar lymph nodes are normal. His left ear-drum is red, dull, and swollen. He is irritable and restless and fights when he is examined. He has—

17. A—chronic otitis media? B—otitis externa? C—acute otitis media? D—tonsillitis? E—mastoiditis?

He needs—

18. A—chloramphenicol? B—sulphaguanidine? C—tetracycline? D—penicillin and sulphadimidine? E—ephedrine tablets?

SUWOTO (20 months, 7 kg) has always been below the road to health. Two months ago he was very ill with a severe cough for five days. He has been moderately ill with a cough since that time. He has not been eating normally and he now weighs one kilo less than he did two months ago. He is thin but his ankles are not swollen. He is still breast-fed. His father is only a labourer but the family always have enough rice. They grow soya beans and sell them so that they have money to buy a little tahu (a food made from soya beans) all the year. SUWOTO shows signs and symptoms of—

19. A—malnutrition? B—malnutrition and infection? C—infection?

Which of these diseases would you look for?

20 Measles B Whooping cough C Asthma D Bronchitis E TB

ZUL (3 months) is wearing a woolly cap and socks, a jersey and a shirt. He is also wearing an 'oto' (a special cloth Javanese children wear). He is wrapped in a blanket. These cover a rash of many small (1 mm) papules and vesicles. Some of them have become secondarily infected. He has—

21. A—eczema? B—a heat rash? C—urticaria? D—measles? E—a drug rash?

ANATOLE (5 years, 19 kg, 38·2 °C) has fever and will not eat. A week ago he cut his foot. The skin round the cut is swollen, red, and tender. A thick yellow discharge is coming from it. There are tender swellings in his groin. Moving his leg is painful. He has—

22 A—TB arthritis? B—tetanus? C—lymphangitis? D—osteomyelitis? E—cellulitis and acute septic lymphadenitis?

He needs—

23. A—procaine penicillin daily for at least three days? B—benzathine penicillin once daily for three days? C—isoniazid (INH) for a year? D—one injection of procaine pencillin? E—streptomycin once daily for three days?

Which of these vaccines could prevent a serious complication of his cut foot?

24. A BCG B Measles C DPT D Polio

DEWI (2 years, 38·9 °C) has had fever for two days. She does not want to eat. She has no other symptoms. Where would you be most likely to find the cause of her fever? In her—

25. A—meninges? B—abdomen? C—urinary tract? D—lungs? E—throat?

SICK CHILDREN TWELVE
Code 2

INDRAN (2 months, 4 kg) was born after a 34 week pregnancy and weighed 1·5 kg. His lips and conjunctivae are pale, but he looks well and is feeding well. His anaemia is probably caused by—

1. A—malaria? B—hookworms? C—folic acid deficiency? D—iron deficiency? E—PEM?

LEOPOLD (4 years, 38·5 °C) has fever, rigors, anaemia, and a large spleen. He is drowsy, he vomits, and has had one fit. The malaria parasites in his district are resistant to chloroquine. Which of these would you give him?

2. A Intravenous chloroquine B Intramuscular sulphadoxine with pyrimethamine C Intravenous pyrimethamine D Sulphadoxine with pyrimethamine by mouth E Intravenous quinine

DOMINIC (18 months, 12 kg, 37·2 °C) would not eat his supper. Soon after he went to bed he started crying. His mother went into his room and found he had vomited. He passed several liquid stools during the afternoon. He is pale and sweating. He has no signs of dehydration, and no abdominal tenderness, rigidity, or guarding. His throat and ears are normal. He is thirsty, but when he is given fluid he vomits. He has never had any attacks like this before. What is his probable diagnosis?

3. A A mild gut infection B Posseting C Meningitis D Cerebral malaria E Acute abdomen

What are you going to do?

4. A Give him an intravenous drip. B Send him to hospital. C Give him glucose–salt solution. D Give him 'Lomotil' (diphenoxylate). E Give him penicillin.

KISWAR (one year) has had mild diarrhoea with blood in it for two weeks. He has not had fever. He drinks and is not dehydrated. He probably has—

5. A—bacillary dysentery? B—amoebic dysentery? C—cholera? D—'Ordinary diarrhoea'? E—giardiasis?

He needs—

6. A—papaverine injections? B—metronidazole? C—sulphaguanidine? D—glucose saline? E—tea only?

KENJI (52 months, 11 kg, 37·3 °C) has had a pain in his left hip for several weeks and has now started to limp. He cannot move his leg normally. His left leg is getting thin. He is mildly 'ill', and sometimes has mild fever. He has not been given BCG. He probably has—

7. A—an acute septic arthritis? B—polio? C—osteomyelitis? D—TB arthritis?

What are you NOT going to say to his mother?

8. A 'Three weeks treatment will cure him.' **B** 'We are going to put him on our special care register.' **C** 'He needs an X-ray of his hip.' **D** 'He needs tablets and injections for a long time.' **E** 'Has anyone in your family got a cough?'

BIMLA (1900 g) was born a few minutes ago. She is pink, she moves her arms and legs and she cries loudly. There is cartilage in her ear, and creases (folds) across the palms of her hands. Her breasts are more than 5 mm in diameter. She is—

9. C—small for dates? **D**—preterm?

CHARITY (6 weeks, 3·5 kg). Her growth curve has been flat for a month. Her mother saw an advertisement which said that bottle feeding is best for modern babies. Since then she has been giving CHARITY milk from a bottle. CHARITY's father is a night watchman and she has four elder brothers and two elder sisters. A half-kilo tin of full cream milk lasts about two weeks. Which of these does NOT harm her nutrition and help to make her weight curve flat?

10. A Her bottle is not sterilized properly. **B** She has half a kilo of full-cream milk in two weeks. **C** She often has diarrhoea. **D** She has three feeds a day. **E** She is fed with full-cream milk.

MOMANYI (36 months, 13 kg, 39·5 °C). Yesterday he said his abdomen hurt. Today he still has pain. He vomited ten minutes ago and passed one loose stool. His spleen is moderately enlarged and there are 'malaria parasites + + +' in his blood slide. He has no abdominal tenderness, rigidity, or guarding. He is moderately anaemic. There are three hookworm ova in a standard stool smear. There is no protein or pus in his urine. His pain is probably caused by—

11. A—malaria? **B**—hookworm anaemia? **C**—dysentery? **D**—an acute abdomen? **E**—urine infection?

TED (5 years, 18 kg) has been brought to the clinic because his left leg is thin and weak. Last year he was ill for a few days with fever and a stiff neck. After the illness his leg was weak. During the months that followed it became thin. He walks with a stick. He cannot straighten his knee. He has no skin lesions, no pain, no thickened nerves, and no anaesthesia. He probably has—

12. A—TB of his leg? **B**—a complication of meningitis or cerebral malaria? **C**—leprosy? **D**—polio? **E**—chronic osteomyelitis?

DHANUSHAN (21 months, 9·5 kg, 36·5 °C, haemoglobin 8 g/dl). His mother is begging in the street while he lies quietly on a pile of rags. His feet are swollen and pieces of skin are coming off his legs. He is mildly anaemic, he has some septic skin lesions and Bitot's spots in both eyes. His corneae are mildly dry but are otherwise normal. You can just feel the edge of his liver. You ask his mother if she will bring him to your clinic. He has—

13. A—kwashiorkor? **B**—the nephrotic syndrome? **C**—marasmus? **D**—pellagra? **E**—keratomalacia?

What treatment does he need MOST?

14. A Penicillin injections **B** An injection of vitamin B **C** Children's iron mixture **D** More food, especially more protein and energy food and vitamin A **E** Ointment for his skin

PURA (10 days, 36·4 °C) has stopped sucking from the breast. He has stopped crying and he cannot open his mouth. His muscles are hypertonic and his head and neck are bent backwards. His umbilicus is sticky, and his respirations are 52 per minute. He has stopped sucking because he has—

15. A—septicaemia? **B**—tetanus? **C**—hypothermia? **D**—pneumonia? **E**—hypoglycaemia?

His disease could have been prevented by—

16. A—immunizing him with DPT? **B**—giving him penicillin? **C**—immunizing his mother? **D**—keeping him warm? **E**—giving him glucose?

MIGUEL (4 years, 15 kg). Two days ago his eyes and skin went yellow. He has had a mild fever for several days and has eaten no food. For the last 2 days his urine has been dark and his stools pale. His spleen is not enlarged and he is not anaemic. When his urine is shaken the froth is yellow. He has had all his immunizations. During the last six months he has also been given treatment for tonsillitis and a discharging ear. He was given pencillin, aspirin, and cough mixture but no other drugs. He probably has—

17. B—malaria? **C**—sickle-cell anaemia? **D**—jaundice caused by drugs? **E**—hepatitis?

CLARA (3 years) screams when she passes urine. She has sore vulva and pus is coming from her vagina. When you put your little finger carefully into her rectum you can feel that there is something hard in her vagina. Her symptoms are probably caused by—

18. A—vulvovaginitis? **B**—a bladder stone? **C**—a foreign body? **D**—a urinary infection? **E**—threadworms?

PIERRE (13 months). His mother thinks his foreskin is too tight because it cannot be pulled back over his penis. His urine comes out drop by drop and makes his foreskin swell. What are you going to tell her?

19. B 'This is normal. The hole in his foreskin will soon get larger.' **C** 'Try to pull back his foreskin every day.' **D** 'He needs a small operation (circumcision) to let the urine come out faster.'

OLUCHIRI (42 months, 13 kg, haemoglobin 9 g/dl) has been having pains in his abdomen for several months. He is thin and has some septic skin lesions. There are a few painless bean-shaped swellings in his groins. He has no abdominal tenderness, rigidity, or guarding. His spleen is not enlarged. There are 43 *Ascaris* ova and 3 hookworm ova in a standard stool smear. What would you tell his mother?

20. A 'Take him to hospital, he needs an operation.' **B** 'He needs some injections (procaine penicillin).' **C** 'Here is a dose of medicine (TCE) for him.' **D** 'His pains will soon go by themselves.' E 'These tablets (piperazine) will soon cure him.'

INGE (3 days) was born at home. Her mother is worried because there are a few drops of blood on her clothes which have came from INGE's umbilicus. Otherwise she is well. What would you say to her mother?

21. A 'Send her to hospital quickly because she may bleed more and need a blood transfusion.' **B** 'This is probably not serious, but I am going to give her some vitamin K.' **C** 'I am going to give her some tetanus antitoxin.' **D** 'She needs a penicillin injection.' **E** 'Put a dry dressing on her umbilicus.'

LATIF is three days old. His skin is peeling, but otherwise he is well. What are you going to tell his mother?

22. A 'His peeling is not serious and will soon stop.' **B** 'Here is some gentian violet for his skin.' **C** 'He is infectious, so keep him away from other babies.' **D** 'He is allergic to your milk. Give him cow's milk from a bottle.' **E** 'Peeling is a sign he was malnourished while he was in the uterus.'

DIDI (6 years, 38·2 °C) has had a discharge of thin pus and blood from the left side of her nose for three days. Her nose is sore and she is not well. Her throat is normal. There are no signs of a foreign body. Her discharge might be caused by—

23. A—nasal diphtheria? **B**—an ordinary upper respiratory infection? **C**—a nosebleed? **D**—herpes? **E**—cancrum oris?

CHIPA (3 years, 12 kg, 38·2 °C) has had many septic crusted lesions on her face and scalp for about a week. Some of them are discharging pus. She has swollen tender lymph nodes in her neck, but no other signs. She is irritable and restless. She has NOT got—

24. A—the general signs of a septic infection? **B**—hyperpyrexia? **C**—lymphadenitis? **D**—a bacterial infection? **E**—the local signs of a septic infection?

If you could only give her one dose of penicillin, which of these would you give her?

25. A Benzyl penicillin **B** Procaine penicillin (PAM) **C** Procaine penicillin forte (PPF) **D** Oral penicillin tablets **E** Fortified benethamine or benzathine penicillin

SICK CHILDREN THIRTEEN
Code 7

AGOSTIN (4 years, 38·8 °C) has had a painful swelling on his thigh for four days. The swelling is in his skin not in his muscles. It is warm and red, and this morning its middle has become yellow and fluctuant. He is ill, and there are some tender swellings in his groin. The swelling is caused by—

1. A—TB? **B**—injury? **C**—osteomyelitis? **D**—acute septic infection? **E**—pyomyositis?

Inside the swelling there are—

2. A—protozoa? **B**—pyogenic bacteria? **C**—viruses? **D**—AAFB? **E**—none of these things?

From what you have read do you think AGOSTIN has—

3. A—lymphangitis? **B**—chronic septic lymphadenitis? **C**—acute septic lymphadenitis? **D**—an infected fracture? **E**—TB lymphadenitis?

Which of these is the most dangerous complication that AGOSTIN might get?

4. A Septicaemia **B** Abscesses in other parts of his body **C** Tetanus **D** Deformity of his thigh **E** Miliary TB

CHERONO (18 months, 8 kg, haemoglobin 8 g/dl) has had diarrhoea and vomiting for one week. She is moderately dehydrated. She has vomited some round white worms about 10 cm long. Which of these would you give her FIRST?

5. A Piperazine **B** Plenty of protein and energy food **C** Tiabendazole **D** An injection of iron dextran. **E** Salt-and-sugar water

NGUGEM (5 years, haemoglobin 13 g/dl) has yellow eyes. He has eaten very little food for about a week and has vomited twice. His urine is dark like tea and his stools are pale. You cannot feel his spleen, and his blood slide is negative. He had one injection of pencillin and some sulphadimidine about a year ago. Several other people in his village have had the same kind of illness during the last few months. He probably has—

6. A—malaria? **B**—syringe jaundice? **C**—infectious hepatitis? **D**—sickle-cell anaemia? **E**—septicaemia?

He was probably infected by—

7. A—an insect? **B**—a virus from another person's gut? **C**—a dirty syringe or needle? **D**—his parents before he was born? **E**—bacteria that can easily be killed by penicillin?

BIKOMBO (3 years, 37·6 °C, haemoglobin 14 g/dl) has a mild cough for three days with a nasal discharge. Her respirations are 36 and there is no insuction. She should be given—

8. A—cough mixture? **B**—penicillin? **C**—amidopyrine? **D**—tetracycline? **E**—children's iron mixture?

ATIENO (2½ years, 16 kg) has been scratching her anus and vulva at night. There is no discharge from her vagina. She probably needs treatment with—

9. A—one dose of piperazine? **B**—tiabendazole for a week? **C**—penicillin? **D**—piperazine for several days? **E**—niclosamide?

MAO (18 months, 7 kg, 37 °C) stopped walking a month ago. He started to walk when he was a year old but three months ago his mother died, so he went to live with his aunt who has five children of her own. He is thin, miserable, and is not eating well. He has no skin lesions and no oedema. He stopped walking because he—

10. A—has an acute infection? **B**—has TB? **C**—has polio? **D**—has kwashiorkor? **E**—is malnourished, and not loved?

What would you tell his aunt?

11. A 'I am sorry, but he will never walk again.' **B** 'Some penicillin injections will make him walk.' **C** 'If he takes these tablets (isoniazid) for a year, he will start walking again.' **D** 'Immunization would have prevented this.' **E** 'He will start walking again when he is loved and wanted and his growth curve starts climbing up his weight chart.'

HILDEGARD (2 days, 2 kg). Her hands and feet are cold, blue, and swollen. The fat under them feels hard. Blood is coming out of her mouth. Her parents have little money and many children. When you take her temperature the mercury does not go up into the scale of the thermometer. She has—

12. **A**—haemorrhagic disease? **B**—TB? **C**—hyponatraemia? **D**—hypothermia? **E**—kwashiorkor?

BICOME (7 years) has had several hard, rough, painless thickenings about 3 mm across on the skin of her hands for several months. They don't itch, they are not anaesthetic and she is not worried by them. She has no lesions in other parts of her body and no other signs. She has—

13. **A**—warts? **B**—leprosy? **C**—scabies? **D**—molluscum contagiosum? **E**—urticaria?

What would you tell her mother?

14. A 'I am going to scrape them out with a needle and put iodine on them.' **B** 'Her hands will recover by themselves in a few months.' **C** 'She needs three penicillin injections.' **D** 'Paint this medicine (benzyl benzoate) on them.'

GUILLAUME (3 years, 14 kg, 39·6 °C) has had a cough and a sore throat for two days. Yesterday he ate very little food and passed a few liquid stools. This morning he vomited. He has a red throat and enlarged tonsils with yellow pus on them. His tonsillar lymph-nodes are enlarged and tender. His ear-drums are normal. His vomiting and diarrhoea were probably caused by—

15. **A**—infected water? **B**—infected food? **C**—the same disease that is causing his other symptoms? **D**—an infection of the lower part of his gut? **E**—fever?

Which of these complications is he LEAST likely to get?

16. **A** Meningitis **B** Acute nephritis **C** Acute otitis media **D** Febrile convulsions **E** Loss of weight

He needs—

17. **A**—promethazine twice daily? **B**—chloramphenicol four times a day? **C**— one injection of 'depot' (benzathine) penicillin? **D**—benzyl penicillin once a day for 3 days? **E**—one injection of procaine penicillin?

NYABOKE (34 months, 9 kg, 38·7 °C) has had fever and abdominal pain for three days. During this time she has not passed any stools. She has not been 'well' for about ten days. She has no abnormal signs except some scabies lesions and a few painless bean-shaped swellings in both her groins. Her throat is normal and her abdomen is not tender. There is 'protein +' and 'pus cells + + +' in her urine. She needs most urgently—

18. **A**—penicillin for five days? **B**—more protein food? **C**—medicine to make her pass faeces? **D**—sulphadimidine for two weeks? **E**—an operation in hospital?

EJNAR (26 months, 7 kg) has oedema of the ankles, and a 'flaking paint rash.' He is also very drowsy. He cries when you try to bend his head forwards. The FIRST thing he needs is—

19. **A**—penicillin? **B**—a lumbar puncture? **C**—paraldehyde? **D**—an injection of B vitamins? **E**—more protein and energy food?

ALPHONSE (7 days) has a swelling beside the inner end of his right eye, which is always discharging tears. When the swelling is gently pressed a yellow substance comes out of a small hole in his lower eyelid. What are you going to tell his mother?

20. **A** 'He will need a small operation.' **B** 'He may have caught this disease from you.' **C** 'He needs penicillin injections.' **D** 'He will become blind if he is not treated properly.' **E** 'The swelling and the tears will go in a few weeks. Gently press the swelling like this …'

SAUD (22 months, 10 kg, 37·1 °C, haemoglobin 9 g/dl) has been brought to the clinic because he is not eating. His ankles are swollen with oedema. His hair is pale and he is mildly anaemic. He has had mild diarrhoea without blood in his stools for several weeks. He has two hookworm ova in a standard stool smear. There is no protein in his urine. Two months ago he weighed 11 kg and three months ago 12 kg. He has—

21. **A**—the nephrotic syndrome? **B**—kwashiorkor? **C**—hookworm anaemia? **D**—amoebiasis? **E**—a urine infection?

CLARICE (3 years, 38 °C) has not eaten normally for two weeks. She has a cough and her right ear-drum is red. Her respirations are 50 per minute and she has mild insuction. She needs—

22. **A**—chloramphenicol? **B**—cough mixture? **C**—streptomycin? **D**—isoniazid? **E**—penicillin?

MARTINUS (1 month, 4 kg, 37·2 °C) has been vomiting milk after each feed for the last week. He is mildly dehydrated. He is very active but is not gaining weight. He seems hungry and his stools are hard. He should be examined to see if he has—

23. **A**—a finger-shaped mass in his abdomen? **B**—meningitis? **C**—a large liver? **D**—a blocked anus? **E**—an infected throat and tonsillar lymphadenitis?

ART (3 years, 13 kg, 37·2 °C) has had a cough and a nasal discharge for five days. His tonsils are not enlarged and there is no pus on them. His ear-drums and his tonsillar lymph nodes are normal. He has—

24. **A**—tonsillitis? **B**—an acute lower respiratory infection? **C**—a cold? **D**—a chronic upper respiratory infection?

He should be given—

25. **A**—penicillin? **B**—tetracycline? **C**—chloramphenicol? **D**—streptomycin? **E**—an aspirin?

SICK CHILDREN FOURTEEN
Code 2

PARVEEN (3 years, 11 kg, 38·0 °C) has not been well for several weeks. She has not been eating normally, and has had mild fever. Yesterday she vomited and this morning she had a fit. She is drowsy. She has a stiff neck but Kernig's sign is negative. Her grandmother has a chronic cough with blood in her sputum. PARVEEN probably has—

1. A—cerebral malaria? B—febrile convulsions? C—a urine infection? D—TB meningitis? E—purulent meningitis?

The most useful special test would be—

2. A—sputum examination for AAFB? B—to measure her haemoglobin? C—a blood slide for malaria parasites? D—to examine her urine for protein and pus cells? E—lumbar puncture?

BRUNO (3 years, 37·5 °C) has had a painful red swelling on his left eyelid for 3 days. The lymph node in front of his left ear is tender. The centre of the swelling is yellow. He has—

3. A—a stye? B—dacrocystitis? C—conjunctivitis? D—a phlycten? E—Trachoma

What would you NOT say to BRUNO's mother?

4. A 'He needs penicillin.' B 'This is not serious.' C 'Squeeze out the pus like this ...' D 'Wash his eyes every day.'

THONG (42 months, 13 kg, haemoglobin 9·5 g/dl) has swollen feet. His eyelids and face are also swollen. His skin is normal, there is protein + + + + in his urine, and ten hookworms in a standard stool smear. His feet are swollen because he has—

5. A—kwashiorkor? B—the nephrotic syndrome? C—severe hookworm anaemia? D—allergy? E—marasmus?

BIENVENIDA (4 years, 14 kg) has been passing worms in her stools. They are round and about 10 cm long, with pointed ends. They are—

6. A—*Taenia*? B—*Ascaris*? C—*Strongyloides*? D—*H. nana*? E—hookworms?

RUCHOYA (3 years, 39·8 °C, Hb 7 g/dl) has vomited several times during the night. He is drowsy and 'floppy' (hypotonic). Early this morning he had two fits. During the night he passed several liquid stools. His spleen is enlarged and his neck is mildly stiff. A blood slide shows 'Malaria parasites + +'. He—

7. B—has meningitis? C—has cerebral malaria? D—has malaria and might have meningitis also? E—has neither of these diseases?

TANYA (7 weeks, 35·6 °C) has a swollen abdomen. She vomited three times during the night and passed several liquid stools. She is pale, slightly jaundiced, and abnormally sleepy. She is not sucking normally and had a fit this morning. The diagnosis that would explain all her symptoms is—

8. A—septicaemia? B—gastroenteritis? C—jaundice? D—acidosis? E—hypothermia?

TANNY (22 months, 9 kg) has been brought to the clinic because she has a cough. She has a mild upper respiratory infection. She also has frothy (bubbly) white spots at the outer edges of both her corneae. Her conjunctivae look dry and there are some small folds in it near her corneae. She cannot see in the dark. Which of these does she need most?

9. A Dry beans B Bananas C Green leaves D Penicillin E Skimmed milk

SHAMMI (5 years, 14 kg, 37·1 °C) was not able to walk when he woke up yesterday morning. Earlier in the week he was ill with fever and was given a penicillin injection into his buttock. Today his right leg is so weak and floppy that he can only move it a little. His leg is not wasted and is not tender. What has probably stopped him walking?

10. A Osteomyelitis B TB C Meningitis D Malnutrition E Polio

His weak leg could have been prevented by—

11. A—immunization? B—eating plenty of protein and energy food? C—giving him penicillin as soon as he started to become ill? D—lumbar puncture? E—wearing shoes?

LUIGI (8 years, 38·1 °C). During the last five days a large painful tender swelling has come on the right side of his face over his upper jaw. He has several carious teeth. The tooth under the swelling hurts when it is hit gently with a spoon. He cannot open his mouth normally. What will you tell his mother?

12. A 'His tooth must be pulled out today.' B 'He has tetanus.' C 'His swelling will go by itself in a few days.' D 'First, I am going to give him some penicillin injections, then his tooth must be pulled out.' E 'Chloramphenicol will cure him.'

SEENAT (8 years, 38·2 °C). During the last three days several tender swellings have come in her left axilla. The largest is about 2 cm in diameter. The skin over them is normal. There is a septic lesion on her left thumb. The swellings in her axilla are—

13. A—acute septic lymphadenitis? B—TB lymphadenitis? C—boils? D—tumours? E—chronic septic lymphadenitis?

Her swellings are caused by—

14. A—fungi? B—viruses? C—protozoa? D—bacteria? E—none of these?

GOPI (3 years, 38·2 °C) has had a painful tender swelling in his left buttock for 3 days. This morning the skin over it has become red, and he has some tender bean-shaped swellings in his right groin. Two weeks ago he was given an injection of penicillin in another clinic because he had a lower respiratory infection. His abscess is probably caused by—

15. A—viruses? B—bacteria? C—protozoa? D—fungi?

The organisms that are causing GOPI's abscess are probably—

16. B—sensitive to penicillin? C—resistant to penicillin?

Abscesses like GOPI's are NOT prevented by—

17. A—boiling syringes? **B**—using a separate sterile needle for each child? **C**—keeping fingers away from the point of a sterilized needle? **D**—using small bottles or ampoules of distilled water? **E**—sterilizing needles with 'sterile' distilled water.

HAYATI (2 years) ate some of her mother's phenobarbitone tablets about half an hour ago. She looks well. Her mother does not know how many tablets HAYATI ate. The nearest hospital is three hours away by bus and the next bus is tomorrow afternoon. What would you do?

18. A Give her paraldehyde to make her vomit. **B** Tell her mother to bring her back any if she has symptoms. **C** Put a spatula down her throat to make her vomit. **D** Send her to hospital in the bus tomorrow afternoon. **E** Give her penicillin to prevent pneumonia.

KATANA (7 years, 37·2 °C) vomited twice yesterday and again in the night. His stools have been normal. He vomited twice like this last year after which he recovered quickly. Each time he vomits he has mild abdominal pain. He is not ill, and his throat, ears, and abdomen are normal. He probably has—

19. A—a chronic gut infection? **B**—TB meningitis? **C**—gut obstruction? **D**—a harmless vomiting attack? **E**—an acute abdomen?

FRANCISCO (2 years, 38 °C) has some yellow crusted lesions on his face and ears, especially near his nose and mouth. They started about a week ago as red macules which became thin vesicles and then pustules. He has tender lymph-nodes under his jaw. He has—

20. A—chickenpox? **B**—boils? **C**—herpes simplex? **D**—scabies? **E**—impetigo?

Which of these is the best local treatment?

21. A Simple ointment **B** Washing off the crusts in potassium permanganate **C** Benzoic acid ointment **D** Benzyl benzoate **E** Calamine lotion

Which of these would be best for him? One injection of—

22. A—benethamine (depot) penicillin? **B**—procaine penicillin? **C**—benzyl penicillin? **D**—streptomycin?

KWANGOLE (5 years) has been vomiting during the day. He started to become ill two days ago with fever, headache, and drowsiness. His neck is stiff and he cannot put his head between his legs. His throat, ears, and abdomen are normal. He has probably been vomiting because he has—

23. A—meningitis or cerebal malaria? **B**—otitis media? **C**—gastroenteritis? **D**—tonsillitis? **E**—an acute abdomen?

His blood slide shows malaria parasites + +. Does he need a lumbar puncture?

24. B Yes **C** No

MWINZAGA (5 years) has been brought to see you at two o'clock on a Sunday morning. He has been vomiting since midday Saturday. He vomits with force and his vomit smells like faeces. He says his abdomen hurts. He is

drowsy, and his abdomen is swollen. There is tenderness and guarding in the lower right side of his abdomen. He has passed no stools for two days. His neck is not stiff. He is vomiting because he has—

25. A—meningitis? **B**—cerebral malaria? **C**—gastroenteritis? **D**—an ordinary vomiting attack? **E**—an acute abdomen?

SICK CHILDREN FIFTEEN
Code 8

AKIRA (6 years, 38 °C) looks very 'ill'. His neck is swollen and you can feel some enlarged tender lymph-nodes under the angles of his jaw. There is a grey–yellow membrane on his tonsils and his pharynx. He is breathing with difficulty and he cannot speak. There is mild insuction. His mouth smells bad. His disease could have been prevented by—

1. A—immunizing him with BCG? **B**—brushing his teeth? **C**—giving him more protein and energy food? **D**—immunizing him with DPT vaccine? **E**—wearing warm clothes?

What would you NOT say to his mother?

2. A 'Don't worry, he has thrush.' **B** 'He must stay in bed for several weeks after he is well.' **C** 'He should go to hospital.' **D** 'We must watch his breathing carefully.' **E** 'His brother and sisters need injections also.'

RAY (4 days) has vomited several teaspoonfuls of bright red blood. What are you going to say to his mother?

3. A 'He is anaemic.' **B** 'This must be blood from cracked nipples.' **C** 'It is blood he swallowed during birth.' **D** 'He must have a vitamin B injection.' **E** 'We must give him vitamin K.'

SUKADI has been brought to the clinic in May 1975. He was born in December 1973. In December 1974 he weighed 5·5 kg, in January 1975 5·4 kg, in February 5·6 kg, in March 5·5 kg, in April 5·5 kg. Today in May he weighs 5·6 kg. His arm circumference is 10·7 cm.

His mother became pregnant when he was three months old, so he was bottle-fed with skim-milk from the clinic. His younger brother died of fever when he was two months old. When he first came to the clinic the midwife there thought he was healthy because nobody made a graph of his weight.

When he was a year old he started to eat rice for the first time with spinach twice a day. Occasionally, he has tempe (a food made with beans).

During the last four months his growth curve has been—

4. A—rising? **B**—falling? **C**—staying nearly flat?

If he had to have an artificial feed when he was three months old, he should have been given—

5. A—skim-milk? **B**—the cheapest full-cream dried milk? **C**—condensed milk? **D**—dried milk with extra lactose? **E**—lactose-free milk?

His mother stopped breast feeding him early. So he should have started to eat rice porridge at the age of—

6. A—4 days? **B**—3 months? **C**—6 months? **D**—9 months?

The birth interval between him and his younger brother was—

7. A—one year? **B**—3 years? **C**—6 months? **D**—9 months?

The birth interval should have been about—

8. B—2 years? **C**—3 years or more? **D**—1 year?

9. He is—

C—above the road to health? **D**—on the road to health? **E**—below the road to health?

Which of these foods would probably be the cheapest way of giving him extra protein food?

10. A Meat **B** Fresh milk **C** Fresh fish **D** Beans or groundnuts **E** Eggs

SHABANA (5 days) has a wet and sticky cord. She is happy and sucking well. The skin round her cord is not inflamed. What are you going to tell SHABANA's mother?

11. A 'Put this antibiotic powder on it.' **B** 'Make a wet dressing for it like this ...' **C** 'She needs injections of penicillin and streptomycin.' **D** 'Put on this ointment.' **E** 'Keep her cord clean and dry. Here is some spirit for it.'

SULAIMAN (3 years) ate about 30 iron sulphate tablets half an hour ago. The nearest hospital is about five hours away by bullock cart. The hospital is expensive and the family are poor. Your syrup of ipecac is finished. What would you tell his mother?

12. A 'I am going to make him vomit the tablets by putting this rubber tube down his throat.' **B** 'Take him to hospital quickly.' **C** 'Iron tablets never harmed any child.' **D** 'Let us wait and see if he gets symptoms.' **E** 'First, we must wash out his stomach.'

MUKAPE (5 years, 7·5 kg) has a deep round 3 cm bad smelling sore on his ankle. There is a thin, yellow discharge from the sore and no skin over it. The sore started as a small injury about three weeks ago and is slowly growing larger. The lymph nodes in his groin are not tender. His lips and conjunctivae are pale. His father has no job and the family are very poor. MUKAPE has—

13. A—a boil? **B**—pyoderma? **C**—impetigo? **D**—a skin ulcer or tropical ulcer? **E**—cellulitis?

His lesion should be treated with—

14. A—gentian violet? **B**—hypochlorite dressings and a bandage, rest, and pencillin? **C**—benzoic acid ointment? **D**—benzyl benzoate? **E**—iodine?

Which of these vaccines might help to prevent one or more of the complications of his lesions?

15. A BCG **B** Polio **C** DPT **D** Measles

What would you NOT tell his mother?

16. A 'Leave his sore open without a dressing.' **B** 'He must take these iron tablets for three months.' **C** 'Penicillin injections will help him.' **D** 'He needs more food, especially more protein food.' **E** 'Treat any more sores on his leg while they are still small.'

TITIEK (36 months, 13 kg, haemoglobin 6 g/dl) has had mild diarrhoea for several months. Sometimes there is blood in her stools. She has had no fever. Her lips and conjunctivae are pale. She is not thirsty, her mouth is wet, and her skin elasticity is normal. A standard stool smear shows '*Ascaris* ova 2, *Trichuris* ova 49, Hookworm ova 6, *Strongyloides* larvae 14'. She should be treated with—

17. A—TCE? **B**—piperazine? **C**—metronidazole? **D**—glucose–salt solution? **E**—tiabendazole?

JAY (10 years) has had a swelling over his spine for several weeks. His back hurts when he walks. He has not been well for several months. He is not eating normally and he has been losing weight. Sometimes he has a mild fever. The lesion in his back is probably caused by—

18. A—osteomyelitis? **B**—TB? **C**—an injury? **D**—pyomyositis?

Which of these would be best for him?

19. A Isoniazid (INH) for three months **B** Penicillin for 3 months **C** Streptomycin for three months, with isoniazid and thiacetazone for a year **D** Penicillin for three days **E** Chloramphenicol and penicillin for six weeks

RAJESH (4 years, 3 kg) has had sore, red, and watery eyes for several days. He has no fever and is otherwise well. Several other people in the village have had the same disease during the last few weeks. He probably has—

20. A—chronic conjunctivitis? **B**—vitamin A deficiency? **C**—trachoma? **D**—acute conjunctivitis? **E**—allergic conjunctivitis?

He needs—

21. A—penicillin injections? **B**—chlortetracycline eye ointment three times a day? **C**—sulphadimidine tablets? **D**—chloramphenicol capsules? **E**—vitamin B tablets?

MANOHAR (18 months) had a cold with fever a week ago. Now he is moderately ill and has tender bean-shaped swellings on both sides of his neck below the angle of his jaw. His tonsils are large and red and there are white spots on them. There are no lesions outside his tonsils. He has—

22. A—diphtheria? **B**—TB lymph nodes of his neck? **C**—mumps? **D**—tonsillitis? **E**—chronic septic lymphadenitis?

SHASHI (36 months, 10 kg) has a sore red vulva. Pus is coming from her vagina. When you put a finger into her rectum you can feel nothing in her vagina. She has not been scratching her anus. She probably has—

23. A—vulvovaginitis? **B**—threadworms? **C**—a foreign body? **D**—thrush? **E**—urinary infection?

When SHASHI's pus is examined, a health-centre laboratory may be able to find the organisms causing—

24. A—worms? **B**—TB? **C**—gonorrhea? **D**—syphilis? **E**—malnutrition?

MWANGI (5 years) has had abdominal pain since yesterday. He had five watery stools during the night and more this morning. He has vomited once. His throat is normal. His eyes are not sunken and his skin elasticity is normal. He drinks thirstily. He has no abdominal tenderness, guarding, or rigidity. He needs—

25. A—a nasogastric drip? **B**—intravenous fluids? **C**—penicillin? **D**—glucose–salt solution? **E**—paracetamol?

SICK CHILDREN SIXTEEN
Code 4

FILBERT (7 years). For the last one or two months he has had several 2-cm, firm, painless swellings down the right side of his neck. There are a few smaller swellings on the left side also. He is not well and is not eating normally. He is becoming thin. His throat and tonsils are normal. The swellings are in his—

1. A—thyroid gland? **B**—mastoid? **C**—lymph nodes? **D**—parotid glands? **E**—skin?

He needs—

2. A—no treatment? **B**—penicillin? **C**—an operation in hospital? **D**—iodine? **E**—streptomycin and isoniazid?

YITZAK was born last night. Both his feet and ankles are bent inwards. You cannot bend his feet so that their outer sides touch the outer side of his legs. He has—

3. A—true talipes? **B**—false talipes?

What are you going to say to his mother?

4. A 'His feet will straighten themselves out in a few months.' **B** 'We must strap his feet straight today.' **C** 'When he starts walking we will put strapping on his feet.' **D** 'His feet need an operation in hospital to bend them straight.'

CHOLIPAH (2 years). Half an hour ago she was burnt with smoking hot oil from a frying pan. The burn covers her right arm and part of her body. At first she was shocked but now she has started to cry. Most of her burn will probably be—

5. B—superficial? **C**—superficial partial thickness? **D**—deep partial thickness? **E**—full thickness?

What would you do?

6. A Treat her in the health centre with dressings of vaseline gauze. **B** Put a sterile dressing on her and send her to hospital. **C** Put gentian violet on her burn and cover it with a dry dressing. **D** Put her hand in cold water.

Which of these complications would you NOT expect to kill her during the next few weeks?

7. B Infection **C** Loss of fluid and protein **D** Loss of iron and energy food.

Which of these complications is likely to be most serious later?

8. A The dark colour of her burnt skin **B** Anaesthesia of the burnt skin **C** Paralysis **D** Contractures **E** None of these

JUMA (6 years, 38·5 °C) has a tender red swelling over the bone behind his left ear. It is fixed to the bone and its edge is difficult to feel. His left ear is discharging pus. There is a perforation in his left ear-drum. He has several carious teeth. The nearest hospital is 8 hours away by camel. He has—

9. A—mumps? **B**—mastoiditis? **C**—lymphadenitis? **D**—a goitre? **E**—a tooth abscess?

10. What would you say to his mother?

B 'He will soon recover. Here are some ear drops for him.' **C** 'Here are 20 tablets (sulphadimidine). Give him 1½ tablets four times a day.' **D** Let me open the swelling with this knife.' **E** 'Take JUMA to hospital quickly, but let me give him an injection first (benzyl penicillin 4 ml).'

UMBERTO (2 years, 8 kg). His mother says that in the evening he falls over things because he cannot see them in the dark. He cannot find his toys in the evenings. What would you tell his mother?

11. A 'He must eat plenty of green leaves such as spinach.' **B** 'Be sure to wash his eyes carefully.' **C** Here is some ointment, put it into his eyes three times a day.' **D** 'He must eat plenty of protein food, such as beans.' **E** 'We must give him capsules of vitamin B.'

INES (8 years, 22 kg). Three months ago she had a cough, fever, and fast breathing. A health worker thought she had pneumonia and gave her penicillin. This did not cure her. She is 'ill' and is still coughing up sputum. She is losing weight even though her mother gives her plenty of food. She has not been immunized. She may have—

12. A—whooping cough? **B**—a foreign body in her bronchi? **C**—TB? **D**—asthma? **C**—bronchiolitis?

The laboratory cannot do any other special tests. Which of these special tests would help most?

13. A Blood for haemoglobin **B** Examining her sputum for viruses **C** Examining her sputum for AAFB **D** Stool for worms **E** Urine for protein

TERESA (4½ years, 37·5 °C, haemoglobin 4½ g/dl) has come to the clinic for her six monthly check. Her lips and conjunctivae are pale. She has not been well and she has had several attacks of fever. Which of these does she probably need most?

14. A Piperazine **B** Pyrantel pamoate **C** TCE (tetrachlorethylene) **D** Chloroquine **E** Tiabendazole

SHUPI (1 week) had a difficult birth. He has a hard swelling over the middle of his clavicle. What are you going to tell his mother?

15. A 'We must put a bandage round his shoulders.' **B** 'The lump will go by itself.' **C** 'If we do not treat him carefully, he will have this swelling all his life.' **D** 'Take him to hospital, he needs an X-ray.' E 'Put hot compresses on the lump.'

CHIPO (4 years, 38·6 °C) has had abdominal pain and a cough since yesterday. He has vomited once. He has large tonsils with pus on them and large tender tonsillar lymph nodes. He has no abdominal tenderness, rigidity, or guarding. His spleen is not enlarged, and his blood slide is normal. There are seven hookworm ova and one *Ascaris* ovum in a standard stool smear. There is no protein or pus cells in his urine. His abdominal pain is probably caused by—

16. A—a urine infection? B—an acute abdomen? C—hookworm infection? D—malaria? E—tonsillitis?

He needs—

17. A—procaine penicillin? B—piperazine? C—chloroquine by mouth? D—an operation in hospital? E—chloroquine by injection?

HERNANTO (9) has a small (1 mm) painful yellow swelling at the outer side of his left sclera close to his cornea. His eye is red and full of tears. He probably has—

18. A—a corneal ulcer? B—a phlycten? C—vitamin A deficiency? D—trachoma? E—a stye?

He probably needs—

19. A—vitamin A capsules? B—chlortetracycline eye ointment? C—isoniazid and streptomycin? D—scopolamine eye ointment?

BIATA (1 month) vomited twice yesterday, once during the night, and once again this morning. In the middle of the night she had a fit. She has stopped sucking, and has a sharp cry. She passed one liquid stool this morning. Her fontanelle is swollen. She has no neck stiffness. There is much falciparum malaria in the district. All these symptoms are most probably caused by—

20. A—meningitis? B—a lower respiratory infection? C—a gut infection? D—tetanus? E—cerebral malaria?

She needs—

21. A—a blood slide for malaria parasites? B—her urine examined for protein and pus cells? C—glucose-salt solution? D— a lumbar puncture? E—subcutaneous chloroquine?

ELENESTO (7 years) has had some round, painless, bald scaly patches on his scalp for several months. They have no scabs, pus, or crusts. Several other children in his school have lesions of the same kind. He has—

22. A—scabies? B—impetigo? C—head lice? D—leprosy? E—ringworm?

He should be treated with—

23. A—benzyl benzoate? B—an antibiotic? C—procaine penicillin? D—dapsone? E—benzoic acid ointment?

His lesions might have been prevented by—

24. B—eating plenty of protein food? C—drinking boiled water? D—plenty of washing in soap and water? E—wearing a hat?

MAGDALENA (4 years, 11 kg) had whooping cough three months ago. She is still coughing and her growth curve is falling. She is not well. She is not eating normally, and she has fever in the evenings. Her throat and tonsillar lymph-nodes are normal. Her whooping cough may have been complicated by—

25. A—measles? B—bronchitis? C—pharyngitis? D—tonsillitis? E—TB?

SICK CHILDREN SEVENTEEN
Code 1

CAUPOLICAN (4 years) has become blind in his left eye during the last two days. The cornea of his left eye is soft, opaque, and ulcerated. The conjunctivae of both his eyes is abnormally folded. There is a frothy (bubbly) white lesion at the outer edge of his right sclera close to the conjunctiva. His right cornea is dry but not yet ulcerated. His LEFT eye shows the lesions of—

1. A—keratomalacia? B—xerophthalmia? C—trachoma? D—acute conjunctivitis? E—phlyctenular conjunctivitis?

His RIGHT eye shows the lesions of—

2. A—phlyctenular conjunctivitis? B—keratomalacia? C—trachoma? D—acute conjunctivitis? E—xerophthalmia?

He needs—

3. A—chlortetracycline eye ointment? B—100 000 units of vitamin A by mouth? C—100 000 units of water miscible vitamin A by injection? D—oily vitamin A by injection? E—isoniazid?

JUAN (3 months, 5·5 kg, 38·2 °C). Three days ago he became drowsy and stopped sucking. He has vomited several times. Earlier this morning he had a fit. His fontanelle is swollen. He has no neck stiffness. Kernig's sign is doubtful. He has probably stopped sucking because he has—

4. A—meningitis? B—tetanus? C—hyperpyrexia? D—epilepsy? E—febrile convulsions?

SOESILO's mother has had red watery eyes most of the time since she was a child. Her eyelids are scarred so that they don't close properly. Some of her eyelashes have turned inwards so that they scratch her eyes. Her corneae are grey and scarred so that she cannot see through them normally. What is her diagnosis?

5. A Second-stage trachoma B Keratomalacia C First-stage trachoma D Fourth-stage trachoma

SOESILO himself is four years old. He now has red watery eyes also, but no other signs. What would you do?

6. A Tell his mother he will soon get well by himself. B Give him sulphadimidine. C Give him penicillin injections. D Ask his mother to put chlortetracycline

ointment into his eyes regularly and observe him carefully. **E** Give him vitamin A only.

BILLY-JEAN (3 years, 39·1 °C) has had several boils during the last few months. Last week she fell and hurt her leg. The pain did not last long, and she could soon walk again. Two days ago she suddenly had a high fever. Yesterday the bone below her left knee became tender and swollen. Now she cannot walk. The skin over the lesion is red. She probably has—

7. **A**—septic arthritis? **B**—polio? **C**—osteomyelitis? **D**—pyomyositis? **E**—cellulitis only?

ACHMAD (35 months, 9 kg) has had an acutely red, painful, watery eye for five days. He has a 1 mm yellow swelling at the outer side of his sclera close to his cornea. He has—

8. **A**—allergic conjunctivitis? **B**—phlyctenular conjunctivitis? **C**—trachoma? **D**—keratomalacia? **E**—a corneal ulcer?

MANUEL (18 months, haemoglobin 13·5 g/dl, 37·1 °C) has stopped sucking from his feeding bottle. He has had diarrhoea for 5 days. His mouth is dry, his eyes are sunken, and his skin elasticity is reduced. He is drowsy, his respirations are 56 per minute and deep. His fontanelle is sunken. He has stopped sucking because he—

9. **A**—has an upper respiratory infection? **B**—is hypothermic? **C**—is dehydrated? **D**—is anaemic?

CHEV (3 years, 12 kg, haemoglobin 8 g/dl) has been brought by his grandfather because both his feet are swelling. He has been living with his grandfather for several months because his mother died when his youngest sister was born. For the last few days he has not wanted to eat. Pieces of skin are peeling off from lesions on his legs. There are a few hookworm ova in his stool. His urine is normal. Last month he weighed 13 kg. Three months ago he weighed 13·5 kg. His feet are swelling because he has—

10. **A**—severe anaemia? **B**—the nephrotic syndrome? **C**—pellagra? **D**—hookworms? **E**—kwashiorkor?

ALEYA (4 years) has been slowly losing weight for several weeks. She is irritable and is not 'well'. She has mild fever and a cough for about two months. Sulphadimidine has not helped her, nor has education about feeding. She is mildly anaemic, but except for this she has no other signs. She may be losing weight because she has—

11. **A**—whooping cough? **B**—TB? **C**—worms? **D**—malaria? **E**—bronchitis?

Which of these questions would help you most with your diagnosis?

12. **A** 'Has she ever passed any worms in her stools? **B** 'Have any of the children in the family got a cough?'

C 'Has she had DPT vaccine?' **D** 'Have any of the older people in the family got a cough?'

Which of these examinations would help you most in your diagnosis?

13. **A** Measuring her arm circumference **B** Looking for a scar on her right shoulder **C** Looking for skin lesions **D** Examining her ears **E** Looking for signs of vitamin deficiency

MWAMGOLE (3·5 years, 14 kg, haemoglobin 6 g/dl) has mild abdominal pain, and scratches her anus because it itches. Her conjunctivae are pale, but she has no other signs. Her stools show—hookworms + +, *Ascaris* + +. Which of these would be your first choice for her?

14. **A** Tetrachlorethylene **B** Piperazine **C** Pyrantel pamoate **D** Bephenium **E** Niclosamide

15. PLATO (2 years) is mildly ill and has vomited twice. He has no abnormal signs. He probably vomited because he has—

A—meningitis? **B**—cerebal malaria? **C**—typhoid? **D**—some infection we cannot diagnose? **E**—an upper respiratory infection?

BITI (48 months, 14 kg, haemoglobin 7 g/dl) has had bloody diarrhoea for several weeks. Her growth curve has been falling. Sometimes, she has pains in her abdomen. She is not thirsty and her skin elasticity is normal. There are 5 hookworm ova, 60 *Trichuris* ova and no amoebae in a standard stool smear. She needs—

16. **A**—tiabendazole and iron? **B**—niridazole and calcium? **C**—niclosamide and iodine? **D**—metrifonate? **E**—TCE?

ONYANGO (3 years, 39·2 °C) vomited twice in the night. He has a sore throat, there is pus on his tonsils, and his tonsillar lymph nodes are enlarged and tender. He has passed a few liquid stools. He has no meningeal signs and his spleen is not enlarged. His ear-drums are normal. He is vomiting because he has—

17. **A**—cerebral malaria? **B**—a harmless vomiting attack? **C**—meningitis? **D**—diphtheria? **E**—tonsillitis?

He needs—

18. **A**—a lumbar puncture? **B**—to be kept warm? **C**—to be cooled down? **D**—to be starved until he is well? **E**—intravenous fluids?

He should also be given—

19. **A**—chloramphenicol? **B**—glucose–salt solution? **C**—streptomycin? **D**—penicillin? **E**—an antipyretic injection?

What would you tell his mother?

20. **A** 'Wrap him in a blanket and don't wash him.' **B** 'Don't put too many clothes on a child with fever.' **C** 'His brother and sisters need injections.' **D** 'Immunization could have prevented this.' **E** 'This is a very dangerous disease.'

MWITA (2 years, 38·8 °C) has vomited twice since yesterday. Early this morning he had a fit. His left ear-drum is red, dull, and swollen. His neck is not stiff and his spleen is not enlarged. His blood slide is normal. He vomited because he has—

21. A—cerebral malaria? **B**—meningitis? **C**—a harmless vomiting attack? **D**—otitis externa? **E**—otitis media?

DIDI (2 months). His mother says she has not got enough milk. What would you tell her?

22. A 'Put him to the breast more often. Bring him to be weighed regularly.' **B** 'Give him this dried skim milk.' **C** 'Put him to your breasts less often.' **D** 'Let me show you how to make a safe bottle-feed.' **E** 'Go on breast-feeding him. Give him a bottle also.'

ADO (3 weeks) sucks weakly, so that his mother's breasts have become engorged and painful. The clinic's breast pump is broken and there are none in shops. What would you tell his mother?

23. A 'Use a nipple-shield like this ...' **B** 'Express your breast-milk for him with your hands like this ...' **C** 'Use a nipple-shell like this ...' **D** 'If feeding him hurts you, give him a bottle.' **E** 'Put hot compresses on your breasts.'

For a few days ADO and his mother are happy. Then the lower part of her left breast becomes painful, tender and swollen. Pus discharges through a hole in the skin. There are tender lymph nodes in her left axilla. Her temperature is 38 °C. What would you tell her now?

24. A 'Let him suck from your right breast. Express the milk from your sore left breast and throw it away.' **B** 'Stop breast-feeding and feed him with a cup and spoon.' **C** 'Let him suck from your sore breast through a nipple shield.' **D** 'Let him go on sucking from both your breasts.' **E** 'Feed him from a bottle until your sore breast is better.'

Which of these would you give her?

25. A Penicillin and chloramphenicol **B** Tetracycline and calcium tablets **C** Penicillin and aspirin **D** Streptomycin **E** Dapsone and aspirin

---

SICK CHILDREN EIGHTEEN
Code 5

ALOYSIUS (1850 g) has just been born. There is no cartilage in his ears and no creases (folds) on the balls of his heels. His breasts are only 1 mm in diameter. He is—

1. D—small for dates? **E**—preterm?

ALOYSIUS—

2. A—has plenty of iron in his body? **B**—can easily keep himself warm? **C**—is more likely to become infected than a baby weighing 3·5 kg? **D**—is unlikely to get jaundice? **E**—lies with his legs bent (flexed)?

Which one of these would NOT be helpful in preventing a serious infection of his eyes?

3. B Tetracycline eye ointment **C** 1 per cent silver nitrate (or proteinate) eye drops **D** Fluorescein eye drops

ALOYSIUS has a soft bruised swelling over most of the top of his skull, it covers several bones, and it has no clear edge. It is—

4. A—cellulitis? **B**—caput succedaneum? **C**—a cephalhaematoma? **D**—a congenital malformation? **E**—a fractured skull?

What would you say to his mother?

5. A 'Let me put a needle into the swelling to let out the blood.' **B** 'He will need an operation when he is older.' **C** 'This is an infected swelling. He needs penicillin.' **D** 'He will have this swelling all his life.' **E** 'This swelling will go by itself in a few days.'

When you rub his cheek he moves his mouth and turns his head towards your finger as if he was going to suck. When you hold him in your arms and lower him, he reaches out his arms as if he was going to fall. This shows that—

6. A—he is probably backward? **B**—his brain has been injured during birth? **C**—he is hungry and wants feeding? **D**—his brain is normal by these tests? **E**—he has tetanus?

Which of these things is NOT necessary. ALOYSIUS should be—

7. A—kept warm? **B**—sucked out quickly if he stops breathing? **C**—bathed every day? **D**—touched with carefully washed hands? **E**—put to the breast as soon as he is born?

One of his hands has six fingers. The extra finger is next to his little finger. It is small and soft and has no bone in it. What are you going to do?

8. A Tie a piece of iodine soaked thread around his extra finger. **B** Send him to hospital to have it cut off. **C** Cut it off yourself. **D** Do nothing until he is three months old and then cut if off. **E** Let his finger dry so that it falls off by itself.

Three days after birth ALOYSIUS has many small red macules on his skin. In the middle of each macule there is a very small white swelling which looks like a pustule. He has—

9. A—impetigo? **B**—erythema neonatorum (a milk rash)? **C**—pyoderma? **D**—measles? **E**—a heat rash?

What will you tell his mother?

10. A 'The rash will go by itself in a few days.' **B** 'Don't put any clothes or blankets on him.' **C** 'He will infect other babies.' **D** 'He needs penicillin.' **E** 'His lesions are caused by breast-feeding, so you must stop breast-feeding.'

Four days after birth ALOYSIUS loses about two teaspoonfuls of blood from his umbilicus. He needs—

11. A—vitamin K by injection? **B**—penicillin and streptomycin? **C**—DPT vaccine? **D**—an antibiotic ointment on his cord? **E**—chloramphenicol?

When ALOYSIUS is a week old his mother brings him to the clinic saying that he is pale and sleepy. He is too weak to suck. He has vomited once and has passed several watery stools. The skin round his umbilicus is red. Which of these diseases are you most frightened of?

12. A Cellulitis **B** Septicaemia **C** Pneumonia **D** Gastroenteritis **E** Haemorrhagic disease

Which of these would be best for ALOYSIUS?

13. A Tetracycline **B** Procaine penicillin and streptomycin **C** Benzathine penicillin and streptomycin **D** Chloramphenicol **E** Benzyl penicillin and streptomycin

He now weighs 1820 g. The dose of streptomycin is 20 mg/kg once daily. How many mg of streptomycin does he need each day?

14. A 3600 mg **B** 90 mg **C** 36 mg **D** 360 mg **E** 900 mg

You have 1 g ampoules of streptomycin. You dissolve one of these in 10 ml of sterile water. ALOYSIUS needs about—

15. A—9 ml **B**—4½ ml **C**—3·6 ml **D**—a third of an ml (0·36 ml) **E**—0·9 ml

He also needs feeding with a—

16. A—bottle? **B**—jug? **C**—cotton wick? **D**—cup and spoon? **E**—tube?

He should be fed—

17. A—expressed breast-milk? **B**—full-cream dried milk? **C**—skim milk? **D**—glucose–salt solution?

ALOYSIUS is in danger from—

18. A—milk allergy? **B**—getting too fat by being given too much milk? **C**—lactose intolerance? **D**—milk getting into his lungs? **E**—milk getting into his ears?

How many times a day should he be fed?

19. A Three times **B** Every three hours **C** Four times **D** Twice **E** Six times

How much feed does he need each time? He is now seven days old.

20 A 34 ml **B** 48 ml **C** 56 ml **D** 64 ml **E** 80 ml

When ALOYSIUS is three months old, which of these vaccines would you give him?

21. A Polio **B** DPT **C** BCG, DPT, and polio **D** Measles **E** Polio and measles

ALOYSIUS recovers. Two months later his mother is worried about his faeces. Sometimes he passes faeces four times on the same day. Sometimes he does not pass any faeces for four days. When he passes faeces he cries and moves about. What are you going to tell her?

22. B 'This is abnormal, all healthy babies pass a soft stool every day.' **C** 'Breast-milk must be making him constipated.' **D** 'Give him this medicine (liquid paraffin).' **E** 'All this is normal, don't worry.'

On her next visit his mother is worried because his fontanelle is too small. His head looks normal. What will you tell her?

23. A 'His fontanelle is normal.' **B** 'He is dehydrated.' **C** 'He has meningitis.' **D** 'He may be backward.' **E** 'Keep his fontanelle covered with a warm cap.'

At his last visit ALOYSIUS has a sore red rash between his buttocks and around his genital organs. He probably has—

24. A—a heat rash? **B**—ringworm? **C**—impetigo? **D**—a nappy rash? **E**—threadworms?

What would you tell her?

25. A 'Here are some tablets (sulphadimidine) for him...' **B** 'Boil his nappies, and leave him without any on as much as possible.' **C** 'Wash him more.' **D** 'Put fewer clothes on him.' **E** 'Give him this sulphur ointment.'

Booklet C——Postests

Booklet C—Postests

C.1. MANUAL POSTEST
Code 4

Do this with your manual open. Do it at any time after you have had time to study the first chapter, the dose tables, and the instructions at the beginning of the index.

1. What disease is described in the section next after chickenpox?

A Herpes simplex **B** Scabies **C** Herpes zoster **D** Tinea versicolor **E** Ringworm

2. What does 9–1 show?

A Words for parts of the body **B** A deformed and disabled child **C** 'My child has diarrhoea.' **D** How to make a dehydration score **E** A drawing of a stool seen through a microscope

3. What does 5:2 show?

A How to decide whether a child is 'well' or 'ill' **B** How to get a clinic ready for integrated care **C** How to make a clinic easy to work in **D** Lymphadenitis and the lymph-nodes **E** A child's lymph-nodes

4. Which of these is reference to a figure in the Laboratory manual?

A L:2 **B** L 6–1 **C** L 7.2 **D** N 6–1 **E** 14.99

5. One of these has a mistake in the alphabet. Which one?

A KLMNO **B** GHIJK **C** VWXYZ **D** NOPQR **E** STVWX

6. Look through the index and find out which ONE of these is wrong.

A Triple vaccine is also called DPT vaccine. **B** *Trichuris* is the same as the roundworm. **C** An ulcer is any break in the skin or mucosa. **D** The worm load is the number of worms that a child has in his body. **E** Stomatitis is a sore mouth.

7. Look through the index until you find which ONE of these is wrong.

A Urticaria is a raised itchy rash. **B** Turbid means cloudy. **C** Tiabendazole is a drug for treating some kinds of worms. **D** Xerophthalmia is a disease caused by lack of vitamin B.

8. Turn to near the end of 15.9. Look under the heading 'Diagnosis'. You will see a list of diseases causing fits. Which of them is the LEAST common cause of fits?

A Febrile convulsions **B** Cerebral malaria **C** Dehydration **D** Hypoglycaemia **E** Meningitis

9. Look up 'itching anus' in the index. Go to the reference you are told to. Read until you get to the first cross reference (such as, for example (16.19). Go to it. Which of these is it?

A Schistosomiasis **B** Her vulva is sore **C** Urinary symptoms **D** Acute nephritis **E** Diagnosing backwardness

10. Look up 'vitamin K' in the index. Go to the section you are told to. Start reading that section until you come to the first cross-reference. Go to that cross-reference. Which of these is it?

A Nappy rash **B** 'He has vomited blood.' **C** Normal faeces **D** 'His eyes are red and sticky.' **E** 'There is blood in his faeces.'

11. Look up sulphadimidine in the index. You will see many references beside it. One of them is to a figure. Go to it. Look at it carefully. How many spoonfuls of sulphadimidine mixture would you give in each dose to a 12 kg child?

A 1 **B** $1\frac{1}{2}$ **C** 2 **D** $2\frac{1}{2}$ **E** 3

12. What is the strength of this sulphadimidine mixture?

A 4 mg **B** 500 mg **C** 500 mg in 5 ml **D** 70 mg in 1 ml

13. How many doses would you give him in 24 hours?

A 1 **B** 2 **C** 4 **D** 5 **E** 6

14. What is the shortest course you would give?

A 2 days **B** 1 day **C** One dose **D** 3 days **E** 4 doses

15. What is the longest course you would give?

A 3 days **B** Two weeks **C** One week **D** 1 day **E** 4 days

16. Look up aspirin in the index. Go to the dose figure for it. How many of the larger of the two tablets would you give to a 13 kg child at each dose?

A 4 **B** 3 **C** 8 **D** $1\frac{1}{2}$ **E** $\frac{1}{2}$

17. What is the size of the larger aspirin tablets?

A 300 mg **B** 200 mg **C** 100 mg **D** 50 mg **E** 75 mg

18. How often should the child take these tablets?

A Twice a day **B** Four times a day **C** Eight times a day **D** Once a week **E** Once a month

19. PRAISETHELORD (2 years, 15 kg) has severe diarrhoea and dehydration. Turn to 9–22. How many ml of intravenous fluid are you going to give him fast?

A 100 ml **B** 200 ml **C** 300 ml **D** 400 ml **E** 500 ml

20. When you have given PRAISETHELORD his fast replacement, how many ml of fluid are you going to give him each hour as slow replacement?

A 100 ml **B** 75 ml **C** 50 ml **D** 25ml **E** 10 ml

21. JAQUES (9 kg) has fever, vomiting, and fits. His blood slide shows 'Malaria parasites + + +'. How much chloroquine does he need?

A 0·1 ml **B** 0·5 ml **C** 0·6 ml **D** 0·9 ml **E** 1·0 ml

22. Look up 'not eating' in the index. Go to the most important reference to it. All these things can stop a child eating EXCEPT one. Which one?

A Malnutrition **B** Unhappiness **C** Sore mouth or throat **D** TB **E** Anaemia

23. AMIN (7 days old) has abnormal movements. Which of these sections is the most helpful in diagnosing whether he has fits or tetanus?

A 15.9 **B** 15.2 **C** 26.24 **D** 15.7 **E** 26.42

24. ROELOFSA (3 years). His mother says he has severe diarrhoea, fever, and vomiting. He will drink but will not eat. Which of these sections would be most useful in diagnosis?

A 26.32 **B** 10.10 **C** 20.15 **D** 9.31 **E** 18.15

25. SALVADOR (4 years) has fever and a cough. Which of these would be most helpful in diagnosis?

D 10.10 **E** 8.20

C.2. OVERALL POSTEST
Questions from all over the microplan: Code 4

1. Which of these is usually a behaviour disease?

A Swelling of the lymph-nodes **B** Cleft palate **C** Bed wetting **D** Malaria **E** Cholera (2.1)

2. Which of these is the LEAST useful treatment for a severe septic infection?

A Penicillin alone **B** Chloramphenicol alone **C** Penicillin and sulphadimidine **D** Ampicillin alone **E** Streptomycin alone (3.21)

3. Which of these vaccines causes a scar?

A BCG **B** DPT **C** Measles **D** Polio (4.6)

4. Which of these signs can be caused by marasmus and by dehydration?

A A dry mouth **B** Loss of skin elasticity **C** A swollen fontanelle **D** Fast breathing **E** Swelling of the ankles (7.9, 9.18)

5. Which of this is NOT true?

A Bottle-feeding needs much water and fuel. **B** Badly managed bottle-feeding causes diarrhoea. **C** Bottle-feeds must be made with boiled water. **D** Feeding-bottles can be sterilized with hypochlorite. **E** Milk which is left over from one bottle feed can safely be used at the next feed. (N 8.1)

6. Which of these diseases is most likely to make a child vomit?

A TB **B** Whooping cough **C** Chronic upper respiratory infections **D** Bronchitis **E** Asthma (8.17)

7. All these children have diarrhoea. Which of them would probably be most difficult to rehydrate?

A TEENY who has fever **B** WEENY who is malnourished **C** HUMPTY who has diarrhoea only **D** DUMPTY who is vomiting (9.23)

8. Which of these is NOT true? Salt-and-sugar water—

A—should be made by mothers in a clinic before they go home? **B**—can be made with ordinary salt and ordinary sugar? **C**—may cause hypernatraemic dehydration if too much salt is given? **D**—should be made with heaped teaspoons of salt and sugar? **E**—can be given down an intragastric tube? (9.21, 9.22)

9. JACINTA (2 years) has fever caused by pneumonia. She is being given penicillin and aspirin. Penicillin is—

A—symptomatic treatment for her fever? **B**—causal treatment for her pneumonia? **C**—both of these? **D**—neither of them? (10.2)

10. A health-centre laboratory can help to diagnose—

A—a heat rash? **B**—urticaria? **C**—a drug rash? **D**—measles? **E**—ringworm? (11.13)

13. If leprosy bacilli infect a child with no immunity he will get—

A—lepromatous leprosy? **B**—borderline leprosy? **C**—tuberculoid leprosy? **D**—indeterminate leprosy? (12.2)

12. TB is caused by—

A—fungi? **B**—worms? **C**—bacteria? **D**—viruses? **E**—protozoa? (13.1)

13. BOGE is having a fit which has already lasted 20 minutes. He comes from a district where falciparum malaria is common. Which of these things would you NOT do?

A Take his temperature. **B** Give him paraldehyde. **C** Give him intramuscular chloroquine. **D** Lie him on his side. **E** Put something between his teeth to stop him biting his tongue. (15.9)

14. The cornea is—

A—the soft pink tissue under the eyelids? **B**—part of the back of the eye? **C**—the white part of the eye? **D**—the window in the front of the eye? **E**—a circle of blue or brown tissue? (16.2)

15. QUEENIE (18 months, 38·2 °C) woke up in the night crying and rubbing her ear. Her ear-drum and the deeper part of the meatus near it are red and dull. She has—

A—a foreign body in her ear? **B**—acute otitis media? **C**—chronic otitis externa? **D**—otitis externa? **E**—carious teeth? (17.9)

16. Children may get tetanus from—

A—large dirty wounds? **B**—chronic otitis media? **C**—infection of the umbilicus? **D**—infected burns? **E**—all of these? (14.3)

17. A child's throat should be examined—

A—at the end of the examination? **B**—at the beginning of the examination? **C**—in the middle of the examination? (18.2)

18. There are no lymph nodes—

A—under the jaws? B—round the eyes? C—in the axilla? D—in the groins? E—behind the ear? (19–1, 19–1b)

19. Which of these is NOT true? An inguinal hernia—
A—comes and goes quickly? B—may go away completely when a child lies down? C—usually cures itself in a few months? D—gets bigger when a child coughs, cries, or runs about? E—may become strangulated? (20.4)

20. USHA's mother says that USHA has passed a worm in her stools. Which of these is it most likely to be?
A *Ascaris* B *Trichuris* C Hookworm D *Strongyloides* E *H. nana* (21.3)

21. All these children have infective hepatitis. Which of them has NOT got one of the danger signs you would be worried about in a child with infective hepatitis?
A BLODWYN with severe jaundice. B GWYNNETH with severe vomiting. C GLYNNIS who is very drowsy. D GWEN who has pale urine and dark stools. E ELUNED who is bleeding from her nose. (22.11)

22. ANEKA has been treated for a urinary infection. She—
A—now has a strong natural active immunity? B—is still infectious? C—is more likely to get infections in other parts of her body? D—should drink fluid as little as possible? E—should be observed carefully because she may get more attacks? (23.4)

23. SAM (3 years) is late walking and talking. His muscles are hypotonic. There is a fold across the inner ends of his eyelids, and the back of his head is flat. He has one fold across the palms of his hands. He has—
A—a kind of backwardness we cannot diagnose? B—cerebral palsy? C—cretinism? D—a birth injury? E—Down's syndrome? (24.13)

24. A baby who starts vomiting between the ages of three and five weeks should be examined for—
A—hiatus hernia? B—intussusception? C—Inguinal hernia? D—pyloric stenosis? E—amoebic dysentery? (26.27)

25. You have examined both these newborn children for jaundice. Which of them is most severely jaundiced?
D TAMSIN whose head only is jaundiced E TOSIN who has jaundiced feet (26.23)

C.3. DOSES POSTEST
This mostly tests the use of the tables and figures in Chapter Three. Study 3-11b on page 34 of the manual carefully first. Do it with the manual open: Code 2

1. PRIMUS (17 kg) has TB and needs isoniazid. How much isoniazid are you going to give him at each dose?
A 200 mg B 75 mg C 100 mg D 150 mg

2. How many 100 mg tablets would you give him at each dose?

A Quarter B Half C Three quarters D One E One and a half.

3. What is the smallest dose he should be getting in mg/kg/day?
A 10 B 20 C 5 D 30 E 50

4. How many tablets would you give him to last until he comes back to see you in a month's time?
A 30 B 35 C 50 D 80 E 100

5. SECUNDUS also has TB and is much more ill than PRIMUS. How many mg/kg/day could you give SECUNDUS?
A 10 B 20 C 30 D 40 E 50

6. How often should he take his isoniazid?
A Twice a day B Once a day C Once a week D Twice a week E Once a month

7. TERTIUS is another child with TB. How long would you treat him with isoniazid for?
A Three days B Three weeks C Two years D One year E Three months

8. QUARTUS (3 months, 5 kg) is wheezing and cyanosed. How much adrenalin would you give him?
A None B 0·1 ml C 0·2 ml D 0·5 ml E 5 ml

9. QUINTUS (3 years, 13 kg) has pyoderma. He lives with his grandmother a long way away and cannot come to see you each day. Which of these would you give him?
A Procaine penicillin B Benzyl penicillin C Benethamine (depot) penicillin D Streptomycin

10. How would you give it?
A As capsules B As tablets C As a mixture D As a powder E As an injection

11. SEXTUS (15 kg) has tuberculoid leprosy. How much dapsone would you give him at each dose?
A 25 mg B Half a tablet C One tablet D One and a half tablets E 2000 mg

12. The shortest time SEXTUS should be treated for is for—
A—one year? B—15 months? C—18 months? D—two years?

13. SEPTIMUS (9 kg) has been treated for pneumonia with sulphadimidine for several days and is not recovering. You have decided to give him chloramphenicol. How much would you give him?
A Half a 250 mg capsule B 250 mg C 500 mg D 1000 mg

14. OCTAVUS (18 kg) has cerebral malaria. Your ampoules of quinine have 60 mg in each ml. How many ml would you give him?
A None B 0·5 ml C 2·5 ml D 3 ml E 4 ml

15. NONUS (19 kg) is drowsy. He has been vomiting and has had one fit. Falciparum malaria is common in the district. Your ampoules of chloroquine have 200 mg in 5 ml. How much would you give him?
A None B 1·9 ml C 2 ml D 3 ml E 4 ml

16. DECIMUS has chronic abdominal pain and diarrhoea sometimes. His stools shows 'Hookworm + +, Ascaris

+ +, Trichuris +, Strongyloides + +.' Which drug would kill all three worms?

A TCE (Tetrachlorethylene) **B** Bephenium **C** Tiabendazole **D** Piperazine **E** Pyrantel pamoate

17. PUBLIUS's mother DOMITIA says she feels weak. She looks anaemic and there are 'hookworms + + +' in her stools. How much TCE (tetrachlorethylene) would you give her?

A 3 ml **B** 5 ml **C** 35 ml **D** 3 ml the first day and 5 ml the second day **E** Any dose between 3 and 5 ml

18. JULIUS (10 kg, haemoglobin 5 g/dl) needs iron dextran by injection. How much would you give him?

A 3 ml **B** 15 ml **C** 10 ml **D** 20 ml **E** 25 ml

19. Baby SERVIUS (2 weeks, 3·5 kg) has stopped sucking. There is a septic sore with a large vesicle on his left arm. He has vomited twice and has diarrhoea. He is also slightly jaundiced. He probably has septicaemia. Which of them would you use?

A Penicillin alone **B** Tetracycline **C** Chloramphenicol **D** Ampicillin **E** Streptomycin alone

20. Which of these drugs would you NOT give SERVIUS?

B Ampicillin **C** Penicillin and streptomycin **D** Pencillin alone **E** Chloramphenicol

21. APPIUS (3 years, 11 kg) has had vomiting and diarrhoea for 3 days. His skin elasticity is much reduced. How much intravenous fluid would you give him fast?

A 20 ml **B** 220 ml **C** 280 ml **D** 350 ml **E** 400 ml

22. After he has had this fluid fast, how many ml of fluid does he need each hour during the next TWO hours?

A 75 ml **B** 100 ml **C** 125 ml **D** 150 ml **E** 200 ml

23. After two hours APPIUS has not yet started to drink. He has passed one liquid stool and his pulse is 130. What would you do?

A Go on with slow replacement. **B** Give him 20 ml/kg of intravenous fluid fast. **C** Stop the drip.

24. After two more hours APPIUS is still passing watery stools and has not passed any urine. What would you do?

A Give him 20 ml/kg of intravenous fluid fast. **B** Go on with slow replacement. **C** Stop the drip. **D** Count his pulse.

25. If APPIUS's pulse had been 160 in Question 23 what would you have done?

C Gone on with slow replacement. **D** Stopped the drip. **E** Given him 20 ml/kg of intravenous fluid fast.

C.4. WEIGHT CHART POSTEST
Code 2

1. In the place marked '1' on the chart I would write—
A—'On the pill.'? **B**—'IUD removed.'? **C**—'Acute diarrhoea.'? **D**—'Twins.'? **E**—'Father has a good job.'?

2. In the places marked '2' on the chart I would write—
B—'Child underweight.'? **C**—'Scabies.'? **D**—'Mother divorced.'? **E**—'Mother would like IUD.'?

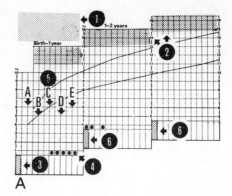

A

3. In the place marked '3' on the chart I would write—
A—the month the child was born? **B**—the day the child was born? **C**—the month in which a clinic is held? **D**—the month a child first became ill? **E**—the month the child first came to the clinic?

4. What do the dots record along the bottom of the weight chart?
A Iron injections **B** Immunization **C** Malaria suppression **D** Home visits **E** Injections of Vitamin A

5. A child should be given porridge for the first time in the month marked on the chart by the arrow at—
A ? **B** ? **C** ? **D** ? **E** ?

6. In the boxes marked '6' on the chart I would write—
A—January? **B**—the child's birth month? **C**—the date of the child's next visit to the clinic? **D**—the child's age? **E**—the month a child first came to the clinic?

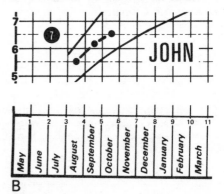

B

7. JOHN weighed—
A—6½ kg at the end of October? **B**—6½ kg in the first week of October? **C**—5 kg in August? **D**—6½ kg in the middle of October? **E**—6 kg in October?

8. Which of these children has the best growth curve?
A FRED **B** SID **C** BURT **D** ALF

9. This growth curve probably shows that a child has—
A—been breast-fed for too long? **B**—been bottle-fed? **C**—not been given enough porridge with added protein food? **D**—not been given enough vitamins? **E**—has kwashiorkor?

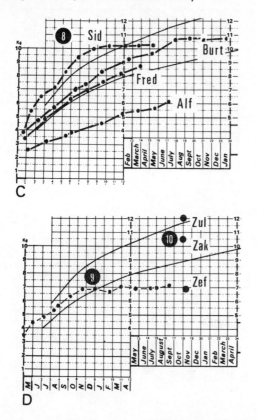

C

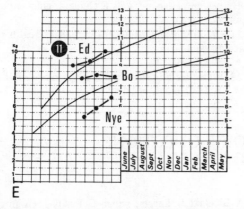

D

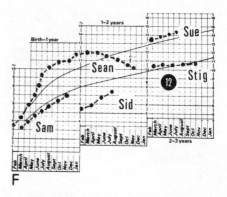

F

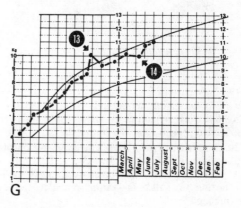

G

diarrhoea and dehydration? **C**—the oedema of kwashiorkor? **D**—very rapid growth? **E**—a very big meal?

14. This part of the growth curve is best explained by—
A—the oedema of kwashiorkor? **B**—better nutrition? **C**—chronic diarrhoea? **D**—a short illness and recovery from it? **E**—the child starting to eat porridge?

10. Which of these children might be malnourished?
A ZUL **B** ZAK **C** ZEF **D** None of them **E** Any of them might be

11. We should be worried about the nutrition of one of these children. Which one?
A BO **B** ED **C** NYE **D** All of them **E** None of them

E

12. One of these children probably needs hospital treatment. Which one?
A SAM **B** SID **C** SUE **D** SEAN **E** STIG

13. This dot is probably caused by—
A—a mistake in weighing or charting? **B**—acute

15. Two things are recorded on Okeke's weight chart. One of them is his weight. The other is his—
A—height? **B**—haemoglobin? **C**—temperature? **D**—treatments? **E**—arm circumference?

16. OKEKE's legs are swollen and he does not eat. His last weighing is best explained by—
A—measles? **B**—acute diarrhoea and dehydration? **C**—the oedema of kwashiorkor? **D**—TB? **E**—his becoming fatter?

17. OKEKE's growth curve in the place shown by the brackets is best explained by—
A—being sent away from his mother and being unhappy? **B**—TB? **C**—eating cassava only? **D**—chronic diarrhoea? **E**—any of these things?

18. Which of these would have made baby UNA grow in the way shown by this part of her growth curve?
A Bottle-feeding with dried skim-milk **B** Bottle-feeding with full-cream milk, 100 ml/kg, three feeds a day **C** Breast-feeding from birth and porridge from the 4th month of life **D** Plenty of vitamins

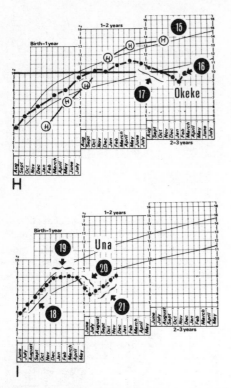

H

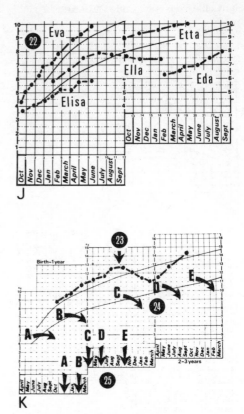

J

I

K

19. This part of UNA's growth curve was probably caused by not giving her enough—

A—fluids? **B**—vitamins? **C**—breast milk? **D**—porridge with added protein food? **E**—minerals?

20. This part of UNA's growth curve was probably caused by lack of food and by—

A—lack of vitamins? **B**—breast-feeding for too long? **C**—starting to walk? **D**—eating porridge too early? **E**—infections?

21. Which of these things would NOT have helped UNA's growth curve to rise in the way shown?

A—breast milk? **B**—extra vitamins? **C**—energy food? **D**—protein? **E**—four meals a day?

22. The mother of one of these children did not have enough breast milk. Which one?

A ELISA **B** EDA **C** ETTA **D** EVA **E** ELLA

23. This child was ill at the place shown by the arrow. Which three diseases are most likely to have caused the growth curve you see?

A TB, measles, or whooping cough **B** Septicaemia, scabies, or ringworm **C** Thrush, tonsillitis, or tapeworms **D** Herpes, impetigo, or boils **E** Cholera, chickenpox, or leprosy

24. Children usually fall off the road to health at the place marked—

A ? **B** ? **C** ? **D** ? **E** ?

25. Breast-feeding should end at the place marked—

A ? **B** ? **C** ? **D** ? **E** or later?

POSTEST MULTIPLE-CHOICE QUESTIONS
OF THE 'CHAPTER SERIES.'

DIFFICULT WORDS POSTEST C
Chapter 1: Code 8

MATCH these words with the explanations for them.
1. De- **2.** Obstructed **3.** Contracted **4.** Transparent **5.** Dilated

A Blocked **B** Larger, wider **C** Easily seen through **D** Without **E** Shorter, narrower

All these words describe a sick child. MATCH them with their explanation.

6. Unconscious 7. Irritable 8. Restless 9. Delirious 10. Drowsy

A Unhappy, easily made angry B Seems to be asleep but cannot be awakened C Always moving about D Abnormally sleepy but can be awakened E Talks nonsense and does not know where he is

MATCH these words with the parts of the body they describe.

11. Buttock 12. Spleen 13. Conjunctivae 14. Anus 15. Axilla

A An organ in the upper left side of the abdomen B The last part of the gut C The space under the arm D Thin wet mucosa inside the eyelids E The parts of our body we sit on

MATCH these words with the explanations for them—

16. Disabled 17. Anaemic 18. Jaundiced 19. Cyanosed 20. Deformed

A Not able to live a normal life B Having yellow eyes and skin C Having blue lips and skin (if he is a child with a light skin) D Having an abnormally shaped body E Lacking haemoglobin

21. Saline is made from water and—
A—sugar? B—salt? C—sodium bicarbonate? D—glucose? E—potassium chloride?

22. ADE has been brought to see you because he cannot see in the dark. He also has mild diarrhoea, and is underweight. His conjunctivae are dry, he has swollen ankles and some skin lesions. You diagnose vitamin A deficiency and kwashiorkor. He is severely ill and needs treatment quickly. His presenting symptom is—
A—kwashiorkor? B—diarrhoea? C—dry conjunctivae? D—not being able to see at night? E—swollen ankles?

23. Which of these is NOT in the head?
A The rectum B The sclerae C The conjunctivae D The scalp E The gums

24. Which of these shows that something does not happen?
A Rarely B Occasionally C Never D Sometimes E Usually

25. What colour is haemoglobin?
A Green B Blue C White D Red E Yellow

DISEASE IN THE CHILD C
Chapter 2: Code 3

1. Which of these two kinds of disease are most often found together in the same child?
A Malnutrition and accidents B Malnutrition and tumours C Infections and accidents D Hereditary diseases and congenital diseases E Malnutrition and infection (2.1)

2. Which of these are the smallest?

A Bacteria B Protozoa C Viruses D Fungi E Worms (2–1)

3. Micro-organisms are killed if they are—
A—heated? B—cooled? C—heated or cooled? (2.2b)

4. Tenderness in a lymph-node is a sign—
A—that infection is staying in the local lesions? B—that there is no need for antibiotics? C—of chronic infection? D—that a child has septicaemia? E—of acute lymphadenitis? (2.4)

5. Which of these is NOT a local sign of acute septic skin infection?
A Redness B Warmth C Swelling D Scaling E Pain (2.4)

6. Which of these diseases almost always kills a child unless he is treated?
A TB B Tonsillitis C Purulent meningitis D Measles E Bronchitis (2.1)

7. Which of these words tells us that a disease lasts a long time?
A Severe B Chronic C Infectious D Preventable E Mild (2.1)

8. BIANCA has a severe hookworm infection. In which of these ways was she probably infected?
A Faeces-to-mouth B By larvae going through her skin C By inhaling infected droplets D By contact E By a dirty needle (2.7)

MATCH these diseases with the kind of organism that causes them—

9. Malaria 10. Thrush 11. Boils 12. Measles
A Bacteria B Protozoa C Viruses D Fungi E Worms (2.2)

13. After lymph has gone through the lymph nodes it goes into—
A—the tissues? B—the heart? C—the arteries? D—the urine? E—lymph vessels and then into the veins? (2–3)

14. OSAMU has secondarily infected scabies. What kind of organism is causing his primary infection?
A Fungi B Insects C Bacteria D Protozoa E Worms (2.6)

15. What kind of organism is causing his secondary infection?
A Fungi B Insects C Bacteria D Protozoa E Worms (2.6)

16. Which of the organisms that are infecting OSAMU can be killed by drugs?
A The primary organism B The secondary organism C Neither of them D Both of them (2.6)

MATCH these with the diseases they prevent—

17. Boiling a child's drinking water 18. Making a child's home safe for him 19. Plenty of washing with soap and water 20. Killing mosquito larvae
A Malaria B Accidents C Skin sepsis D Diarrhoea E TB (2.7)

21. ANNA has an abscess on her left elbow. It is probably caused by—

A—viruses? B—fungi? C—protozoa? D—worms? E—bacteria? (2.4)

22. When you examine ANNA you should look for lymphadenitis in her left—

A—shoulder? B—groin? C—hand? D—axilla? E—neck? (2–5)

23. ANNA has a pale skin. If she had acute lymphangitis, where would you expect the red lines on her skin to go—

B—down towards her hand? C—round her arm? D—towards her axilla and her hand? E—up towards her axilla? (2–4)

24. One of the steps in making the community diagnosis is to decide how manageable a disease is. Which of these best explains the 'manageability' of a disease?

A How easy it is to prevent or cure B How easy it is to prevent C How easy it is to cure D How many children die from it E How infectious it is (2.10)

25. In some hot districts it is the custom to pour cold water over the body of a child with a fit. Is this—

A—a bad custom? B—a good custom? C—a harmless custom? D—a custom it is hard to be sure about? (2.9)

DRUGS C
Chapter 3: Code 7

MATCH these diseases with the drugs you would use to treat them—

1. Septicaemia in babies **2.** Acute otitis media **3.** Trachoma **4.** TB **5.** Amoebic dysentery

A Thiacetazone and isoniazid B Penicillin and sulphadimidine C Chlortetracycline eye ointment D Penicillin and streptomycin E Metronidazole (3.14, 3.17, 3.21, 3.22, 3.26)

MATCH these diseases or symptoms with the drugs that can be used to treat them—

6. TB **7.** Malaria **8.** Fever **9.** *Ascaris* **10.** Fits

A Paracetamol B Chloroquine C Aminosalicylate (PAS) D Piperazine E Paraldehyde (3.2, 3.23, 3.25, 3.28, 3.42, 3.44)

MATCH these diseases with drugs you would use to treat them with—

11. A severe allergic reaction after injecting antitetanus serum (ATS) **12.** Cholera **13.** Anaemia **14.** Xerophthalmia **15.** Poisoning with iron tablets

A Folic acid B Vitamin A C Ipecacuanha D Glucose-salt solution E Adrenalin (3.35, 3.37, 3.47, 3.17)

16. CANDY is being given sulphadimidine because she has a urinary infection. What would you tell her mother?

A 'Give her plenty of fluids.' B 'Rest her bladder by giving her less fluid.' C 'She may infect other children.' D 'Don't give her too many of these tablets or her teeth will go yellow.' E 'Three days treatment is enough.' (3.14, 23.4)

17. With which drug are large doses LEAST dangerous?

A Chloroquine B Adrenalin C Penicillin D Thiacetazone E Quinine (3.14, 3.22, 3.25, 3.40)

18. In a standard teaspoon there are—

A—4 ml? B—3 ml? C—6 ml? D—5 ml? E—10 ml? (3–1)

19. Which of these is the only really safe way of giving an intramuscular injection?

A Giving each child a separate sterile needle, and using the same syringe for ten children only. B Using a separate sterile syringe and sterile needle for each child. C Sterilizing syringes and needles with sterile distilled water. D Sterilizing syringes and needles in spirit. E Sterilizing syringes and needles in a refrigerator. (3.5)

20. All these drugs, EXCEPT one, are useful for treating worm infections. Which one?

A Metrifonate B Niclosamide C Pyrantel pamoate. D Bephenium E Metronidazole (3.26)

21. KAWAMBWA (1 month) has a severe septic infection. What would you give him?

A Penicillin B Penicillin and streptomycin C Chloroquine D Penicillin and isoniazid E Streptomycin (3.21, 26.24)

22. Which of these drugs most often causes a severe allergic reaction?

A Streptomycin B Isoniazid C Sulphadimidine D Tetracycline E Penicillin (3.14)

23. BILLY (10 kg) needs chloramphenicol. The dose is 50 mg/kg/day and it has to be given four times a day. How much does he need at each dose?

A 125 mg B 100 mg C 250 mg D 500 mg E 500 mg

24. Which of these drugs has to be given for the longest time?

A Streptomycin B Sulphadimidine C Dapsone D Isoniazid E Iron (3.20, 3.24, 3.33)

25. Which of these can dissolve some kinds of plastic syringe?

A Phenobarbitone B Paracetamol C Promethazine D Pyrimethamine E Paraldehyde (3.44)

HEALTHY CHILD C
Chapter 4: Code 8

1. Which of these diseases may be common in the children coming to a clinic without causing symptoms?

A Meningitis B Pneumonia C Tonsillitis D Vitamin A deficiency E Acute otitis media (4.11)

2. Which of these would you NOT do every time a healthy child comes to a clinic?

A Examine his abdomen B Weigh him C Tell his mother when to come again D Praise his mother E Make sure his mother learns something (4.12)

3. If a disease is very common in a district all the children in a clinic may need treating even if they have not got symptoms. Which of these drugs is NEVER used to treat every child in this way?

A Pyrimethamine B Piperazine C Vitamin A D Pyrantel pamoate E Isoniazid (4.11)

4. When healthy children come to the clinic I would—
A—examine them with all their clothes on? B—look for signs of vitamin C deficiency? C—chart their weights? D—care for them all in exactly the same way? E—only give them one immunization at each visit? (4.12, 4.13)

5. Your clinic is busy and full. Which of these children LEAST needs to be seen again soon?

A The child from a problem family B The child with ringworm C The bottle-fed child D The child in the special-care register E The very young child (4.14)

MATCH these vaccines with the sentences which describe them

6. Measles 7. Polio 8. DPT 9. BCG 10. Tetanus toxoid

A Prevents a disease which causes muscle wasting. B Should be given at the age of nine months. C Prevents a disease which causes coughing and vomiting. D Is given to pregnant mothers to protect their children. E Causes a scar. (4.2, 4.6, 4.8, 4.8b, 4.9)

Each of these vaccines protects a child against one (or more) diseases. MATCH each vaccine with the way the disease often presents—

11. Measles 12. Polio 13. The 'D' part of DPT vaccine 14. BCG 15. Tetanus toxoid.

A A weak leg B Loss of weight, cough, and mild fever for several weeks C Not sucking, not able to open his mouth, muscle spasms D A sore throat with membrane on the tonsils E Cough, fever, and red eyes for a few days (4.2, 4.6, 4.8, 4.8b, 4.9)

16. Which of these vaccines should NOT be put in the freezing part of a refrigerator?

A DPT B Polio C Measles D BCG (4.10)

17. Which of these vaccines would you NOT expect to cause fever?

C Measles D DPT E Polio (4.8, 4.8b, 4.9)

18. Which of these vaccines must be given intradermally?

A Polio B BCG C Measles D DPT E Tetanus toxoid (4.6)

19. Which of these vaccines should be given with a 1 ml tuberculin ('Microstat') syringe?

A DPT B Measles C BCG D Polio E Tetanus toxoid. (4.2, 4.6, 4.8, 4.8b, 4.9)

20. If a live vaccine is not kept cold in a refrigerator in the right way, it—

A—must be cooled again for 24 hours before being used? B—can be used for up to a week? C—causes the disease it should prevent? D—becomes useless after a few hours? E—becomes harmful? (4.10)

21. Which of these vaccines is dead?

B DPT C BCG D Polio E Measles (4.6, 4.8, 4.8b, 4.9)

22. What kind of immunity protects the child of an immune mother from measles or malaria until he is about six months old?

B Natural active immunity C Artificial passive immunity D Natural passive immunity E Artificial active immunity (4.2)

23. Measles vaccine is—

A—only given to a child once? B—dangerous if it is given to a child less than 6 months old? C—usually given to children at the age of 3 years? D—usually given to children at birth? E—the least easily killed of all the vaccines? (4.8a)

24. EUGENE (6 months) was given BCG a few weeks ago. He now has an ulcer at the place where he was immunized, and some painless swellings in his axilla. Which of these would you give him?

A Penicillin B Sulphadimidine C A dry dressing on the ulcer D Streptomycin E Isoniazid (4.6)

25. KABAN was given his first DPT injection last week, and another DPT injection this week. He will get—

A—more immunity than other children. B—no immunity? C—dangerous side effects? D—less immunity than other children immunized at the right time? (4.5)

SICK CHILD C
Chapter 5: Code 7

MATCH these diseases with the signs they cause—

1. Lower respiratory infection 2. Kwashiorkor 3. Meningitis 4. Diarrhoea

A Loss of skin elasticity B Thin pale hair C Fits D Insuction E Enlarged tonsillar lymph-nodes (5.17)

MATCH these specimens with the special tests that a health centre laboratory can do on them—

5. Blood 6. Urine 7. CSF 8. 'Sellotape' swab

A Threadworms B Pandy's test C Ova of *Schistosoma haematobium* D AAFB E Haematocrit (5.19)

9. A 'local events calendar' helps us to find a child's—

A—weight for height? B—diagnosis? C—weight? D—weight for age? E—arm circumference? (7.1)

10. When you examine young children you should—

A—sit at the other side of the table from the child's mother? B—always feel their fontanelle? C—leave the easiest part of the examination until last? D—keep their clothes on as much as possible? E—examine them on their mothers' knees? (5.2)

11. Before you start weighing children, you should make sure that—

A—all the children have emptied their bladders? B—there is no cloth or plastic sheet on the balance? C—children are not crying? D—you have enough time to do all the weighing yourself? E—the balance is set to '0'? (5.3)

12. If a mother can get antenatal care, advice about family planning and care for a well or sick child in the same place she gets—

A—intensive care? **B**—continuity of care? **C**—individual care? **D**—integrated care? **E**—curative care? (5.2)

13. Which of these has the steps in caring for a sick child in the WRONG order?

A Management, family planning, explanation **B** Weighing, history **C** History, examination, special tests **D** Special tests, diagnosis, management **E** Family planning, recording, and reporting (5.1)

14. When children are being cared for in a clinic—

A—waiting mothers should be standing outside? **B**—mothers and children should see the same health worker at each visit? **C**—workers must spend the same length of time on each child? **D**—very sick children should be examined last? **E**—you should weigh every child yourself? (5.2)

15. Which of these CANNOT be used as a milestone for development?

A Smiling **B** Standing **C** Sucking **D** Walking **E** Talking (24.10, 5.10)

16. Which of these is part of a child's nutrition history?

A 'Is he breast-fed?' **B** 'Can he talk?' **C** 'Have any of his brothers or sisters died?' **D** 'Has he been to hospital?' **E** 'Has he had whooping cough?' (5.11)

17. Which of these are likely to be most dangerous? Symptoms which—

B—the child has had before and recovered from before? **C**—are getting worse? **D**—are getting better? **E**—have lasted a long time? (5.6)

18. A child is LEAST likely to be severely ill if he—

A—is cyanosed? **B**—is in coma? **C**—is hypothermic? **D**—cries loudly when he is examined? **E**—has stridor and insuction? (5:2)

19. Which of these children is well?

A GRACIELA who is having fits. **B** PABLO who is talking and laughing. **C** NARCISA who has a temperature below 35 °C. **D** FELIPA who seems to be asleep but cannot be woken up. **E** JUANA who is irritable and restless. (5:2)

20. A child is probably only mildly ill if he—

A—has had fits? **B**—is delirious? **C**—has sunken eyes? **D**—is in shock? **E**—fights when he is examined? (5.15)

21. Which part of a child would you examine last?

A The part of his body which is causing symptoms **B** The part that will make him fight most **C** The lower part of his body **D** The easiest part to examine **E** The parts of him which are not causing symptoms (5.16)

22. When would you examine a child's breathing?

A After his throat has been examined **B** While he is crying **C** While he is running about **D** At the end of the examination **E** While he is quiet before you do anything to him (5.17)

23. Which of these diseases needs treatment for the shortest time?

A Tonsillitis **B** TB **C** Leprosy **D** Anaemia (5.24)

24. EULALIA was born this morning. Her mother is very poor and she wants another child. When should this other child be born? After—

A—two years? **B**—two and a half years? **C**—three years or more? **D**—one and a half years? **E**—one year? (5.25)

25. Koplik's spots are diagnostic for—

A—thrush? **B**—chickenpox? **C**—ringworm? **D**—vitamin A deficiency? **E**—measles? (5.20)

RECORDING AND REPORTING C
Chapter 6: with revision: Code 8

MATCH these worms with the drugs used for treating them—

1. Strongyloides **2.** Threadworms **3.** Hookworms **4.** Tapeworms

A Piperazine **B** Thiacetazone **C** Niclosamide **D** Tiabendazole **E** Tetrachlorethylene (3.22, 3.27, 3.28, 3.29, 3.30 (Revision))

5. Home-based records—

A—do not need to be kept in a plastic bag? **B**—save the time of the workers in a clinic? **C**—don't teach families anything? **D**—should be left at home when a child comes to a clinic? **E**—should be left at home when a child goes to hospital? (6.2)

6. Health workers should—

A—use all the records they are using already and also any new ones? **B**—use only those records which help somebody to decide something? **C**—not let patients see their own records? **D**—make records which only they themselves can understand? (6.1)

7. A health worker should keep—

A—as few records as are absolutely necessary? **B**—as many records as possible? **C**—copies of all the records he gives to the patients? (6.1)

8. Which of these things would you be LEAST likely to record on a child's weight chart?

A His father's job **B** What kind of family planning is being used **C** His mother's haemoglobin **D** When he had severe diarrhoea **E** Immunization against measles (6.2, 7.1)

9. Which of these is NOT useful for treating acute septic infections?

A Ampicillin **B** Tetracycline **C** Benzathine penicillin **D** Chloramphenicol **E** Chloroquine (3.13 (Revision))

10. Which of these is the LEAST likely reason for putting a child on the special-care register?

A Twins **B** Malnutrition **C** Backwardness **D** Tonsillitis **E** TB (6.3)

11. A special-care register helps health workers to—
A—make better diagnoses? B—care for more children?
C—care for all the children in a clinic better? D—give better care to children who are acutely ill? E—visit the children who most need visiting? (6.3)

12. SARANYA (2 years) has a severe lower respiratory infection and needs penicillin. Unfortunately, your penicillin is finished. Which of these drugs could you use instead?
A Chloramphenicol B Dapsone C Sulphadoxine with pyrimethamine D Pyrantel pamoate E Metrifonate (3.11)

13. Which of these is the shorthand for a disease?
A DSM B PPF C AFB D PEM E BCG (6:1)

14. Which of these drugs is NOT used on the skin?
A Benzyl benzoate B Pyrimethamine C Gammexane
D Calamine E Gentian violet (3.48 (Revision))

15. Which of these is a way of giving injections?
A HW B FH C IM D BS E HB (6:1)

16. About how many of the people in your district are children under five? About one child in every—
A—6 people? B—8 people? C—10 people? D—4 people? E—12 people? (6.10)

17. The average number of times each child in the community comes to a clinic each year is a measure of—
A—output? B—the health of the community? C—how sick children are? D—input? E—coverage? (6.7)

18. Which of these CANNOT be used to sterilize something?
A Boiling water B Sterile water C A pressure cooker
D A flame E Steam (2.2b, 6.13)

19. Children in the special-care register should be—
A—seen on separate days from the other children?
B—given a special record to take home with them?
C—visited if they do not come to the clinic? D—given a different kind of weight chart from the other children?
E—punished if they do not come to the clinic? (6.3)

20. A pressure cooker should—
A—be heated while the handles are separated (apart) from one another? B—be used three quarters full of liquid? C—be heated slowly at first and then more strongly later? D—always have some water in it? E—be opened when it is full of steam? (6.13)

21. Sterilizing in a pressure-cooker is better than sterilizing by boiling because—
A—it sterilizes more slowly? B—it uses less fuel? C—it uses more water? D—it cleans instruments? E—instruments are covered with water? (6.13)

22. A pressure-cooker should—
A—be used with its vent closed from the time that sterilization starts? B—not be cooled too quickly? C—be heated with the lid off to begin with? D—never be filled to the top with water? (6.13)

23. Organisms are most easily killed by—
A—steam at 120 °C? B—hot air at 120 °C? C—water at 100 °C? D—water at 0 °C? E—water at 37 °C? (6.13)

24. The antibiotics that we commonly use in a clinic kill—
A—fungi? B—worms? C—the bacteria causing septic infections? D—viruses? E—all of these? (3.11, 3.12, 3.13 (Revision))

25. When you sterilize equipment in a pressure-cooker, you should start counting the time from the moment you—
A—put the weight on the vent? B—light the stove?
C—start heating? D—turn the heat down when steam starts coming out strongly from under the weight? E—put the lid on? (6.13)

NUTRITION C
Chapter 7: Code 4

1. Which of these children is in the greatest danger from malnutrition. The child whose growth curve is—
A—above the road to health and has been flat for one month? B—following the lower line closely? C—above the road to health but falling? D—on the road to health and rising? E—below the road to health and rising? (7.1)

2. The arm circumference of a healthy two-year-old child should be—
A—under 10 cm? B—over 18 cm? C—between 12 and 14 cm? D—under 14 cm? E—over 14 cm? (7.13, N 1.5)

3. Which of these things is LEAST likely to cause PEM in a child?
A Breast-feeding him until he is two years old (as well as giving him other foods) B Whooping cough C Many attacks of diarrhoea D Customs which prevent him or his mother eating protein foods E Too many people in the district and not enough land (7.2)

4. Underweight children—
A—learn as well as other children in school? B—get more severe infections than healthy children? C—grow up taller than healthy children? D—are easily diagnosed by looking at them? E—are above the road-to-health on their weight charts? (N 2.1)

5. Which child is likely to have the lowest weight for his age?
D The child with kwashiorkor E The child with marasmus (7.9, 7.10)

6. Which of these contains the LEAST protein?
A Rice B Cassava C Maize D Millet E Groundnuts (N 3–5)

7. Which vitamin deficiency is most often seen in malnourished children? Deficiency of—
A—vitamin C? B—vitamin D? C—vitamin E? D—vitamin A? E—vitamin K? (7.11)

PLEASE DO NOT WRITE ON THESE QUESTIONS SOMEONE ELSE MAY NEED THEM

8. Supplementary foods, such as dried skim-milk—

A—should be given to all the children coming to a clinic? **B**—can be given to mothers instead of health education? **C**—should be given to mothers to make them bring their children to the clinic? **D**—should be mixed with a child's ordinary food? **E**—should be given to a child instead of his ordinary food? (7.6)

9. A mother should breast-feed her baby until he is—

A—a year old? **B**—at least 18 months old? **C**—at least two years old? **D**—3 years old? (7.2)

10. A mother tells you that dried skim-milk gives her malnourished child diarrhoea. What would you tell her?

A 'Dried skim-milk never does this.' **B** 'Your child is intolerant to lactose.' **C** 'Feed it to him in a feeding-bottle.' **D** 'His diarrhoea will soon stop.' **E** 'Mix this dried skim-milk into his porridge; don't give it to him to drink.' (7.6, 9.14)

11. Which of these is NOT caused by a lack of protein and energy food?

A Keratomalacia **B** Marasmus **C** Kwashiorkor **D** The 'underweight child'. **E** Marasmic kwashiorkor (16.13)

12. Badly managed bottle-feeding is most likely to cause—

A—kwashiorkor? **B**—vitamin B deficiency? **C**—marasmus? **D**—worms? **E**—rickets? (7.9)

MATCH these descriptions with the foods that fit them—

13. The best energy food **14.** Contains too much sugar for feeding to babies **15.** A staple food **16.** Prevents xerophthalmia

A Evaporated milk **B** Maize **C** Cooking oil **D** Sweetened condensed milk **E** Green leaves (N chapters 3 and 4)

17. Which of these is NOT true?

A Milk which is left over from one bottle-feed can be used at the next feed. **B** Bottle-feeding needs much water and fuel. **C** Badly managed bottle-feeding causes diarrhoea. **D** Bottle-feeds must be made with boiled water. **E** Feeding-bottles can be sterilized with hypochlorite. (N 8.1)

18. Which of these contains the highest percentage protein?

A Dried beans **B** Dried fish **C** Eggs **D** Fresh fish **E** Meat (N 3–6)

19. Plant proteins—

A—are more expensive than animal protein? **B**—are found in plenty in foods such as cassava and sago? **C**—when mixed together are almost as good as animal protein? **D**—are necessary to give a child energy? **E**—are not important for the nutrition of village families? (N 3.5)

20. Malnutrition—

A—is made worse by infection? **B**—cannot be prevented? **C**—can only be treated by injections of drugs? **D**—has the same causes in every community? **E**—is more common in its severe forms than in its mild forms? (7.5, 7.8)

21. We most often see malnourished children—

A—at school? **B**—before birth? **C**—during the early months of breast-feeding? **D**—while a child is changing over from breast-feeding to adult food? **E**—when a child is fully able to feed himself with adult food? (7.1)

22. Mothers should be taught about—

A—what the letters PEM mean? **B**—joules? **C**—bulk? **D**—lactose? **E**—the underweight child? (10.11)

23. Children with kwashiorkor—

A—can be cured with vitamins? **B**—are always very severely wasted? **C**—are hungry? **D**—are usually happy? **E**—can sometimes be on the road-to-health or even above it? (7.10)

24. Nutrition education—

A—should be done by specially trained workers only? **B**—should only be done on special days each month? **C**—does not need evaluation? **D**—is the most important step in treating a malnourished child? **E**—does not need recording? (2.11 N Chapter 10)

25. A severely malnourished child is LEAST likely to need treatment for—

A—TB? **B**—worms? **C**—diarrhoea? **D**—malaria? **E**—asthma? (7.11)

COUGH C
Chapter 8: Code 6

1. One of these kinds of organism most often causes secondary infection in the respiratory tract. It can be treated with the common antibiotics. Which is it?

A Viruses **B** Worms **C** Bacteria **D** Protozoa **E** Fungi (8.3)

2. Acute infections of the lower respiratory tract—

A—often kill children? **B**—can usually be treated with cough mixture only? **C**—can be treated with one injection of procaine penicillin? **D**—are more serious in older children than in babies? **E**—are more common than infections of the upper respiratory tract? (8.1)

3. In children TB usually presents as—

A—chest pain? **B**—wheezing? **C**—stridor? **D**—a chronic cough with blood-stained sputum? **E**—loss of weight? (8.1)

4. Which of these are NOT parts of the lower respiratory tract?

A The bronchioles **B** The nasal cavities **C** The trachea **D** The alveoli **E** The bronchi (8.2)

5. Children with pneumonia—

A—can be treated with cough mixture only? **B**—must be sent to hospital? **C**—breathe faster than normal? **D**—should be given fluids only until they are well? **E**—wheeze? (8.15)

6. HALFDAN (2 years, 11 kg, 37·0 °C) has a discharging nose and a cough. He is eating normally. Which of these would you give him?

A Ampicillin B Tetracycline C Penicillin D Ephedrine tablets E None of these things (8.7)

7. Which of these is NOT a sign of a lower respiratory disease?

A Insuction B Cyanosis C Wheezing D A large spleen E Moving nose (8.9)

8. SULAIMAN (3 years) has had a cough for about ten days. He now coughs in spasms. After a spasm of coughing he makes a loud noise as he breathes in and then vomits. He has—

A—diphtheria? B—TB? C—obstructive laryngitis? D—whooping cough? E—chronic lower respiratory infection (8.17)

9. Which of these would have prevented SULAIMAN's disease, or made it less severe?

A Boiling his drinking water B Penicillin injections C More protein and energy food D BCG vaccine E DPT vaccine (8.17)

10. Postural drainage—

A—can be done by mothers at home? B—can be used to treat upper respiratory infections? C—is only useful in young babies? D—needs special equipment? E—cures a post nasal drip? (8.5)

11. NAKALIMA (4 years) had a cough and a nasal discharge a few days ago. Her cough has got worse, her breathing has become difficult, and she has begun to wheeze. She is irritable and restless. Last year she had two attacks like this. What is her diagnosis?

A Whooping cough B Asthma C Bronchiolitis D Bronchitis (8.13)

TAM (2 years, 17 kg, 37·2 °C). Four weeks ago he had a nasal discharge, a cough, and a mild fever. A health worker thought he had a cold, and gave him chloramphenicol capsules for three days. He often has colds, his mother always wants treatment for them, and he has often been given chloramphenicol before.

Last week he became very ill with a very severe sore throat, anaemia, and a high fever. He was sent to hospital but he died in a few days. The doctor there said that he died because his white cells had been harmed. He died because—

12. A—colds should not be treated with chloramphenicol? B—a two-year-old child is too young to be given chloramphenicol? C—he was not given chloramphenicol for long enough? D—he did not go to hospital soon enough? E—he was given chloramphenicol capsules instead of chloramphenicol syrup? (3.18)

13. Which of these diseases is most likely to cause severe stridor, cyanosis, and insuction?

A Tonsillitis B Bronchiolitis C Asthma D Bronchitis E Obstructive laryngitis (8.11)

14. Diphtheria sometimes causes—

A—asthma? B—bronchiolitis? C—obstruction of the larynx? D—bronchitis? E—pneumonia? (8.11)

15. The most common cause of wheezing in an older child is—

A—pneumonia? B—TB? C—a foreign body in his bronchus? D—asthma? E—worms in his lungs? (8.13)

16. Which of these children would you give chloramphenicol to?

A MERIDA (4 years) who has been whooping for two weeks. B MUTEBA (2 months) has fever and a cough. Her older brother has whooping cough. C MILLIAM (18 months) who has tonsillitis. D MAIKO (2 years) who has asthma. E MAKINA (2 years) who has an upper respiratory infection. (8.17)

17. JOKO (2 years) has sudden spasms of very severe coughing and cyanosis. He is well for a few hours and then has another attack. Which of these diseases would explain his symptoms? It is also the least common of these diseases. He has been immunized with DPT.

A Obstructive laryngitis B Foreign body in his bronchus C Measles D Bronchitis E Bronchiolitis (8.18)

18. Which of these diseases causes the LEAST insuction?

A Obstructive laryngitis B Pneumonia C Dehydration with acidotic breathing D Asthma E Bronchiolitis (8.9)

19. Which of these is NOT a complication of whooping cough?

A Marasmus B TB C Pneumonia D Measles E Fits (8.17)

20. Most children who come to a clinic with a cough should be given—

A—cough mixture or nothing? B—depot penicillin? C—sulphadimidine? D—tetracycline? E—ephedrine? (8.20)

21. KULISTINA (3 years) has started coughing today. Some of her friends have whooping cough. She will probably start whooping in about—

A—6 weeks? B—three weeks? C—ten days? D—three days? E—one day? (8.17)

22. PETERO has stridor. The most important sign to look for is—

A—a red throat? B—fast breathing? C—moving nose? D—wheezing? E—insuction? (8.20)

23. Which of these diseases causes the most difficulty breathing out?

A Pneumonia B Asthma C Obstructive laryngitis. D Diphtheria E Bronchitis (8.13)

24. Which of these is NOT one of the danger signs that you would teach mothers to watch for when their children have a cough?

A Fast breathing B Moving nose C Going blue (cyanosis) D Obstruction of the nose (8.20)

25. KEAMOKA (8 months) is coughing and wheezing. He is cyanosed and has insuction. His respiratory rate is 56. He has—

A—an upper respiratory infection? B—septicaemia? C—asthma? D—bronchiolitis? E—diphtheria? (8.14)

DIARRHOEA C
Chapter 9: Code 5

1. Infections outside the gut most easily cause diarrhoea in—

A—girls? B—adults? C—school children? D—children between 2 and 6 years? E—children under 2 years? (9.10)

2. Which of these things is LEAST likely to cause diarrhoea?

A A food which has been spoiled by organisms growing in it B Infections inside the gut C Tetanus D Malaria E Tonsillitis (9.2 to 9.13)

3. When a child has dysentery he has—

A—diarrhoea with abdominal pain? B—yellow frothy diarrhoea? C—watery diarrhoea? D—diarrhoea with blood and mucus in his stools? E—rice water stools? (9.3)

4. The most sudden and severe dehydration is caused by—

A—amoebic dysentery? B—cholera? C—bacillary dysentery? D—giardiasis? E—malnutrition? (9.7)

5. ICABOD (1 month) has diarrhoea and fever. Which of these things is LEAST likely to be causing his symptoms?

A Septicaemia B An infected artificial feed C A septic skin infection D A gut infection E Too much breast milk (9.10, 26.32)

6. ZOYA (4 years, 11 kg) has had mild diarrhoea for several months. She is not dehydrated. Her mother says that if she gives her more food she passes more liquid stools. She has therefore stopped feeding Zoya so that her stools should get less. What would you tell ZOYA's mother?

B 'Here is some medicine (sulphaguanidine).' C 'She is losing much fluid in her stools. Give her this glucose–salt solution.' D 'You must feed her well. She may pass more stools, but she will also take more food into her body.' E 'Stop giving her solid food until her diarrhoea is cured.' (9.13)

7. Marasmus and dehydration can both cause—

A—a swollen fontanelle? B—hyperpyrexia? C—loss of skin elasticity? D—a dry mouth? E—a fast, weak pulse? (9.12)

8. Heavy infections with any of these worms EXCEPT one may cause diarrhoea. Which one?

A Hookworms B *Schistosoma mansoni* C Trichuris D *Strongyloides* (9.5)

9. The breathing of a child with acidotic breathing is different from a child with pneumonia because it is—

A—less regular? B—deeper? C—shallower? D—more regular? E—noisy? (9.18)

10. Dehydration makes a young child's fontanelle—

A—sink and pulsate less? B—sink and pulsate more? C—swell and pulsate more? D—swell and pulsate less? (9.18)

11. A child's skin should be tested for elasticity—

A—at the side of his abdomen? B—on his arms? C—on his head? D—over his ankles? E—at his umbilicus? (9.18)

12. Which of these is NOT true?

A Diarrhoea can cause malnutrition. B Salt-and-sugar water is a better rehydration fluid than glucose–salt solution. C All children with acute watery diarrhoea are dehydrated. D Too much salt or sugar in a rehydration fluid is dangerous. E The worst treatment for diarrhoea is to stop giving fluids. (9.21)

13. Glucose–salt solution also contains—

B—potassium chloride and sodium carbonate? C—sodium chloride and potassium chlorate? D—sodium chloride and potassium bicarbonate? E—sodium bicarbonate and potassium chloride? (9.21)

14. Which of these is NOT true? Salt-and-sugar water—

A—should be made by mothers in a clinic before they go home? B—can be made with ordinary salt and ordinary sugar? C—should be made with heaped tablespoons of salt and sugar? D—may cause hypernatraemic dehydration if too much salt is used? E—can be given down an intragastric tube? (9.21, 9.22)

15. Which of these is NOT a danger sign in a dehydrated child?

A Sunken eyes B Vomiting C Not drinking D A wet mouth E Diarrhoea getting worse (9.18)

16. INNA (15 months) is still breast-fed and is having a drip into her arm. Which of these would you NOT say to her mother?

A 'The fluid in the bottle should have reached this mark by this evening (you show her where).' B 'Give her porridge as soon as she can eat.' C 'Nurse her on your knee if you want to.' D 'Let her drink this fluid (glucose–salt solution) as soon as she can.' E 'Don't let her suck from your breasts because she is having this drip.' (9.27)

17. ZOYENKA (3 years) is severely dehydrated. While she is having an intravenous drip she starts to have rigors. Her rigors are probably caused by—

A—the fluid or the drip set not being perfectly clean? B—her severe dehydration? C—too little salt in the fluid she is being given? D—too much fluid being given? (9.29b)

18. An intragastric drip—

A—is cheaper when given with half strength Darrow's solution? B—cannot be given to a child who is vomiting? C—is only useful for mildly dehydrated children? D—can be given with glucose–salt solution or salt-and-sugar water? E—must be given with new equipment each time? (9.24)

19. MAGALITA (9 months) has had severe watery diarrhoea for several days. Her diarrhoea stops when she is given glucose–salt solution, but it starts again when she is breast-fed. She is not dehydrated now. Her mother is very poor. What would you tell her mother?

A 'Give her bottle feeds.' B 'Take her off the breast. Express your breast milk. Give her porridge only for a few days. She will probably be able to breast feed in a few more days or a week.' C 'She has an infection which is causing lactose intolerance. Take this medicine (chloramphenicol).' **D** 'Stop breast-feeding and give her ordinary food.' **E** 'Give her lactose-free milk.' (9.29)

20. Which of these kinds of rehydration are LEAST likely to cause swollen eyelids if you give too much fluid?

A Intravenous rehydration **B** Nasogastric rehydration **C** Oral rehydration (9.24, 9.27)

21. ABAS (2 years, 38·5 °C) has mild diarrhoea, fever, a cough and large tonsils with pus on them. He is not dehydrated and has no other abnormal signs. What treatment would you give him?

A Glucose saline **B** Tetracycline **C** Penicillin **D** Salt-and-sugar water **E** Kaolin mixture (9.10)

22. Which of these are MOST useful for treating diarrhoea in children?

A Antibiotics **B** Opium **C** Purgatives **D** Enterovioform **E** Fluids (9.30)

23. LILOKALANI has diarrhoea. Her mother can stop giving her extra fluids when—

A—her stools are no longer liquid? **B**—she starts eating? **C**—her mouth is wet? **D**—her eyes are no longer sunken? **E**—she has had 5 cups of fluid? (9.31)

24. ALPHONSE (4 years) has diarrhoea, vomiting and 'hotness of the body'. He is drowsy and moderately dehydrated. There is much falciparum malaria in the district. His mother will not take him to hospital, and there are no sterile fluids in the health centre. What would you say to his mother?

A 'We can only treat him for malaria.' **B** 'The only thing you can do is to go on giving him fluids by mouth.' **C** 'We can help him by giving him fluid into his abdomen.' **D** 'We can help him by giving him fluids through a tube down his nose and treating him for malaria.' (9.9)

25. Which of these would you give ALPHONSE?

A Chloroquine tablets **B** Subcutaneous chloroquine **C** Penicillin **D** Tetracycline **E** Subcutaneous quinine (9.9)

FEVER C
Chapter 10: Code 7

1. The rectal temperature of a healthy child is between—

A—34·5 and 35 °C? **B**—35 and 35·5 °C? **C**—35·5 and 36°C? **D**—36·0 and 37·5 °C? **E**—37·5 and 40 °C? (10.1)

2. If a sick child shivers and says he feels cold his temperature is—

A—too high? **B**—going up? **C**—going down? **D**—staying the same? **E**—too low? (10.1)

3. A child is diagnosed as having hypothermia when his temperature is below—

A—35·5 °C? **B**—34·5 °C? **C**—35 °C? **D**—36 °C? **E**—34°C? (10.1)

4. Which of these children are LEAST good at keeping their bodies at a normal temperature?

A Low-birth-weight babies **B** Normal babies **C** Children 5 months old **D** Children 1 year old (10.1)

5. The mouth is about half a degree hotter than the— **D**—rectum? **E**—axilla? (10.1)

6. If a child's axillary temperature is 39 °C, his rectal temperature is—

B—38 °C? **C**—40 °C? **D**—38·5 °C? **E**—39·5 °C? (10.1)

7. If you cannot make the mercury in a rectal thermometer go up into the scale the child has—

B—hypothermia? **C**—hyperpyrexia? **D**—a normal temperature? (10.1)

8. Which of these is NOT true?

A We can treat measles with quinine. **B** Children with measles need feeding. **C** Urinary infections often present as fever. **D** Typhoid fever is caused by bacteria. **E** Malaria can cause hyperpyrexia. (10.2)

9. JOSE has measles which presented with fever and a febrile convulsion. He is being treated with paracetamol. Paracetamol is—

A—specific treatment for the measles? **B**—specific treatment for the fits? **C**—an antibiotic to prevent secondary infection? **D**—symptomatic treatment for the fever? **E**—preventive treatment for the rash? (10.3)

10. SEIJI (3 years) has fever. There is much malaria in the district. He needs all these things EXCEPT—

A—chloroquine? **B**—cooling with wet cloths? **C**—plenty of fluids? **D**—as much food as he will eat? **E**—to be kept warm with plenty of clothes? (10.3)

11. Which of these is LEAST likely to PRESENT as fever?

A Urinary infection **B** Tonsillitis in young children **C** Typhoid **D** Malaria **E** Bronchitis (10.5)

12. Which of these is caused by a virus?

A Urinary infections **B** Malaria **C** Typhoid **D** Measles **E** Cellulitis (10.6)

13. Which of these diseases is most often complicated by TB?

A Measles **B** Typhoid **C** Otitis media **D** Pharyngitis **E** Scabies (10.6)

14. If you look at a child's blood with a microscope, you can find the organisms which cause—

A—pneumonia? **B**—malaria? **C**—measles? **D**—typhoid? **E**—sickle-cell anaemia? (10.7)

15. Which of these diseases leaves a child with a strong natural active immunity?

A Otitis media **B** Urinary infections **C** Measles **D** diarrhoea **E** Pneumonia (10.6)

16. Which of these diseases is most likely to be complicated by otitis media?

A Measles **B** Pneumonia **C** Malaria **D** Impetigo **E** Diarrhoea (10.6)

17. LUKE (4 years) has cerebral malaria. He could have any of these signs or symptoms EXCEPT—

A—fits? **B**—shock? **C**—sore red eyes? **D**—coma? **E**—vomiting? (10.7)

18. Where would you look for Koplik's spots?

A On the tonsils **B** On the tongue **C** On the skin **D** Inside the cheeks **E** On the palate (10.6)

19. Which of these is spread by infected droplets which go from one person to another through the air?

A Diarrhoea **B** Measles **C** Typhoid **D** Malaria **E** Urinary infections (10.8)

20. In a malarious area a child with severe measles may need any of these things EXCEPT—

A—'MEASLES' written on his weight chart? **B**—chloroquine? **C**—vitamin A? **D**—an antibiotic? **E**—stopping breast-feeding? (10.6)

21. A child with fever, anaemia, and a large spleen probably has—

A—measles? **B**—malaria? **C**—hookworms? **D**—TB? **E**—a urinary infection? (10.7)

22. FATNESS (3 years 40 °C) has been in coma since this morning. Yesterday she had diarrhoea. During the night she vomited and had a fit. She comes from a malarious area. Which of these things does she need LEAST?

A Intravenous quinine or subcutaneous chloroquine **B** Intravenous fluids **C** Cooling with water **D** A lumbar puncture **E** To be nursed on her back (10.7)

23. SUCHI has had fever for seven days. She passes urine often, and each time she passes it she screams with pain. Her infection is probably in her—

A—bladder? **B**—gut? **C**—lungs? **D**—spleen? **E**—blood? (10.10)

24. If a child has fever and fits caused by malaria, his blood slide—

B—always has '+ + + +' parasites? **C**—usually has parasites but may have none? (10.7)

25. Which of these is NOT true? The rash of measles—

A—forms macules and papules? **B**—may cause desquamation (peeling)? **C**—comes first behind the ears? **D**—comes on the fourth day of a child's fever? **E**—is paler when measles is severe? (10.6)

SKINS C
Chapter 11: Code 8

MATCH these with the diseases they prevent—

1. Washing children and their clothes and bedclothes?
2. Vitamin B? **3.** Treating small cuts and sores carefully?
4. Eating more protein and energy food?

A Pellagra **B** Xerophthalmia **C** Kwashiorkor **D** Scabies **E** Chronic ulcers (7.10, 11.17, 11.10, 11.23)

5. Septic skin diseases can be prevented by—

A—wearing clothes? **B**—washing? **C**—ointment? **D**—vitamins? **E**—immunization? (11.1)

6. Which of these diseases harms a child's skin, but not the rest of his body?

A Measles **B** Scabies **C** Chickenpox **D** Impetigo of the newborn **E** Cellulitis with lymphadenitis and lymphangitis (11.19)

7. Which of these diseases usually causes a few large plaques or patches?

A Ringworm **B** Measles **C** Heat rash **D** Herpes zoster **E** Scabies (11.13)

8. SEBASTIAN (2 years) has severe itching and scratches himself all night. He has NOT got—

A—scabies? **B**—eczema? **C**—leprosy? **D**—lice bites? **E**—mosquito bites? (12:1)

9. Some skin diseases go through several stages, one after the other. Which of these has the stages in the RIGHT order?

A Pustule, papule **B** Crust, pustule, scar **C** Scar, pustule **D** Papule, macule, crust **E** Macule, papule, vesicle (11.2)

10. Dry, scaly lesions can be caused by—

A—a heat rash? **B**—impetigo? **C**—urticaria? **D**—ringworm? **E**—chickenpox? (11.13)

11. Which of these diseases usually causes lesions which are the same on both sides of the body?

A Leprosy **B** Creeping eruption **C** Boils **D** Herpes zoster **E** Pellagra (11.23)

12. A vesicle is a—

A—lesion filled with clear fluid? **B**—lesion filled with pus? **C**—lesion that cannot be felt when it is touched? **D**—dry lesion? **E**— red lesion? (11.2)

13. KNUT (4 years, 38·5 °C) has spreading skin sepsis. The most important treatment for him is—

A—vitamin injections? **B**—washing his lesions in potassium permanganate? **C**—an antiseptic ointment on his skin? **D**—an antibiotic by injection or by mouth? **E**—an antipyretic injection? (11.3)

14. Impetigo—

A—does not harm small babies? **B**—can be treated with benzathine (depot) penicillin? **C**—is best treated with chloramphenicol? **D**—is a chronic disease? **E**—can be treated with benzoic acid ointment? (11.4)

15. KAMALKURMANI (3 years) has a line of vesicles going down one side of her arm, but no lesions anywhere else. Her arm is painful where the vesicles are. She had pain and fever before the vesicles came. Her lesions—

A—will spread all over her body? **B**—are caused by bacteria? **C**—are caused by the same virus that causes chickenpox? **D**—are urticarial? **E**—are caused by insect bites? (11.17)

16. Which of these would you NOT use on the skin?

A Lysol **B** Hypochlorite **C** Permanganate **D** Gentian violet **E** Benzoic acid ointment (3.11, 3.48)

17. TARMAYA has some small, hard, round, smooth solid papules on her skin. There is a small hole in the middle of each of these papules. They—

A—itch? **B**—are very serious? **C**—are not infectious? **D**—will cure themselves in a few days? **E**—will cure themselves in a few months and do not need treatment? (11.19)

18. Which of these diseases is caused by bacteria?

A—scabies? **B**—impetigo? **C**—ringworm? **D**—pellagra? **E**—warts? (11.4)

19. SABINE's uncle has herpes zoster. She might get—
A—smallpox? **B**—herpes simplex? **C**—chickenpox?
D—pellagra? **E**—eczema? (11.17)

20. PROSERPINA (5 years) has diarrhoea. She also has lesions on the parts of her neck, arms, and legs where the sun shines. Both these symptoms could be caused by—
A—impetigo? **B**—scabies? **C**—kwashiorkor? **D**—pellagra? **E**—eczema?

21. Urticaria are lesions which—
A—cannot be felt with a finger? **B**—itch? **C**—go septic?
D—have a dark red centre? **E**—last a long time? (11.24)

22. Hypochlorite can be used to treat—
A—creeping eruption? **B**—warts? **C**—drug rashes?
D—secondarily infected scabies? **E**—pellagra? (11.7)

23. RATMANAYA (4 years) has scabies. A health worker should—
A—treat everyone who lives in the same house?
B—treat her with benzoic acid ointment? **C**—leave the medicine on her skin for an hour then wash it off?
D—treat her with zinc and caster oil ointment? **E**—give her an antihistamine? (11.10)

24. Which of these diseases causes skin lesions and mental symptoms?
A Eczema **B** Urticaria **C** Pellagra **D** Creeping eruption **E** Scabies (11.23)

25. Penicillin will NOT help—
A—pyoderma? **B**—impetigo? **C**—a lesion in which there is pus? **D**—leprosy? **E**—secondarily infected ringworm? (3.15)

LEPROSY C
Chapter 12: Code 5

1. LOUIS has several skin lesions which might be leprosy. Which of these would be a sign that they are leprosy?
A Fever and lymphangitis **B** A short history of a few days **C** Dark coloured lesions **D** Itching **E** A tender thickened ulna nerve (12.3)

2. The most common kind of leprosy in children is—
B—borderline leprosy? **C**—indeterminate leprosy?
D—lepromatous leprosy? **E**—tuberculoid leprosy? (12.2)

3. Which of these is NOT true about leprosy and TB? Both—
A—are chronic diseases? **B**—are caused by AAFB?
C—can spread from a mother to her child? **D**—can be cured with the same drugs? **E**—can usually be treated without a patient going to hospital? (12.1)

4. SANTIKO has some lesions which are probably indeterminate leprosy. They will most probably—
A—become lepromatous? **B**—cure themselves in a few months? **C**—become tuberculoid? **D**—become borderline? **E**—spread all over his body? (12.2)

5. The nearest help is 50 km away through the jungle. What would you do for SANTIKO?
A Treat him with benzoic acid ointment? **B** Start him on clofazimine? **C** Observe him carefully and treat him if the lesions do not go? **D** Start him on clofazimine and dapsone? **E** Start him on dapsone only? (12.4)

6. Which of these children should start their leprosy treatment with two drugs?
C MEGA with tuberculoid leprosy. **D** GIGA with lepromatous leprosy. **E** TERA with indeterminate leprosy. (12.4)

7. RUTH may have lepromatous leprosy. Which of these would be the best place to take a skin scraping from?
A The palms of her hands **B** Her scalp **C** The lobes of her ears **D** Her fingers **E** Her lips (12.2)

8. When you examine a child for thickening of his nerves you should—
A—compare one side of his body with the other?
B—feel the nerve at the outside of his elbow? **C**—feel for thickened nerves in the lesion? **D**—feel below and inside his knee? (12.3)

9. Leprosy lesions are—
A—always hypopigmented? **B**—often hypopigmented? **C**—completely white? **D**—usually painful?
E—always raised above the normal skin? (12.3)

10. Leprosy makes a child's muscles weak and thin because organisms are growing in his—
A—nerves? **B**—muscles? **C**—skin? **D**—bones?
E—brain? (12.1)

11. A skin scraping is most likely to be positive if it is taken from—
A—a lepromatous lesion? **B**—a borderline lesion?
C—an indeterminate lesion? **D**—a tuberculoid lesion? (12.3)

12. YOLANDA is deformed and disabled by leprosy. Drug treatment can—
A—cure him? **B**—stop his deformity and disability becoming worse? **C**—make injured nerves grow again? (12.1)

13. Leprosy is most common in—
A—children under the age of one year? **B**—malnourished children? **C**—children who also have other skin diseases? **D**—children between one and five years?
E—school children? (12.3)

14. If leprosy bacilli infect a child with no immunity he will get—
B—indeterminate leprosy? **C**—lepromatous leprosy?
D—borderline leprosy? **E**—tuberculoid leprosy? (12.2)

15. REB's lesions are hypopigmented, but not completely white. He—
C—certainly has leprosy? **D**—may have leprosy?
E—has certainly not got leprosy? (12.3)

16. AAFB can be found in a skin scraping—
A—only in TB of the skin? **B**—in all leprosy lesions?
C—in most children with indeterminate leprosy? **D**—in most tuberculoid lesions? **E**—in most lepromatous lesions? (12.3)

17. Leprosy—

A—is an ordinary disease that can be treated by ordinary health workers in ordinary clinics? **B**—must always be treated in special leprosy hospitals? (12.5)

18. SIGIT's lesions itch. They—

C—might be leprosy? **D**—are not leprosy? (12.3)

19. LUCKY has some large chronic macules. His lesions—

B—might be leprosy? **C**—are not leprosy? (12.3)

20. AAFB in the sputum shows that a patient has—

C—TB? **D**—leprosy? (12.1, 13.1)

21. Leprosy—

C—must be diagnosed early? **D**—need not be diagnosed early because modern treatment quickly cures a child? (12.1)

22. Lepromatous lesions—

A—contain no bacilli? **B**—do not harm the face or the ears? **C**—are always anaesthetic? **D**—have a sharp edge between them and the skin around them? **E**—are usually swollen above the level of the skin? (12.4)

23. Leprosy causes disability because it harms a child's—

A—nerves? **B**—skin? (12.1)

24. Dapsone can cause all these side effects EXCEPT—

A—mental symptoms? **B**—anaemia? **C**—pain in the nerves? **D**—diarrhoea? **E**—fever? (3.24, 12.4)

25. INEKE is newborn, her mother has leprosy. Her mother needs to be told all these things EXCEPT one. Which one?

A 'INEKE will probably not get leprosy.' **B** 'INEKE should be cared for by someone else, or she will catch your leprosy.' **C** 'We will put her on our special-care register.' **D** 'Go on taking your tablets.' **E** 'She does not need leprosy tablets.' (26.66, 12.4)

TB C
Chapter 13: Code 1

1. TB is—

A—a chronic bacterial disease? **B**—an acute viral disease? **C**—a chronic viral disease? **D**—an acute bacterial disease? **E**—a chronic fungal disease? (13.1)

2. A child with TB usually has—

D—one symptom only? **E**—several symptoms?

3. TB most often harms the—

A—stomach? **B**—bladder? **C**—lungs? **D**—muscles? **E**—heart? (13.2)

4. Where would you most often expect to see lymphnodes enlarged by TB?

A In a child's neck **B** In his axilla **C** In his groin **D** Under his jaw (13.2, 19.3)

Which of these is true?

C All patients with TB are infectious **D** Patients are only infectious if live TB bacilli are leaving their bodies (13.3)

6. A primary TB infection USUALLY causes—

C—severe symptoms? **D**—no symptoms? **E**—mild symptoms? (13.2)

7. Which of these children is most likely to have TB? The child who—

A—has had mild fever and a cough for a week? **B**—has had tender swellings in his neck for 3 days? **C**—does not recover several weeks after whooping cough? **D**—has otitis media? **E**—has a chronic upper respiratory infection? (13:1)

8. TB usually presents as the child who—

B—is 'not well' and has had mild fever and loss of weight for several weeks? **C**—has chronic abdominal swelling? **D**—has had a high fever for 4 days? **E**—passes blood in his stools? (13:1)

9. Which of these children have MOST immunity to TB?

A ZOE who is newborn. **B** ZELLA with marasmus. **C** ZACHARY (3 years) with a rising weight curve. **D** ZIMMA with kwashiorkor. **E** ZEPHRAIMY who is underweight and is recovering from measles. (13.2)

10. An adult with infectious TB is usually—

C—completely well? **D**—so ill that he has to stay in bed? **E**—well enough to work? (13.3)

11. Which of these diseases is LEAST likely to cause difficulty when you are trying to diagnose TB?

A Malnutrition **B** Cerebral malaria **C** Chronic pyogenic lower respiratory infection following measles **D** Chronic urinary infection **E** Chronic pyogenic lower respiratory infection following whooping cough (10.7)

12. A child who has been given BCG—

C—will not become ill with TB? **D**—is less likely to become ill with TB than a child who has not been given BCG? (13.4)

13. BCG vaccine contains—

A—toxoids? **B**—living organisms? **C**—dead organisms? **D**—antibiotics? (4.6, 13.4)

14. Which of these is not used for preventing or treating TB?

A Thiacetazone **B** BCG **C** Penicillin **D** Isoniazid **E** PAS (13.5)

15. Which of these two drugs are often mixed together in the same tablet?

A Thiacetazone and streptomycin **B** PAS and streptomycin **C** PAS and thiacetazone **D** Thiacetazone and isoniazid (3.21, 13.6)

16. Which of these is true?

A TB in children seldom presents as a cough with blood stained sputum. **B** A different kind of TB organism infects children. **C** TB is a more chronic disease in children. **D** Children get TB meningitis less often than adults. **E** Children infect one another whereas adults do not. (13.3)

17. A child with TB should be treated with isoniazid for—

B—three weeks? **C**—six months? **D**—three months? **E**—one year? (13.6)

18. MAURICE (7 years) has TB meningitis. He was probably infected by—

A—another child at school? **B**—an adult with TB meningitis? **C**—an adult with a chronic cough? **D**—eating infected food? **E**—his younger sister who has been coughing for two weeks? (13.3)

19. Which of these children is most likely to have TB?

A WILLY (6 months) who has had a cough for 3 days with respirations of 80 per minute. **B** LIZ (5 years) with chronic abdominal pain who has gained a kilo in the last six months. **C** JOHN (18 months) who is always coughing and wheezing and who has gained 3 kg during the last nine months. **D** FRED (2 years, 38·2 °C) who has not been well for 4 weeks and who has lost two kilos in weight. (13:1)

20. ADSONI (3 years) had pneumonia four months ago. He was treated with penicillin and he recovered a little, but he still had a cough and fever and was losing weight. He was given INH for 3 months, and is now much better. Should he—

A—stop his INH? **B**—go on with it for a year? (13.7)

21. Which of these diseases is LEAST common in unimmunized children?

A 'Ordinary diarrhoea' **B** Measles **C** Whooping cough **D** Tonsillitis **E** TB (13.1)

22. Which of these drugs does NOT help TB?

A Sulphadimidine **B** Streptomycin **C** Aminosalicylate (PAS) **D** Isoniazid **E** Ethambutol (3.14)

23. Which of these diseases kills children slowest?

A Cerebral malaria **B** TB **C** Tetanus **D** Septicaemia **E** Diarrhoea with dehydration (13.1)

24. TARIMO (3 years). His elder brother (21 years) is sputum positive. TARIMO himself has no symptoms. He should be—

A—given BCG and put on the special-care register? **B**—told that there is no need to worry and sent home? **C**—given streptomycin, thiacetazone, and isoniazid? **D**—given PAS (aminosalicylate) only? **E**—given streptomycin only? (13.7)

25. JOEL (4 years) has TB. He might have presented in any one of these ways EXCEPT as—

A—chronic swelling of the lymph nodes of his neck? **B**—a chronic cough? **C**—a sore throat? **D**—loss of weight? **E**—not eating? (13.1)

ACCIDENTS C
Chapter 14: Code 6

1. All these children have swallowed phenobarbitone tablets. Which of them should be made to vomit?

A HUA who swallowed tablets several hours ago and is in coma. **B** MAO who swallowed some tablets yesterday and is awake. **C** CHIAO who swallowed them an hour ago and is awake. **D** All of them. **E** None of them. (14.6)

2. Which of these kills the LEAST number of children in a poor rural area?

A Accidents **B** Infection **C** Malnutrition (2.1, 14.4)

3. Which of these is the best way of preventing accidents?

A Boiling water **B** Better nutrition **C** Building more clinics **D** Early treatment **E** Health education (14.1)

4. NICOLA (5 years) is severely shocked. She has—

A—rapid movements of her arms and legs? **B**—a fast weak pulse? **C**—a warm, dry skin? **D**—a temperature above 37·5 °C? **E**—fast, shallow breathing? (14.2)

5. A mother should prevent her child being poisoned with tablets by—

A—punishing him if he plays with bottles? **B**—putting the lid on the tablet bottle? **C**—keeping them locked up? **D**—hiding them? **E**—putting them in a cupboard? (14–9)

6. TERESINA has burnt the palm of her hand. It is now healing well. What would you say to her mother about preventing contractures?

B 'We must bind up her hand in this splint.' **C** 'Opening her hand will hurt her. Rest it and it will open as it heals.' **D** 'Here is some medicine to make her hand open.' **E** 'Be sure to open out her hand several times a day.' (14.3)

7. TANCREDI has been badly burnt by boiling fat. He is most likely to be killed by—

A—toxins from the fat? **B**—pneumonia? **C**—haemorrhage? **D**—infection? **E**—the heat of the burn? (14.3)

8. Which of these burns are most likely to need a skin graft?

A A superficial burn **B** A superficial partial thickness burn **C** A deep partial thickness burn **D** A full thickness burn **E** A burn on which there are vesicles (14.3)

9. A child in coma should lie on his front or his side because—

A—he breathes more easily? **B**—his stomach falls forward and stops him vomiting? **C**—this cures his coma? **D**—this cures the complications that coma causes? **E**—this helps to prevent saliva going into his lungs? (14.8)

10. Which of these does NOT need to be sewn up?

A Cut skin where the edges meet easily and will stay together **B** Cut skin where the edges are wide apart **C** Cut nerves **D** Cut tendons (14.4)

11. SAMSURI has cut his arm in a car accident. We can find out if a nerve has been cut by—

A—looking for the cut end of the nerve? **B**—testing for anaesthesia below the cut? **C**—testing for anaesthesia above the cut? **D**—asking if the cut is painful? (14.4)

12. ED has cut his foot with a spade and there is earth in it. What would you do FIRST—

A—wash it well with water to remove the earth? **B**—disinfect it with alcohol or peroxide? **C**—give intramuscular penicillin? **D**—give tetanus toxoid? **E**—stitch it up? (14.4)

13. Stitches should—

A—cause the cut edges of the skin to overlap? B—be loose enough to leave a space for the blood to drain through? C—be put into the skin before it is washed? D—be as tight as possible without causing pain? E—be just tight enough to bring the edges of the skin together? (14.4)

14. We can give a child an artificial passive immunity with—

A—DPT? B—tetanus toxoid? C—tetanus antitoxin? (4.2, 14.4)

15. In a compound fracture—

A—the bone is broken in two places? B—there are injuries to other parts of the body? C—there is bleeding into the tissues? D—there is a wound which goes through from the skin to the broken bones? E—the bones are bent into an abnormal shape? (14.5)

16. Which of these is LEAST dangerous if a child eats too many of them?

A Pyrimethamine tablets B Multi-vitamin tablets C Vitamin A capsules D Iron tablets E Dapsone tablets (14.6)

17. We can safely make a child vomit if he has eaten—

B—poisonous leaves? C—kerosene? D—a strong acid? E—a strong alkali? (14.6)

18. A safe way to make a child vomit is to—

A—hold him upside down? B—give him salt and water to drink? C—rub the back of his throat with a spatula? D—pinch his nose and press his stomach? E—put a spatula under his tongue? (14.6)

19. Which of these burns heals by the epidermis growing over it from the edges?

B A superficial partial-thickness burn C A deep partial-thickness burn D A full-thickness burn E A superficial burn (14.3)

20. KAMALA (4 years) is in coma. His greatest danger is from—

A—saliva going into his lungs? B—anaemia? C—septicaemia D—fits? E—malnutrition? (14.8)

21. Which of these is LEAST likely to cause coma?

A Cerebral malaria B Meningitis C Amoebic dysentery D Severe dehydration E Head injury (14.8)

22. Which of these is MOST likely to cause coma if a child eats too many tablets?

A Piperazine B Vitamin B C Dapsone D Iron E Phenobarbitone (14.8)

23. A child with a large full thickness burn does NOT need—

A—very careful dressing? B—vitamin B injections? C—immunization against tetanus? D—hospital treatment? E—replacement of the fluid he loses through the burn? (14.3)

24. ALLONIA (4 years) is in severe shock. This is LEAST likely to have been caused by—

A—a road accident? B—severe diarrhoea and dehydration? C—septicaemia? D—tonsillitis? E—cerebral malaria? (14.2)

25. MARKKU (2 years) fought when he was being given a penicillin injection and the needle broke off deep inside his leg. What would you do?

B Make an incision in his leg and try to take out the needle with forceps. C Wait for the needle to come out by itself. D Send him for help. (3.5)

FITS C
Chapter 15: Code 5

1. A late sign of meningitis is that a child's fontanelle—

A—opens? B—closes? C—moves up and down? D—sinks? E—swells? (15.6)

2. Which of these would make you think that a child was having the spasms of tetanus?

A Movements in one arm only B Upward-looking eyes C Crying with pain D Falling to the ground E Losing consciousness (15.1)

3. CSF is—

A—another name for lymph? B—part of the blood? C—found inside all the bones? D—the fluid around the brain and spinal cord? E—pus which forms when children have meningitis? (15.2)

4. Pandy's test measures—

A—glucose? B—protein? C—sugar? D—cells? E—bacteria? (15.2)

5. If we do a lumbar puncture badly and allow bacteria to get into the CFS, a child's greatest danger is—

A—haemorrhage? B—septicaemia? C—a spinal cord abscess? D—pain? E—meningitis? (15.3)

6. Needles for lumbar puncture should be sterilized by—

A—keeping them in hypochlorite? B—keeping them in lysol? C—wiping them with iodine? D—boiling them? E—flaming them? (15.3)

7. Lumbar puncture in young children—

A—must always be done with a special needle? B—should never be done in a health centre? C—can be done with an ordinary intramuscular needle? D—must be done in hospitals, because only hospitals can test CSF? E—does not require sterile equipment? (15.3)

8. Normal CSF NEVER—

A—looks slightly turbid? B—gives a very mildly positive Pandy's test? C—has less than 35 mg/dl of protein? D—gives a negative Pandy's test? E—has less than five cells per microlitre? (15.2)

9. When you do a lumbar puncture you should NOT—

A—ask a helper to hold the child's head and legs? B—ask the helper to hold the child's back straight? C—put the CSF into two bottles? D—put the needle into the space below the third lumbar spine? E—touch the needle with iodine-covered fingers? (15.3)

10. Pandy's test is done by—

A—dropping CSF into Pandy's solution? **B**—dropping Pandy's solution into CSF? **C**—looking at the CSF against something white? **D**—using the phenol from the bottom of the bottle of Pandy's solution? (15.3b)

11. TRAN has purulent meningitis. What would you NOT expect in his CSF?

A 20 mg/dl of protein **B** Pandy's test positive + + + **C** Pus cells **D** Bacteria **E** Turbid CSF (15.3b)

12. OBEDIENCE (3 years, 37·0 °C) came to the health centre three days ago. She had not been well for about 12 days before that. She had not been eating, she had vomited twice and she had had three fits. Her neck was stiff. Her CSF was slightly turbid and Pandy's test was positive. Purulent mengingitis was diagnosed and she was treated with penicillin and chloramphenicol. After four days treatment she is now worse than when treatment started. This is probably because she—

A—was given penicillin and chloramphenicol? **B**—has TB meningitis? **C**—has virus meningitis? **D**—came too early for treatment? **E**—had three fits? (15.6)

13. Which of these things would you NOT expect a health centre laboratory to do with a specimen of CSF?

A Look for turbidity. **B** Do Pandy's test. **C** Count the cells. **D** Look for bacteria in a stained film of CSF. **E** Grow the bacteria. (15.3b)

14. Organisms can get to a child's meninges in all these ways. Which one is most easily preventable?

A From his nose **B** From his ears **C** On a dirty lumbar-puncture needle **D** Through his blood (15.6)

15. MANFRED (7 years) has had several fits during the last year. When he has these fits he does not have fever. In between fits he has been well. He has—

A—TB meningitis? **B**—virus meningitis? **C**—cerebral malaria? **D**—epilepsy? **E**—febrile convulsions? (15.8)

16. MANFRED's fits could be completely or partly prevented by giving him—

A—pyrimethamine? **B**—paracetamol? **C**—promethazine? **D**—paraldehyde? **E**—phenobarbitone? (15.8)

17. BOGE is having a fit which has already lasted 20 minutes. He comes from a district where falciparum malaria is common. Which of these things would you NOT do?

A Give him intramuscular chloroquine. **B** Take his temperature. **C** Give him paraldehyde. **D** Lie him on his side. **E** Put something between his teeth to stop him biting his tongue. (15.9)

18. All these children have had fits today. They all should have a lumbar puncture. Which of them needs a lumbar puncture MOST urgently?

A HOANG with swollen tonsils with pus on them. **B** COLOUTHUR with whooping cough. **C** MONAWAR with severe diarrhoea. **D** RAUF with fever and vomiting and a stiff neck. **E** LEON with fever and vomiting and P. falciparum + + + in his blood today. (15.9)

19. All these children have a cough, fever, and one fit.

They all should have a lumbar puncture. Which of them needs a lumbar puncture MOST urgently?

A JITKA (3 years, 38·7 °C) who has an upper respiratory infection. **B** EDESIO (9 months) who has rapid respirations and a swollen fontanelle. **C** ZENILDA (3 years, 39 °C) who has rapid respirations and no meningeal signs. **D** AUSSANY (4 years) who has had whooping cough for 3 weeks and who has a conjunctival haemorrhage. **E** UILHO who has a cough, red eyes, and Koplik's spots. (15.9)

20. All these children have had a fit today. All EXCEPT one of them should have a lumbar puncture. Which of them does NOT need a lumbar puncture?

A NIDIA who has had mild fever for 10 days. **B** AMPARO who has fever and a positive Kernig's sign. **C** ISABEL (6 years, 37·2 °C) who has had several epileptic fits during the last year, and is now quite well. **D** NEY who is paralysed in his right arm and leg since the fit. **E** JARBAS (38·5 °C) who is drowsy. (15.9)

21. 'Any child who has had a fit should, if possible, have a lumbar puncture, unless he is known to have epilepsy, *and* has no fever.'

C True **D** False (15.9)

22. Kernig's test is the name for a test in which a child—

B—has a swollen fontanelle? **C**—cannot put his head between his knees? **D**—has a stiff neck? **E**—cannot straighten his knee with his hip bent? (15.9)

23. Children with purulent meningitis need large doses of—

A—penicillin? **B**—isoniazid? **C**—aspirin? **D**—streptomycin? **E**—tetracycline? (15.6)

24. GUILELMA (8 months) has meningitis. Which of these signs would you NOT expect her to have?

A Fever **B** 'Not sucking' **C** Abnormal movements of her body **D** Bitot's spots **E** Vomiting (15.6)

25. Which of these will be LEAST helpful in deciding why a child has fits?

A Examining his throat **B** Measuring his arm circumference **C** Taking his temperature **D** Testing his skin for elasticity **E** Examining his ears (15.9)

EYES C
Chapter 16: Code 4

1. Which of these would you LEAST expect to cause a corneal ulcer?

A Vitamin A deficiency **B** An injury **C** A stye **D** Severe acute conjunctivitis **E** A foreign body (16.5)

2. Which of these is NOT true? Acute conjunctivitis—

A—can be caused by bacteria or viruses? **B**—is infectious? **C**—is more common where there is a lack of soap and water? **D**—can make a child's eyes swell so much that he cannot open them? **E**—is a disease of older children only? (16.8)

3. Which of these does NOT cause a red painful eye?

A Xerophthalmia **B** Foreign body **C** Corneal ulcer **D**

Acute conjunctivitis **E** Phlyctenular conjunctivitis (16.3)

4. A common cause of blindness can be prevented if children eat—

A—bananas? **B**—green leaves? **C**—cassava porridge? **D**—salt? **E**—minerals? (16.14)

5. The white part of the eye is called—

A—the iris? **B**—the pupil? **C**—the cornea? **D**—the conjunctiva? **E**—the sclera? (16.2)

6. The iris is—

A—a gland which makes tears? **B**—a circle of brown (or blue) tissue? **C**—part of the back of the eye? **D**—the white part of the eye? **E**—the clear front part of the eye? (16.2)

7. The hole in the iris is called—

A—the cornea? **B**—the retina? **C**—the conjunctiva? **D**—the pupil? **E**—the sclera? (16.2)

8. Which of these is NOT true about keratomalacia?

A Treatment is urgent. **B** Blindness comes on suddenly in a few days. **C** Keratomalacia is preventable. **D** Treatment will easily make a blind child see again. **E** Keratomalacia means softening of the cornea. (16.3)

9. A painful septic swelling on a child's eyelid is called—

A—a hypopyon? **B**—a stye? **C**—a phlycten? **D**—a follicle? **E**—trachoma? (16.3)

10. If a foreign body might have gone inside a child's eye, he should be—

A—observed carfully for two weeks? **B**—given procaine penicillin for three days? **C**—treated with chlortetracycline eye ointment? **D**—treated with scopolamine eye ointment and a pad and bandage? **E**—sent for help immediately? (16.5)

11. Fluorescein is used for—

A—diagnosing ulcers? **B**—diagnosing styes? **C**—treating conjunctivitis? **D**—diagnosing xerophthalmia? **E**—treating trachoma? (16.5)

12. When capsules of vitamin A (200 000 units for children of 1–6 years) are given for prevention, they should be given—

A—every month? **B**—every 2 months? **C**—every 6 months? **D**—every year? **E**—once only? (16.13)

13. Corneal ulcers are—

A—an important complication of chickenpox? **B**—an early sign of trachoma? **C**—lesions where the corneal mucosa has been harmed? **D**—white lesions on the cornea? **E**—lesions which should be treated with hypochlorite in the same way as chronic ulcers on the skin? (16.7)

14. Corneal ulcers are dangerous because—

A—foreign bodies can go through them? **B**—organisms easily go through them into the blood and cause septicaemia? **C**—they make the eye red and swollen? **D**—organisms can get through them into the eye? **E**—they are very painful? (16.7)

15. Conjunctivitis—

A—is caused by lack of vitamins? **B**—can cause corneal ulcers? **C**—is rare? **D**—is seldom infectious? **E**—is usually in one eye only? (16.7)

16. A child with trachoma needs treatment for—

B—six days? **C**—six weeks? **D**—one year? **E**—six months? (16.9)

17. N'SOUGAN (3 years) has very severe acute conjunctivitis with much swelling of the eyelids. You should treat him as if it was—

A—caused by gonococci? **B**—impetigo of the newborn? **C**—septicaemia? **D**—trachoma? **E**—a corneal ulcer? (16.8)

18. Trachoma is treated with—

A—penicillin eye-drops? **B**—chlortetracycline eye ointment? **C**—chloramphenicol? **D**—sulphadimidine eye-drops? **E**—scopolamine eye ointment? (16.9)

19. POLLY (6 years) has red, watery eyes with pinkish grey swellings underneath her upper lids. The edges of her corneae are grey and there are new blood vessels in them. She has—

A—gonococcal conjunctivitis? **B**—keratomalacia? **C**—second stage trachoma? **D**—allergic conjunctivitis? **E**—phlyctenular conjunctivitis? (16.9)

20. Trachoma is caused by—

A—organisms which are half way between viruses and bacteria? **B**—viruses? **C**—a bacteria? **D**—protozoa? **E**—fungi? (16.9)

21. Pannus can be caused by—

A—TB? **B**—xerophthalmia? **C**—allergic conjunctivitis? **D**—trachoma? **E**—trachoma and allergic conjunctivitis? (16.9)

22. Vitamin A deficiency is most common in children—

A—in the uterus? **B**—in the first month of life? **C**—over the age of five years? **D**—below the age of one year? **E**—between the age of one year and five years? (6.13)

23. RODRIGO (18 months). His mother says he cannot find his toys in the dark and he often falls over things. He could be cured by eating—

A—coconut? **B**—bread? **C**—cassava porridge? **D**—sugar? **E**—cassava leaves? (16.13)

24. HENRIQUE (18 months). Both his eyes are dull and dry. There is a small ulcer on his right cornea. He—

A—should be treated with penicillin eye-drops? **B**—should be treated by eating yellow fruits and vegetables? **C**—has severe keratomalacia? **D**—needs an injection of vitamin A? **E**—has mild xerophthalmia? (16.13)

25. Children with vitamin A deficiency usually present—

A—as night blindness? **B**—as ordinary blindness? **C**—with corneal ulcers? **D**—with red eyes? **E**—with symptoms of malnutrition or infection? (16.13)

1. Which of these things is NOT true? A chronically discharging ear—
A—always heals itself after a few years? B—may cause meningitis? C—may become infected with tetanus bacteria? D—may cause mastoiditis? E—may make a child deaf? (17.10)

2. The middle ear is a small air-filled space inside—
C—the muscles of the top of the neck? D—the brain? E—the bone of the skull? (17.2)

3. The mastoid air space joins on to—
A—the brain? B—the inner ear? C—the middle ear? D—the outer ear? E—the meninges? (17.2)

4. The handle of the maleus is in—
A—the ear-drum? B—the outer ear? C—the inner ear? D—the Eustachian tube? E—the mastoid air spaces? (17.2)

5. When you examine the ear of an older child with an auriscope you should pull his ear gently—
B—upwards and forwards? C—downwards and backwards? D—upwards and backwards? E—forwards and downwards? (17.3)

6. Which of these can you use for treating otitis media?
A Penicillin B Sulphadimidine C Ampicillin D Any of these E None of these

7. Otitis media does NOT present as—
A—fever? B—fits? C—difficulty breathing? D—vomiting? E—pulling at the ear and crying? (17.9)

8. When you syringe a child's ear you should—
A—try to block the meatus with the end of the syringe? B—point the syringe upwards and forwards? C—use hot water? D—use cold water? E—pull his ear downwards? (17.6)

9. The middle ear usually becomes infected by organisms which—
C—go up the Eustachian tube? D—come from the blood? E—go through the drum? (17.9)

10. QUENTIN has otitis media. Otitis media is an important complication of—
A—mumps? B—otitis externa? C—infected teeth? D—lower respiratory infections? E—upper respiratory infections? (17.9)

11. Moving a child's ear hurts him if he has—
A—acute otitis media? B—otitis externa? C—chronic otitis media? D—tonsillitis? E—mumps? (17.9)

12. Chronic otitis media is—
A—easily cured by careful cleaning? B—easily cured by antibiotic ear-drops? C—easily treated with penicillin? D—difficult to cure? E—easily cured by penicillin injections, cleaning, and ear-drops? (17.10)

13. Which of these children do NOT need to have their ears examined?
A RORY with meningeal signs. B RHODA with anaemia and a large spleen. C REX with fever and a sore throat.

D RUBY with a swelling behind her ear. E RITA with fever and fits. (17.9)

14. The most important complication of chronic otitis media is—
A—acute lymphadenitis? B—acute otitis media? C—mastoiditis? D—otitis externa? E—lower respiratory infection? (17.11)

15. Otitis media should be treated—
A—as soon as there is any mastoid tenderness? B—if the child seems deaf? C—if moving his ear-lobe is painful? D—as early as possible? E—when his ear has begun to discharge pus? (17.9)

16. BENEDICT (1 year) pulls and scratches at his ear every few days. He has no fever, does not cry, and is 'well'. His meatus is normal. He probably has—
A—no serious lesion? B—otitis externa? C—acute otitis media? D—chronic otitis media? (17.9)

17. When an ear drum has perforated during acute otitis media it—
B—always heals? C—never heals? D—never heals unless antibiotics are given? E—is more likely to heal if antibiotics are given? (17.10)

18. Any of these things may make a child partly or completely deaf EXCEPT—
A—acute otitis media? B—severe chronic otitis media? C—mild otitis externa? D—a foreign body in his ear? E—too much streptomycin? (17.12)

19. When a child with acute otitis media is given antibiotics he should be given them for about—
C—two days? D—five days? E—one month? (17.9, 17.10)

20. Chronically discharging ears—
A—cannot be prevented? B—can be prevented by diagnosing and treating otitis media early? C—can be prevented by giving penicillin to all children with colds? D—can be prevented by immunization? E—can always be cured by the right antibiotic? (17.10)

21. None of these children have been immunized. Which of them most needs DPT vaccine?
A DATSON with acute otitis externa. B WATSON with a boil in his ear. C GADSON with a foreign body in his ear. D MATSON with acute otitis media. E PATSON with chronic otitis media. (17.10)

22. AMINA (4 years) has not been able to open her mouth since yesterday. Sometimes she has muscle spasms and her head bends backwards. She does not lose consciousness. She has no signs except a discharging right ear and a large perforation. She has—
A—tetanus? B—a brain abcess? C—mastoiditis? D—meningitis causing fits? E—otitis externa? (17.10, 18.16)

23. FIFI (4 years) has pain and discharge from her ear. She has a glass bead in it. What would you use first to try to remove it?
A Lying her on her side and shaking her B An ear syringe C A bent wire D Forceps E A swab (17.13)

24. Acute otitis media becomes chronic otitis media after a child has had a discharging ear for—

A—3 weeks? B—6 months? C—3 years? D—3 days? (17.10)

25. Which of these diseases does NOT cause pain in or near the ear?

A Carious teeth B Mumps C Meningitis D Otitis media (17.14)

MOUTH AND THROAT C
Chapter 18: Code 7

1. Tonsillitis is LEAST likely to present as the child who—

A—will not eat? B—is vomiting? C—has abdominal pain? D—has yellow eyes? E—has fever? (18.1)

2. When a young child's throat is examined, he should be—

A—standing up? B—sitting on his mother's knee? C—lying down on a couch? D—sitting on a chair? (18.2)

3. When I examine a child's throat I should use—

C—a spatula which can be boiled? D—a spatula which is sterilized in antiseptic? (18.2)

4. A child's tonsillar lymph-nodes are—

A—in his neck below the angles of his jaw? B—in front of his ears? C—under the front of his jaw? D—at the sides of the lower part of his neck? E—at the back of his neck? (18.2)

PLEASE DON'T WRITE ON THESE QUESTIONS SOMEONE ELSE MAY NEED THEM

---

5. A child's throat should be examined—

C—at the beginning of the examination? D—in the middle of the examination? E—at the end of the examination? (18.2)

6. A child's throat should be examined—

B—only when he has a cough? C—whenever he is 'ill'? D—only when he has symptoms in his throat? E—only when he has fever? (18.2)

7. Which of these diseases does NOT cause lesions in a child's mouth or lips?

A Measles B Vitamin A deficiency C Cancrum oris D Most fevers lasting more than a week E Deficiency of one of the B vitamins (18.3)

8. Which of these children would you most expect to have thrush?

A RANDA who is newborn B DAYO who is a schoolboy C ADE who is breast-fed D COMLAN who has ringworm E BOYO with a high fever for 3 days, red eyes, and some small white spots inside her cheeks (18.4)

9. PITIRIM (3 weeks) is sucking very weakly from the breast and has mild diarrhoea. He has lesions in his mouth which look like milk curds stuck to the inside of his cheek. He has—

A—herpes stomatitis? B—Vincent's stomatitis? C—diphtheria? D—thrush? E—lactose intolerence? (18.5)

10. One of these is a virus disease which can cause a sore on a mother's lip and a sore mouth in her baby. Which disease it it?

A Vincent's stomatitis B Impetigo C Thrush D Herpes zoster E Herpes simplex (18.6)

11. Penicillin or sulphadimidine are helpful for treating—

A—thrush? B—herpes simplex? C—virus infections of the throat? D—mumps? E—tonsillitis? (18.11)

12. JON's mother had 3 injections of tetanus toxoid with her last pregnancy. She is pregnant again. How many injections does she need now?

A Four B Three C Two D One E None (18.16)

13. RAWYA (4 years, 11 kg) has some dirty bad-smelling ulcers on her gums and inside her cheeks. One of them is starting to spread through to her cheek where a black lesion has started to form. Which of these is NOT true?

A Treatment is easy. B She is malnourished. C Her disease could have been prevented. D She may need an operation later. E She may become very deformed. (18.8)

14. Sores at the corner of a child's mouth can be caused by lack of—

A—vitamin A? B—one of the B vitamins? C—vitamin C? D—energy food? E—protein? (18.10)

15. Which of these children would you give an antibiotic to?

A ANTOYO with a nasal discharge and a cough. B AUW with fever and no other signs. C BADYA with pus on his tonsils and tonsillar lymphadenitis. D BAKTI with a red throat and a temperature of 37·8 °C. E BAMBANG with a cough for one week and no other signs. (18.11)

16. Which of these organisms does NOT make a toxin? The organism which causes—

A—thrush? B—diphtheria? C—tetanus? (4.2)

17. LADIPO (2 years, 38·5 °C) has a cough and has vomited twice. His tonsils are large and there is pus on them. His tonsillar lymph-nodes are large and tender. What would you give him?

A Chloramphenicol B Cough mixture C Penicillin D Ampicillin E Streptomycin (18.11)

18. Many children with coughs or sore throats can be treated with cough mixture, or paracetamol and need no other drug?

D True E False (18.11)

19. Which of these diseases can be prevented by immunization—

A—bronchitis? B—diphtheria? C—tonsillitis? D—pharyngitis? E—upper respiratory infections? (18.12)

20. A membrane is more likely to be caused by diphtheria if—

B—it is easily scraped off? C—it is white? D—it is

inside the cheeks? **E**—it is on the tonsils and the back of the pharynx? (18.12)

21. Which of these is LEAST likely to make a child stop eating?

A Tonsillitis **B** Scabies **C** TB **D** Acute malaria **E** Being taken away from his mother (18.14)

22. In an older child the most important presenting symptom of tetanus is—

A—spasms? **B**—an infected wound? **C**—a sore throat? **D**—fits? **E**—not being able to open his mouth? (18.16)

23. Which of these CANNOT be used either to prevent or treat tetanus?

A Tetanus toxin **B** Tetanus toxoid **C** Tetanus antitoxin **D** DPT vaccine **E** Penicillin (4.2, 18.16)

24. If I had to treat a newborn child with tetanus at home, I should teach his mother to feed him—

B—by cup and spoon? **C**—by nasogastric tube? **D**—with a feeding-bottle? **E**—by letting him suck from the breast? (18.16)

25. Which of these children is most likely not to eat normally? The child with—

A—marasmus? **B**—molluscum contagiosum? **C**—vitamin A deficiency? **D**—anaemia? **E**—kwashiorkor? (7.10)

SWELLINGS C
Chapter 19: with revision: Code 3

1. Hernias may be found—
A—over the ankles? **B**—in front of the ear? **C**—in the middle of the neck? **D**—behind the ear? **E**—at the umbilicus? (19.9)

2. Mastoiditis can cause swellings—
A—above the ear? **B**—over the jaw? **C**—behind the ear? **D**—in front of the ear? **E**—in the neck? (19.1, 17.11)

3. Tenderness in a lymph-node is a sign that lymphadenitis is—
A—acute? **B**—chronic? (19.2)

4. Which of these would you expect to cause a swelling over a child's spine?
A A goitre **B** An enlarged lymph-node **C** A hernia **D** An enlarged parotid gland **E** A TB abscess (24–7)

5. A hydrocoele makes a swelling in a child's—
A—penis? **B**—abdomen? **C**—groin? **D**—scrotum? (19.9, 26.59)

6. TAREK has several firm, painless, 1 cm, bean-shaped swellings in both his groins. They are probably caused by—
A—acute lymphadenitis? **B**—TB lymphadenitis? **C**—chronic septic lymphadenitis? **D**—normal lymph-nodes? (19.2)

7. Completely healthy lymph nodes are—
B—difficult to feel or see? **C**—easy to see? **D**—easy to see and feel? (19.2)

8. A child with fever, a septic skin lesion, and enlarged tender lymph-nodes needs—
A—an antiseptic ointment only? **B**—aspirin and an antibiotic? **C**—aspirin only? (19.2)

9. Which of these is most common?
A TB lymphadenitis **B** Chronic septic lymphadenitis **C** Acute septic lymphadenitis (19.2)

10. Where would you MOST often expect to find the swelling caused by oedema—
A—at the side of the neck? **B**—over the wrists? **C**—on the scalp? **D**—over the ankles? **E**—over the front of the neck? (7.10)

11. Mumps is a virus disease of—
A—the parotid glands? **B**—the muscles of the face? **C**—the lymph nodes? **D**—the thyroid gland? **E**—the tonsils? (19.3)

12. Which of these children is LEAST ill?
A LUDWIG who is unconcious. **B** LULU with severe insuction. **C** LUISE with molluscum contagiosum. **D** LORENS with oedema of his feet. **E** LUX with a temperature of 34 °C. (11.19)

13. Lack of iodine causes swellings of—
A—the lymph-nodes? **B**—the parotid glands? **C**—the liver? **D**—the testicles? **E**—the thyroid? (19.5)

14. JAMES is being treated for pneumonia. His mother has brought him for a follow-up visit. Which of these things would you do FIRST?
A Count his respirations. **B** Show his mother that you recognize him and tell her how pleased you are to see her. **C** Look at his weight chart. **D** Examine his chest with a stethoscope. **E** Take his temperature. (5.28 (Revision))

15. Swelling of the ankles and eyelids can be caused by severe—
A—cyanosis? **B**—fever? **C**—anaemia? **D**—jaundice? **E**—dehydration? (19.7)

16. Which of these children would you expect to have the most protein in his urine?
A TOM with kwashiorkor. **B** DICK with hookworm anaemia. **C** SID with acute nephritis. **D** HARRY with the nephrotic syndrome. (19.8, 23.7)

17. Lymph nodes can be found in all these places EXCEPT—
A—in front of the ear? **B**—in the axilla? **C**—in the groin? **D**—on the palms of the hands? **E**—along the sides of the neck? (2–5, 19–1)

MATCH these diseases with the things that are used to diagnose or treat them—
18. Foreign body in the nose **19.** Corneal ulcer **20.** Pneumonia **21.** Malnutrition
A A watch **B** A piece of bent wire **C** A piece of fluorescein paper **D** A tongue depressor **E** A tape measure (17.13, 16.7, 8.15, 7.13 (Revision))

MATCH these things with the signs they would prevent—
22. DPT vaccine **23.** Keeping children's growth curves rising **24.** Measles vaccine **25.** BCG vaccine

A Koplik's spots B A phlycten C Tenderness of the bone behind the ear D Membrane on the tonsils and a swollen neck E A hole in the cheek (18.8, 18.12, 16.13, 16.11 (Revision))

ABDOMEN C
Chapter 20: with revision: Code 2

1. TUNDE (3 years) has abdominal pain. You should examine him when his abdominal muscles are—
C—contracted? D—relaxed? (20.2)

2. Which of these children is MOST likely to have an acute abdomen?
A MABEL with blood-stained stools and dehydration. B MAUREEN with constipation and no other symptoms. C MARIAM with diarrhoea, vomiting, and abdominal pain. D MAY with diarrhoea and vomiting. E MARY with vomiting and abdominal pain. (20.13)

3. A child with an acute abdomen needs—
A—hospital care quickly? B—penicillin? C—streptoymcin? D—glucose–salt solution by mouth? E—as much food as he can eat? (20.2)

4. Which of these is NOT a sign of peritonitis?
A Rigidity B Tenderness C Diarrhoea D Guarding E Rebound tenderness (20.2)

5. DARRAGH (20 months) is vomiting. Which of these signs would make you think she has meningitis?
A Sunken fontanelle B Neck stiffness C Abdominal guarding D Swollen abdomen E Abdominal pain (15.6)

6. A health worker should examine a child's abdomen with—
A—his fist? B—his hand flat on the child's abdomen? C—only the tips of his fingers touching the child? D— his thumb and first finger? (20.3)

7. The spleen is on—
C—the right? D—the left? (20.3)

8. An enlarged spleen can be caused by—
A—typhoid? B—measles? C—urinary infections? D—pneumonia? E—meningitis? (20.3)

9. BENT has a swelling in his groin which gets bigger when he coughs, cries, or runs about. When he lies down it goes away. It is—
A—a swelling caused by cellulitis? B—an abscess? C—a hernia? D—a goitre? E—a hydrocoele? (20.6)

10. We must be sure to diagnose acute abdomens because—
A—they are infectious? B—they easily become chronic? C—they are a common cause of diarrhoea? D—they can easily be treated in a health centre? E—they kill children quickly? (20.2)

11. A strangulated hernia is dangerous because it may cause—
A—obstruction of the gut? B—acute diarrhoea? C—bleeding into the gut? D—typhoid? E—dysentery? (20.4, 20.5)

12. Which of these children is most likely to need an operation?
D KOK with an inguinal hernia. E BOK with umbilical hernia. (20.5, 20.7)

13. TAKAKO (1 year) has an umbilical hernia. What would you say to his mother?
A 'His hernia will probably go by itself as he grows older.' B 'He needs an operation quickly.' C 'Keep his hernia flat by putting a binder round him.' D 'Here is some medicine for him.' E 'These injections will cure him.' (20.7)

14. The first sign of malnutrition is—
A—oedema? B—an arm circumference of 10 cm? C—diarrhoea? D—a growth curve that does not climb normally? E—a flaking paint rash? (7.1 (Revision))

15. Which of these is LEAST likely to cause abdominal pain?
A Urinary infection B Scabies C Malaria D Hepatitis E Peritonitis (20.11)

16. JOHN has peritonitis. In his peritoneum he has—
A—blood? B—the food he ate a few hours ago? C—fluid or pus? D—bile? E—faeces? (20.2)

17. AKIMASA has had abdominal pains for several months. Which of these special tests would be most helpful?
B Blood for parasites C Urine for sugar D Blood for haemoglobin E Stool for parasites (20.12)

18. Which of these is the best symptomatic treatment for vomiting?
A Promethazine B Paracetamol C Glucose–salt solution D Food E Phenobarbitone (20.14)

19. Which of these children is most likely to have an acute abdomen? The child with—
A—abdominal pain, vomiting, and diarrhoea? B—vomiting and fever without abdominal pain? C—constipation and abdominal pain for several months? D—abdominal pain, vomiting, and constipation for one day? (20.14)

20. Which of these would make you think that a child's vomiting was caused by gut obstruction?
A Diarrhoea B Blood in his vomit C Undigested food in his vomit D Pale vomit E Vomit which looks and smells like stools (20.14)

21. The most important result of vomiting is—
A—fever? B—dehydration? C—anaemia? D—malnutrition? E—jaundice? (20.15)

22. FRITZ (2 years) has had diarrhoea and vomiting for two days. He is mildly dehydrated. There is a little blood in his vomit. What would you tell his mother?
A 'This is not serious.' B 'He has haemorrhagic disease.' C 'He has a stomach ulcer.' D 'He has hookworms.' (20.15)

23. Which of these most often causes bloody diarrhoea?

A Amoebiasis **B** Giardiasis **C** Cholera **D** Food poisoning **E** Lactose intolerance (9.4 (Revision))

24. Which of these diseases does NOT cause signs inside the mouth?

A Herpes simplex virus **B** Meningitis **C** Thrush **D** Measles **E** Dehydration (15.6 (Revision))

25. Which of these children would you treat FIRST?

B MIKO who has pneumonia with insuction. **C** MARKO who has dehydration with sunken eyes. **D** MITO with sulphadimidine allergy with fever and a rash. **E** MIRO who has penicillin allergy with wheezing and cyanosis. (3.2 (Revision))

WORMS C
Chapter 21: with revision: Code 3

1. Which of these worms is most likely to cause bloody diarrhoea if a child's worm load is heavy?

A *T. solium* **B** *T. saginata* **C** *Ascaris* **D** Threadworms **E** *Trichuris* (21.4)

2. AJIT has 45 *Ascaris* ova and 65 hookworm ova in a standard stool smear. You have piperazine and tetrachlorethylene (TCE) but no other worm drugs in your clinic. He should be given—

A—TCE first, then piperazine? **B**—piperazine first, then TCE? **C**—both drugs together? **D**—TCE only? **E**—piperazine only? (21.3)

MATCH these patients with the special tests that will be most useful in diagnosis—

3. MALA with severe anaemia. **4.** PABLO (3 years, 38 °C) who had two fits last night. **5.** PEDRO'S uncle who has a chronic cough with blood-stained sputum. **6.** CARLOS with severe anal itching.

A Standard stool smear **B** Urine for protein **C** 'Sellotape' ('Scotch tape') swab **D** Smear for AAFB **E** Pandy's test (21.1, 21.3, 13.13, 15.3 (Revision))

7. USHA'S mother says that USHA has passed a worm in her stools. Which of these is it most likely to be?

A *Trichuris* **B** *Ascaris* **C** *Taenia* **D** *Strongyloides* **E** *H. nana* (21.2)

8. Which of these worms lives in the veins of the bladder?

A Threadworms **B** *Schistosoma haematobium* **C** *Ascaris* **D** *Trichuris* **E** *Strongyloides* (21.1)

9. Tiabendazole is NOT useful for treating—

A—the worms causing creeping eruption? **B**—*Schistosoma haematobium*? **C**—*Strongyloides*? **D**—*Trichuris*? (21.7)

10. Which of these is round, smooth, and about 20 cm long with pointed ends?

A *H. nana* **B** *Taenia* **C** *Trichuris* **D** *Ascaris* **E** *Strongyloides* (21.3)

11. Which of these helps to prevent hookworm infection?

A Wearing shoes **B** Washing hands after passing stools **C** Drinking boiled water **D** Wearing socks **E** Using handkerchiefs (21.1)

12. The stools of a child with *Ascaris* infection are—

A—paler than the stools of a healthy child? **B**—harmless because *Ascaris* ova die quickly? **C**—dangerous because *Ascaris* ova can live in the soil a long time and infect other children? **D**—harmful because *Ascaris* ova go into a child through his skin? (21.3)

13. Each worm larva grows into—

D—many adult worms? **E**—one adult worm? (21.1)

14. Which of these worms would you treat with piperazine for several days?

A Schistosomes **B** Threadworms **C** Ascaris **D** Tapeworms (21.5)

15. Which of these worms is more than a metre long, flat, and made of many pieces (segments)?

A Hookworms **B** *Trichuris* **C** *T. solium* **D** *Ascaris* **E** *H. nana* (21.4)

16. Hookworm infection can be caused by—

A—eating uncooked meat? **B**—playing in infected water? **C**—eating dirty food? **D**—sitting on infected ground with bare buttocks? **E**—eating earth with hookworm ova in it? (21.1, 22.5)

MATCH these signs with the diseases that cause them—

17. Deep breathing **18.** Macules, papules, vesicles, and pustules **19.** Severe inspiratory stridor **20.** Arm circumference of 10 cm

A Marasmus **B** Chickenpox **C** Obstructive laryngitis **D** Severe dehydration **E** Bronchitis (9.18, 11.16, 8.11, 7.13 (Revision))

21. In which of these can a child make his worm load heavier by infecting himself with his own faeces on his own hands?

A *Strongyloides* **B** Hookworms **C** *T. saginata* **D** *Schistosoma haematobium* **E** Threadworms (21.5)

22. Which of these worms has to go through a pig before it can infect a child?

A *Schistosoma haematobium* **B** *Ascaris* **C** *H. nana* **D** *T. solium* **E** *T. saginata* (21.4)

23. Which of these organisms is LEAST likely to cause fever?

B Viruses **C** Protozoa **D** Bacteria **E** Worms (21.3)

24. GUL has an *Ascaris* infection. He should be given—

A—one dose of tablets? **B**—tablets once a day for a week? **C**—one dose of tablets and a purgative? (21.3)

25. Which of these worms is most likely to cause abdominal pain and diarrhoea?

A *T. solium* **B** *H. nana* **C** *T. saginata* **D** Hookworms **E** *Schistosoma haematobium* (21.4)

ANAEMIA C
Chapter 22: Code 6

1. Oxygen is carried round the body by—
C—the red cells? D—the white cells? E—the liquid part of the blood? (22.1)

2. The blood of an anaemic child has—
A—too little haemoglobin? B—too many red cells? C—too few white cells? D—too much haemoglobin? E—too many white cells? (22.1)

3. The hand–foot syndrome is helpful in diagnosing anaemia caused by—
A—hookworms? B—schistosomes? C—lack of iron? D—lack of folic acid? E—sickle cells? (22.8)

4. Anaemia is usually—
A—a child's presenting symptom? B—found when he is examined for something else? (22.1)

5. Which of these children is most likely to lack iron?
A The small-for-dates baby. B The baby with *Ascaris* ova + + + in his stool. C The child with hookworm ova + + + in her stool. D The baby who has had a difficult birth. E The baby who is not gaining weight. (22.5)

6. VICTOR is a healthy full-term newborn baby. His haemoglobin is about—
A—8 g/dl? B—10 g/dl? C—12 g/dl? D—14 6 g/dl? E—18 g/dl? (22.2)

7. MERCEDES (2 years) has a haemoglobin of 4 g/dl. She is—
B—mildly anaemic? C—moderately anaemic? D—severely anaemic? (22.2)

8. Children with the sickle-cell trait usually—
A—die during the first year of life? B—are not able to go to school? C—are severely anaemic? D—have no symptoms? (22.8)

9. When an anaemic child is treated his haemoglobin curve should—
C—stay above the red (10 g/dl) line on his weight chart? D—fall down the chart? E—climb up the chart? (22.2)

10. Which of these is an important cause of anaemia?
A Malaria B Measles C Diphtheria D Pneumonia E Tonsillitis (22.7)

11. Which of these worms is the most serious cause of anaemia?
A *Strongyloides* B *Schistosoma haematobium* C *Ascaris* D *T. Solium* E *T. Saginata* (22.3)

12. Haemoglobin contains protein and—
A—iron? B—iodine? C—sodium? D—potassium? E—calcium? (22.1)

13. Each red cell lives for—
A—about 12 days? B—the rest of a child's life? C—about one day? D—about 12 months? E—about 120 days? (22.1)

14. HILDE has a haemolytic anaemia. Which of these would help her most?

A Iodine B Calcium tablets C Folic acid D Iron E Vitamin K (22.3)

15. Which of these children is most likely to lack iron?
A PASTOR who is three years old. B LUMEN who is a school child. C RAUL (newborn) who was born after a 39-week pregnancy. D VALOIS (newborn) who was born after a 35-week pregnancy. (22.4)

16. Which of these is used again many times and is NOT destroyed in the body?
B Iron C Energy food D Folic acid E Haemoglobin (22.3)

17. A child should be given 'Children's iron medicine' for at least—
A—three weeks? B—three months? C—three days? D—three years? (22.4)

18. A child should stop taking iron medicine—
A—as soon as his haemoglobin is normal? B—six months after his haemoglobin is normal? C—two months after his haemoglobin is normal? (22.4)

19. The cheapest way for a child to get the folic acid he needs is for him to eat—
A—milk? B—maize? C—eggs? D—dark green leaves? E—liver? (22.6)

20. Which of these foods contains both folic acid and vitamin A?
A Cassava leaves B Cassava roots C Millet D Sugar E Rice (22.6)

21. A large spleen can be a sign of—
A—hookworm anaemia? B—an iron deficiency anaemia? C—a haemolytic anaemia? D—the anaemia caused by malnutrition? (22.7)

22. Which of these is NOT a symptom of infective hepatitis?
A Abdominal pain B Tiredness C Fever D Dark urine E Dark stools (22.11)

23. SAMARABAHAWE is jaundiced. He probably has hepatitis. What are you going to tell his mother?
A 'Penicillin cures jaundice.' B 'He needs plenty of fluids and any food he will eat.' C 'He is not infectious.' D 'Bacteria are harming his liver.' E 'He can go on taking any medicines you have been giving him.' (22.11)

24. DIDRIK has jaundice, vomiting, fever, pale stools, and dark urine. When might he have been given the injection that has caused these symptoms?
A Yesterday B Last week C Three weeks ago D Three months ago E One year ago (22.11)

25. Which of these things does the spleen do?
A Secrete bile B Store food C Make new red cells D Remove old red cells from the blood E Make folic acid (10.7)

1. When a patient has to pass urine often he has—
B—urgency? C—frequency? D—haematuria? E—dysuria? (23.1)

2. ACHMAD's urine was left on the clinic table all night. It can now be examined for—
B—bacteria? C—pus cells? D—red cells? E—none of these things? (23.2)

3. Which of these kinds of urine is MOST likely to be normal?
A Pale urine B Dark urine C Red urine D Urine with protein in it (23.1)

4. Which of these is most likely to make a child pass pale urine?
A Hot weather B Drinking much fluid C A urinary infection D Fever E Nephritis (23.1)

5. WENDY's urine has 'Protein +, pus cells + + +, and bacteria +' in it. She probably has—
A—schistosomiasis? B—acute nephritis? C—a stone? D—the nephrotic syndrome? E—a urinary infection? (23.2)

6. Which of these things most easily spoils a specimen of urine?
B Letting bacteria grow in urine before it is examined C Taking the middle part of the stream of urine D Taking too much urine E Putting the specimen in a refrigerator (23.2)

7. ABDUL has 240 pus cells in a microlitre of his urine. Has he got a urinary infection?
D Yes E No (23.2)

8. Which of these is LEAST likely to be caused by infection of a child's urinary tract?
A Fever B Dysuria C Frequency D A swollen fontanelle E Urgency (23.1)

9. In children over the age of one year, urinary infections are—
A—more common in boys? B—more common in girls? C—equally common in boys and girls? D—very rare in boys and girls? (23.4)

10. Which of these is LEAST likely to be a symptom of urinary infection?
A Rigors B A child who has become dry starting to wet himself again C Vomiting D Abdominal pain E Constipation (23.4)

11. All these children have fever. Whose urine most needs examining?
A AGUS with abdominal pain. B AKAT with headache. C ALEX with a sore throat. D AMAT with ear pain. E ALPHONSE with severe pain in his lower leg. (23.4)

12. Penicillin is usually NOT useful for treating—
A—acute septic lymphadenitis? B—severe skin sepsis? C—urinary infections? D—pneumonia? E—tonsillitis? (23.4)

13. Chronic urinary infections—

A—are easy to diagnose in a health centre? B—do not need treatment? C—can destroy a child's kidneys? D—seldom cause harm? E—cause sugar to come in the urine? (23.4)

14. When a child is having one of these drugs he needs to drink plenty of water. Which drug?
A Tetracycline B Chloramphenicol C Penicillin D Sulphadimidine E Ampicillin (23.4)

15. *Schistosoma haematobium* lives mostly in the veins of—
A—the large intestine? B—the bladder?

16. 10 days treatment with penicillin is helpful for treating children with—
A—schistosomiasis? B—acute urinary infection? C—stone? D—chronic nephritis? E—acute nephritis? (23.7)

17. All these children have fever. Which would you expect to have pus cells in their urine?
A MARY with dysuria. B MARTY with rapid respirations. C MAXINE with a swollen fontanelle. D MASE with Koplik's spots. E MOBY with bloody diarrhoea. (23.4)

18. ATYEP's urine is mildly red with blood. Which of these diseases might he have?
A The nephrotic syndrome B Acute nephritis C Severe dehydration D Hyperpyrexia (23.7)

19. Which of these worms is most likely to cause haematuria?
A *Taenia solium* B *Taenia saginata* C *Schistosoma haematobium* D *Thrichuris* E *Schistosoma mansoni* (23.8)

20. Which of these diseases causes the most protein in the urine?
A The nephrotic syndrome B Acute nephritis C Schistosomiasis D Urinary infection E Kwashiorkor (23:1)

21. Which of these passes through a snail during its life cycle?
A *Taenia solium* B *Taenia saginata* C *H. nana* D *Schistosoma haematobium* E *Giardia lamblia* (23.8)

22. Where might you find a foreign body in a child? In—
A—his bronchus? B—his ear? C—his nose? D—her vagina? E—in any of these places? (23.10)

23. Which of these is LEAST likely to be a symptom of vulvovaginitis?
B Itching C Redness D Dysuria E Haematuria (23.10)

24. Which of these 3-month-old children needs to be circumcised?
A CLAUD who has a urinary infection. B CLEM who cannot pass urine because he has a stone in his bladder. C CUBA whose mother thinks that the hole in his foreskin is too small, but who passes a normal stream of urine. D SEVESE whose foreskin swells when he passes urine. E TAU whose foreskin cannot be pulled back. (23.11)

25. A urinary infection which causes fever is most likely to be caused by—

A—viruses? **B**—fungi? **C**—worms? **D**—protozoa? **E**—bacteria? (23.4)

NOT WALKING C
Chapter 24: Code 2

1. XANTHE is two years old. Her mother says that she is not walking. Which of these is the FIRST thing you will want to know?

A Are her muscles hypotonic? **B** Are her legs equally strong on both sides? **C** Can she touch her toes? **D** Has she stopped walking or did she never start to walk? **E** Did she have a birth injury? (24.1)

2. KOK is 18-months old. He was walking well until 3 days ago, but he has now stopped. This could be caused by any of these diseases EXCEPT—

A—kwashiorkor? **B**—osteomyelitis? **C**—pyomyositis? **D**—poliomyelitis? **E**—cerebral palsy? (24.1)

3. BARDI (15 months) started walking when he was a year old. A week ago he had a mild fever and he stopped walking. This might be caused by—

A—poliomyelitis? **B**—cerebral palsy? **C**—cretinism? **D**—Down's syndrome? **E**—some other disease which causes backwardness? (24.1)

4. Polio does NOT cause—

A—weakness? **B**—wasting? **C**—anaesthesia? **D**—deformity? **E**—disability? (24.4)

5. When a spastic child with cerebral palsy is picked up his legs usually—

A—open wide apart? **B**—cross each other like a pair of scissors? **C**—bend at his hips? **D**—are hypotonic? (24.15)

6. Polio most often paralyses the muscles in a child's—

A—arms? **B**—legs? **C**—diaphragm? **D**—thorax? (24.4)

7. The most serious complication of polio is paralysis of the muscles in a child's—

A—larynx? **B**—abdomen? **C**—pharynx? **D**—diaphragm? **E**—bronchi? (24.4)

8. Polio usually presents as the child who—

A—has stopped walking? **B**—has a thin, weak arm? **C**—is not eating? **D**—is not breathing normally? **E**—has a high fever? (24.4)

9. HERNOKO (3 years) became severely paralysed by polio two weeks ago. What would you say to his mother?

A 'Few children with polio learn to walk again.' **B** 'His weak muscles will be strong again in a few days.' **C** 'You must soon find ways of giving his weak muscles work to do.' **D** 'Unfortunately it is not possible to prevent contractures.' (24.4)

10. Which of these is a symptom of acute osteomyelitis?

A A large spleen **B** A swollen fontanelle **C** A positive Kernig's sign **D** Muscle wasting **E** Tenderness over a bone (24.5)

11. HIOE (5 years, 37·6 °C) has started to limp. He has not been well for several months, he is not eating normally and he sometimes has a mild fever. When you examine him you cannot bend (abduct) his left hip outwards in the same way as his right hip. Which of these diseases is most likely to be causing his symptoms?

A TB of the hip. **B** Septic arthritis **C** Polio **D** Osteomyelitis **E** Pyomyositis (24.6)

12. Backwardness most commonly presents as the child who—

A—is underweight for his age? **B**—has weak hypotonic muscles? **C**—started to walk and then stopped? **D**—is not walking at the age when he should walk? **E**—cries a lot? (24.9)

13. When we try to decide if a child is backward or not we should use—

A—several milestones? **B**—one milestone only? (24.10)

14. SAM (3 years) is late in walking and talking. His muscles are hypotonic. There is a fold across the inner ends of his eyelids and the back of his head is flat. He has one fold across the palms of his hands. He has—

A—a kind of backwardness we cannot diagnose? **B**—cerebral palsy? **C**—cretinism? **D**—Down's syndrome? **E**—a birth injury? (24.13)

15. Which of these things is LEAST likely in a cretin?

A A wide open mouth **B** One fold across the palms of his hands **C** A big tongue **D** A nose with a flat bridge **E** Thick dry skin (24.14)

16. Children with cerebral palsy usually—

A—recover if we give them the right antibiotics? **B**—become normal by the time they are adults? **C**—have about the same amount of disability all their lives? **D**—become more and more disabled until they finally die? **E**—infect other children? (24.15)

17. Goitres and backward children can both be caused by lack of—

A—iron? **B**—fluorine? **C**—vitamins? **D**—calcium during pregnancy? **E**—iodine? (24.14)

18. Which milestone do normal children reach by 18 months?

A Speaking sentences **B** Sitting **C** Walking **D** Smiling (24–8)

19. Which of these diseases causes the most severe pain?

A Down's syndrome **B** Leprosy **C** Chronic polio **D** Osteomyelitis (24.5)

20. If a newborn child is abnormally slow starting to breathe he may get—

A—cretinism? **B**—hyperglycaemia? **C**—pneumonia? **D**—cephalhaematoma? **E**—cerebral palsy? (24.12)

21. Which of these diseases can cause cerebral palsy?

A Thrush **B** Meningitis **C** Bronchitis **D** Malnutrition **E** Pneumonia (24.12)

22. Which of these diseases CANNOT be prevented in a child by injecting or immunising his mother during pregnancy?

A Diphtheria **B** Tetanus of the newborn **C** Iodine embryopathy (24.14b)

23. Which of these diseases is most likely to cause deafness?

A Iodine embryopathy **B** Down's syndrome **C** Cerebral palsy **D** Polio (24.14b)

24. We can diagnose the cause of backwardness in—
A—most backward children? **B**—a few backward children only? **C**—all backward children? (24.9)

25. Backward children are helped most by—
A—drugs? **B**—hospital treatment? **C**—injections? **D**—operations? **E**—careful teaching by their families? (24.11)

OTHER SYMPTOMS C
Chapter 25: with revision: Code 5

MATCH these drugs with the way they are usually given—
1. Tetrachlorethylene **2.** Children's iron mixture **3.** Isoniazid **4.** Depot penicillin
B One injection **C** Once a day for not less than three months **D** Once a day for a year **E** One dose by mouth (3.15, 3.33, 3.20, 3.27)

MATCH these diseases with the advice that you would give to a child's mother—
5. Acute abdomen **6.** Tuberculoid leprosy **7.** Folic-acid-deficiency anaemia **8.** Polio
A 'Move his weak leg through its full movements several times every day.' **B** 'He must drink plenty of fluids.' **C** 'He must eat plenty of green vegetables.' **D** 'He must take these tablets (dapsone) for several years.' **E** 'Take him to hospital quickly.' (21.4, 22.6, 19.3, 20.2, 22.5, 19.22 (Revision))

9. Which of these children need extra fluids?
A RAMA who is having penicillin. **B** RANI who is having sulphadimidine. **C** RITA who is having chloramphenicol. **D** RORY who is having dapsone. **E** RAM who is having paraldehyde. (3.14 (Revision))

10. YESIDE (2 years) has swallowed a marble. What are you going to tell her mother?
A 'Feed her as usual.' **B** 'We must send her for help.' **C** 'Here is some medicine to help her pass it.' **D** 'It will probably get stuck in her gut.' **E** 'She must not eat anything until she has passed it.' (25.5)

MATCH these diseases with the signs they cause—
11. Gonorrhoea **12.** Chronic polio **13.** Whooping cough **14.** Cretinism
A Inflamation of the vulva of young girls **B** Muscle wasting **C** Constipation **D** Diarrhoea **E** Conjunctival haemorrhage. (23.10, 24.2, 24.14)

15. Which of these diseases is LEAST likely to make a child's spleen enlarge?
A Sickle-cell anaemia **B** Malaria **C** Typhoid **D** Iron-deficiency anaemia (22.4 (Revision))

16. EFFENDI (12 months, 6·5 kg). His mother says that he will only suck from the breast and will not eat any food. What are you going to tell her?

A 'He probably does not need extra food yet.' **B** 'Stop breast-feeding him.' **C** 'Give him a feeding bottle.' **D** 'Try to give him porridge after he has sucked all the milk he can get.' **E** 'Give him porridge when he is hungry, before he feeds from the breast.' (25.3)

17. Which of these things helps to cause prolapse of the rectum?
A Protein energy malnutrition **B** Anal fissure **C** Lack of vitamins **D** Hookworms **E** Gonorrhoea (25.7)

18. A worker in a health centre is LEAST able to remove a foreign body if it gets into a child's—
A—throat? **B**—ear? **C**—nose? **D**—bronchi? **E**—vagina? (8.18 (Revision))

19. GONDO's nose has started bleeding. What would you say to him?
A 'Keep on blowing your nose.' **B** 'Sit up, lean forwards, bite onto this wooden spatula, and hold your nose closed with your fingers.' **C** 'Let me put this cotton wick into your nose.' **D** 'Lie down on this couch.' **E** 'Bend your head back so that the blood can run out of your nose.' (25.10)

20. Which of these is LEAST likely to be serious?
A Stridor **B** Vomiting **C** Constipation **D** A discharging ear **E** Oedema (25.1)

21. You can use penicillin for treating—
A—thrush? **B**—amoebic dysentery? **C**—cellulitis? **D**—worms? **E**—TB meningitis? (3.15 (Revision))

22. Which of these is LEAST likely to be a symptom of a behaviour disease in a five year old child?
B Stammering **C** Tantrums **D** Bed wetting **E** Not being able to walk (25.2)

23. SOEWARNO has had a blood-stained discharge from one side of his nose for two weeks. He has no fever and is otherwise well. The most likely diagnosis is—
A—foreign body? **B**—stomatitis? **C**—TB? **D**—amoebiasis? **E**—thrush? (25.11)

24. Which of these is NOT a broad spectrum antibiotic?
A Ampicillin **B** Penicillin and sulphadimidine together **C** Chloramphenicol **D** Pyrantel parmoate **E** Tetracycline (3.13 (Revision))

25. Prolapse of the rectum—
A—is less common in malnourished children? **B**—can usually be treated in a clinic? **C**—seldom returns after being replaced? **D**—is seldom ulcerated and bleeding? **E**—is the only cause of a red swelling at the anus? (25.7)

NEWBORN BABY C
Chapter 26: Sections 1 to 22: Code 7

1. Which of these things is NORMAL for a baby who was delivered an hour ago?
A Hypotonia **B** Insuction **C** Grunting **D** Coughing when his mouth is sucked out (26.1)

2. When you resuscitate a newborn baby you should put your mouth over his—

A—nose? **B**—nose and mouth? **C**—mouth? (26.3)

3. Which of these is a normal pulse for a baby about an hour old?

A 60 **B** 80 **C** 140 **D** 200 **E** 100 (26.1)

4. You have just delivered a baby and he has not started to breathe. What would you do FIRST?

A Suck out his throat **B** Tie his cord **C** Give mouth-to-mouth resuscitation **D** Inject vitamin K **E** Hit the soles of his feet (26.3)

5. Which of these is the best antibiotic for septic infections in newborn babies?

A Streptomycin **B** Chloramphenicol **C** Tetracycline **D** Penicillin **E** Penicillin and streptomycin (26.24)

6. If a baby's cord is tied too close to his umbilicus—

A—he may become anaemic? **B**—he may get tetanus? **C**—his gut may be harmed? **D**—he may get septicaemia? **E**—he may get an umbilical hernia? (26.2)

7. When you give a baby mouth-to-mouth resuscitation you should—

A—bend the baby's head forwards? **B**—blow from your cheeks? **C**—blow strongly? **D**—blow air into his stomach and his lungs? **E**—blow from your lungs? (26.3)

8. A newborn baby with a cold which is obstructing his nose has difficulty feeding because—

A—he cannot breathe and feed at the same time? **B**—feeding makes him cough? **C**—he has a sore tongue and cannot suck? **D**—he cannot swallow? **E**—he does not want to suck? (26.4)

9. ZACHARY (1 day) has a cephalhaematoma. What would you do?

A Send him to hospital **B** Inject penicillin **C** Remove the blood from the swelling with needle **D** Give him vitamin K and leave the swelling to go by itself **E** Put hot compresses on the swelling (26.4)

10. Which of these is NOT a congenital malformation?

A No hole in his anus (imperforate anus) **B** An extra finger **C** Club foot (talipes) **D** Cleft palate **E** Cephalhaematoma (26.4)

11. Which of these is a NORMAL sign in a newborn baby?

A A high sharp cry **B** Not passing urine for 48 hours **C** A blue body **D** A swollen fontanelle **E** A Moro reflex (26.6)

12. If a baby is bottle-fed, he is—

A—less likely to be constipated? **B**—less likely to get diarrhoea? **C**—less likely to get marasmus? **D**—more likely to become malnourished? **E**—less likely to get other infections? (26.7)

13. If a newborn baby sucks from the breast soon after birth—

A—this helps milk to come into the breasts? **B**—he becomes tired? **C**—he sucks colostrum which is harmful? **D**—his mother's nipples become sore? **E**—he wastes his mother's time because there is no milk in his mother's breasts? (26.7)

14. When a baby stops sucking, his mother's breasts—

A—stop making milk immediately? **B**—take several days to stop making milk? **C**—make more milk? **D**—become less engorged? (26.8)

15. Breast pumps—

A—cannot be used if a nipple is flat? **B**—should not be sterilized in hypochlorite? **C**—have to be kept clean in the same way as a feeding-bottle? **D**—cause pain if a nipple is cracked? **E**—cannot be used with engorged breasts? (26.8)

16. Nipple shields—

A—allow a baby to suck from a breast with a cracked nipple or flat nipple? **B**—must be used as long as breast-feeding lasts? **C**—need not be sterilized? **D**—should be worn by a mother during pregnancy? **E**—can be used with feeding bottles? (26.9, 26.11)

17. JOHN'S mother has a painful, tender swelling in her left breast. It is not fluctuant. Her temperature is 38·2 °C and there are some tender lymph-nodes in her axilla. What would you tell her?

A 'Injections will not help.' **B** 'Don't press the milk out of your sore breast.' **C** 'Let him suck from both your breasts.' **D** 'Stop breast-feeding and give him a bottle.' **E** 'We must make a small incision to let out the pus.' (26.12)

18. Which of these makes cow's milk most like mother's milk?

A Adding one part of water to three parts of milk **B** Adding three parts of water to one part of milk **C** Adding a heaped teaspoonful of sugar to a cupful of milk **D** Doing A and C **E** Doing B and C (26.14)

19. PABLO is one day old. His mother is worried because there is very little milk in her breasts. What would you tell her?

A 'Give him an extra feed before you put him to your breasts.' **B** 'Let him suck from your breasts as often as he wants to.' **C** 'He needs plenty of water to drink.' **D** 'Normally there is plenty of milk on the first day after delivery.' **E** 'He probably needs a bottle.' (26.13)

---

20. How much feed does a bottle-fed baby need every day for each kilo he weighs?

A 100 ml **B** 200 ml **C** 275 ml **D** 125 ml **E** 150 ml (26.16)

21. If a baby needs extra water, you should give it—

A—before he has sucked from the breast? **B**—after he has sucked from the breast? (26.17)

22. A newborn baby weighing 1800 g—

A—coughs easily? **B**—fights bacteria well? **C**—seldom

192

becomes anaemic? **D**—lies with his arms and legs bent (flexed)? **E**—easily becomes jaundiced? (26.22)

23. The most common reason why a two-month-old baby does not grow is because he—

A—is not getting enough milk? **B**—has kwashiorkor? **C**—has some congenital abnormality? **D**—is anaemic? **E**—is constipated? (26.21)

24. A very weak baby who cannot suck should be fed with—

B—a jug? **C**—a tube? **D**—a feeding-bottle? **E**—a cup and spoon? (26.22)

25. HEINRICH is 10 days old. His mother says that when he was born he sucked normally, but yesterday he stopped sucking. Which of these is the LEAST likely diagnosis?

A Hypothermia **B** Septicaemia **C** Tetanus **D** A lower respiratory infection **E** Cleft palate (26.20)

NEWBORN BABY C
Chapter 26: Section 23 to the end: Code 1

1. Haemolytic disease of the newborn usually causes jaundice—

A—on the first day? **B**—between the second and the fifth day? **C**—after the fifth day? (26.23)

2. Which of these is a sign that a baby's jaundice is severe?

A Pale urine **B** Fast breathing **C** Sunken fontanelle **D** Jaundice in his eyes only **E** Not sucking normally (26.23)

3. Jaundice is LEAST likely to be dangerous if it comes—

A—in the first 24 hours? **B**—after the fifth day? **C**—between the second and the fifth day? (26.23)

4. Tetanus of the newborn usually presents as—

A—not sucking? **B**—erythema round the umbilicus? **C**—fits? **D**—muscle spasms? **E**—a stiff neck? (26.20)

5. ZENOBIA (Birth weight 3·7 kg) was born 4 days ago after a difficult delivery. She did not breathe immediately and needed resuscitation. She is pale and hypotonic and sucks weakly. This morning she had a fit. She probably has—

A—meningitis? **B**—septicaemia? **C**—tetanus? **D**—a brain injury during birth? **E**—epilepsy? (26.6)

6. If the weather is cold, or if a baby is small, sick, or wet he is likely to get—

A—hyperpyrexia? **B**—cyanotic attacks? **C**—septicaemia? **D**—hypothermia? **E**—an upper respiratory infection? (26.23)

7. A newborn baby is too young to be able to produce one of these signs. Which one?

A Vomiting **B** Diarrhoea **C** A positive Kernig's sign **D** Jaundice **E** Fits (26.26)

8. CHANDRA (1 month) is vomiting. Which of these is he LEAST likely to have?

A A gut infection **B** An obstruced anus **C** Septicaemia **D** Pyloric stenosis **E** Meningitis (26.47)

9. A newborn child with true talipes—

A—can only be treated in hospital? **B**—needs a plaster-of-Paris splint? **C**—must have his leg put into adhesive strapping as soon as possible? **D**—should be treated when he is about six months old? **E**—can never be made to walk normally? (26.52)

10. Which of these things is normal for a baby during the first three months of his life?

A Passing soft stools **B** Passing one stool every four days **C** Crying and pulling up his legs as if he is in pain when he passes stools **D** Passing a stool every time he feeds **E** All of these things (26.29)

11. ZAREER (2 days) passed no meconium during birth and has not passed any since. What would you say to his mother first?

A 'This is normal.' **B** 'Let me try to pass this rubber tube into his rectum.' **C** 'Take him for help immediately.' **D** 'There is no need to do anything unless he starts vomiting.' **E** 'He needs a laxative.' (26.31)

12. BORDAN (2 months) has diarrhoea, a dry mouth, and a sunken fontanelle. He is breast-fed and can still suck. He should—

A—stop breast-feeding until his diarrhoea has stopped? **B**—be given an intravenous drip immediately? **C**—stop breast-feeding completely? **D**—be given oral glucose–salt solution between breast feeds? **E**—be given an artificial feed? (26.32)

13. You have not got enough vitamin K for every baby to have an injection. Which baby needs it LEAST?

A A very small baby **B** A baby weighing 3 kg **C** A baby who has had a difficult birth **D** A baby who has bled from his cord (26.33)

14. Which of these is NOT useful for preventing tetanus neonatorum?

A Immunizing mothers with tetanus toxoid? **B** Cutting the cord with sterile scissors? **C** Giving a baby DPT vaccine as soon as he is born? **D** Keeping the cord clean after it has been cut? **E** Tying the cord with sterile string? (26.37)

15. MIRIAM (2 days) has severe swelling of her eyelids and pus discharging from her conjunctivae. She probably has—

A—'sticky eye'? **B**—chemical conjunctivitis? **C**—viral conjunctivitis? **D**—gonococcal conjunctivitis? **E**—conjunctivitis caused by a birth injury? (26.40)

16. IAN (2 days) has a swelling close to the inner end of his right eye which is wet with tears. What are you going to tell his mother?

A 'Gently press (massage) the swelling and it will go in a few weeks.' **B** 'The tube that takes away his tears is blocked. I must open it with a needle.' **C** 'He needs penicillin injections.' **D** 'He will have this swelling all his life.' (26.41)

17. Fits in a newborn baby can be caused by a lack of—
A—folic acid? **B**—vitamin A? **C**—iron? **D**—blood?
E—glucose? (26.42)

18. YASSER (3 days) has many small red macules on his skin. In the middle of each macule is a white papule which does not contain pus. He has—
A—measles? **B**—impetigo of the newborn? **C**—erythema neonatorum (milia, the milk rash)? **D**—pemphigus neonatorum? **E**—a heat rash? (26.43)

19. AJIT (7 days) has large rapidly spreading vesicles and erythema on his face and chest. He is not sucking well and is abnormally sleepy. Some of the vesicles are filling with pus. What would you tell his mother?
B 'His rash will cure itself in a few days.' **C** 'His rash will not harm other babies.' **D** 'He must have injections (penicillin).' **E** 'This blue medicine (gentian violet) will cure him.' (26.47)

20. MAXIM (3 months). His mother is worried because his head is larger on one side than the other. What are you going to tell her?
A 'We must bind up his head so as to make it grow in the right way.' **B** 'His head will get normal as he grows older.'**C** 'His head will always be this shape.' **D** 'He should always sleep on the same side.' (26.51)

21. ALEXANDER (3 weeks) has some lesions which look like small pieces of white cloth fixed to his cheeks and tongue. What is his diagnosis?

A Vincent's stomatitis **B** Herpes stomatitis **C** Milk curds **D** Diphtheria **E** Thrush (26.55)

22. DOUGAL (7 days) has large breasts. One of them is secreting a few drops of milk. What would you tell his mother?
A 'Leave them and they will cure themselves.' **B** 'He needs some injections.' **C** 'His breasts will be large all his life.' **D** 'Squeeze them and they will get smaller.' **E** 'Bottle-feed him.' (26.56)

23. ELDRED was born two days ago and has not passed any urine. What would you tell his mother?
A 'Here is some medicine (chlorthiazide) to make him pass urine.' **B** 'Take him to hospital quickly.' **C** 'This is normal, he will pass urine tomorrow or the next day.' **D** 'Give him glucose–salt solution to drink.' (26.57)

24. All these children have just been born after a difficult labour and a forceps delivery. Which of them is most likely to have a permanent deformity?
A TOPAZ with Erb's palsy? **B** EMERALD with a facial palsy? **C** DIAMOND with a hydrocoele? **D** RUBY with a cephalhaematoma? (26.60, 26.61)

25. MELISSA (1 month) cries soon after feeds. She pulls up her legs and looks as if she is in pain. She—
A—will probably cry like this until she is at least a year old? **B**—is probably seriously ill? **C**—probably has colic? **D**—needs a feeding-bottle? **E**—is constipated? (26.65)

Dedication

The end of a book is perhaps a better place for a dedication than the beginning. This one concerns the effort and struggle required of all of us to achieve even a very little in such a difficult field as this, and the proper assignment of any small merit as may possibly be granted to our labours.

To all who live and fight for this work, and whose joy is in the job well done.

Non nobis Domine, non nobis sed nomine tua da gloriam. Super misericordia tua et veritate tua.   Psalm 115